Environmental Contaminants and Human Health

Environmental Contaminants and Human Health

Guest Editors

Lin Xu

Penghui Li

Xingchen Zhao

MDPI

Basel • Beijing • Wuhan • Barcelona • Belgrade • Novi Sad • Cluj • Manchester

Guest Editors
Lin Xu
Research Center for Eco-Environmental Sciences
Chinese Academy of Sciences
Beijing
China

Penghui Li
School of Environmental Science and Safety Engineering
Tianjin University of Technology
Tianjing
China

Xingchen Zhao
School of Environmental Science
Shandong University
Qingdao
China

Editorial Office
MDPI AG
Grosspeteranlage 5
4052 Basel, Switzerland

This is a reprint of the Special Issue, published open access by the journal *Toxics* (ISSN 2305-6304), freely accessible at: https://www.mdpi.com/journal/toxics/special_issues/NVO09614ZR.

For citation purposes, cite each article independently as indicated on the article page online and as indicated below:

Lastname, A.A.; Lastname, B.B. Article Title. *Journal Name* **Year**, *Volume Number*, Page Range.

ISBN 978-3-7258-5993-1 (Hbk)
ISBN 978-3-7258-5994-8 (PDF)
https://doi.org/10.3390/books978-3-7258-5994-8

Contents

toxics

Article

Effects of Benzo[a]Pyrene Exposure on Lung Cancer: A Mechanistic Study of Epigenetic m6A Levels and YTHDF1

Siyi Xu †, Jie Li †, Sheng Yang, Panpan Yang, Yiru Niu, Yiling Ge and Geyu Liang *

Key Laboratory of Environmental Medicine Engineering, Ministry of Education, School of Public Health, Southeast University, Nanjing 210009, China; 15851876530@163.com (S.X.); lijies7@163.com (J.L.); 101300318@seu.edu.cn (S.Y.); yangpanpan199912@163.com (P.Y.); niuyiru666@163.com (Y.N.); geyiling11@163.com (Y.G.)

* Correspondence: lianggeyu@163.com

† These authors contributed equally to this work.

Abstract: Benzo[a]pyrene, as the primary component of air pollutants, has been implicated in the pathogenesis of non-small-cell lung cancer (NSCLC). As an m6A reader that facilitates mRNA translation, YTHDF1 serves as a crucial regulator in tumor progression. Therefore, we established Benzo[a]pyrene(B[a]P)-induced bronchial epithelial malignant transformed cells (HBE-P35) to simulate the precancerous lesions of NSCLC and investigated the regulatory axis of YTHDF1 in both HBE-P35 and A549 lung cancer cells. A high level of m6A expression was detected in both HBE-P35 and A549 cells. Over-expression of YTHDF1 was observed in NSCLC tissues and correlated with poor overall survival in NSCLC patients. TMT labeling-based proteomic analysis and clinical lung tissue microarray assays demonstrated that CDK6 and MAP3K6 were positively correlated with YTHDF1 expression. MeRIP and RIP analyses revealed that YTHDF1 mediates the m6A-dependent regulation of CDK6 and MAP3K6 protein expression. The acquisition and deletion of miR-139/145-5p, along with luciferase reporter gene assays, demonstrated that miR-139-5p can target YTHDF1. Therefore, we conclude that YTHDF1 regulates CDK6 and MAP3K6 through m6A in B[a]P-induced HBE-P35 and A549 cells, providing a potential target for lung cancer treatment.

Keywords: m6A; YTHDF1; benzo[a]pyrene (B[a]P); lung cancer; HBE-P35; A549; MAP3K6; miR-139-5p; TMT labeling

1. Introduction

Lung cancer ranks among the most prevalent malignancies globally. Despite recent advances in diagnostic and therapeutic strategies, lung cancer remains the second most common malignancy by incidence (11.4%) and the foremost cause of mortality (18%), according to the Global Cancer Statistics 2020 [1]. Therefore, there is a pressing need for extensive research aimed at identifying potential biomarkers for early diagnosis and developing targeted therapeutic strategies [2].

Benzo(a)pyrene (B[a]P), belonging to the polycyclic aromatic hydrocarbon family, predominantly exists in cigarette smoke, food [3], and atmospheric pollutants. The initial study of benzo(a)pyrene commenced in 1974 [4], with subsequent investigations exploring the relationship between B[a]P and the development of lung cancer [5–7]. Benzo(a)pyrene-trans-7,8-diol-9,10-epoxide (BPDE), a metabolite of B[a]P, is a well-known mutagen and carcinogen [8,9]. In 1996, Denissenko et al. exposed HeLa cells and human bronchial epithelial (HBE) cells to various concentrations of BPDE, finding strong adduct signals on guanine residues at positions 157,248, and 273 of the TP53 gene, indicating that different concentrations of BPDE caused mutations in the TP53 gene in both HeLa and HBE cells at these sites [10]. B[a]P contributes to lung cancer initiation, progression, and metastatic dissemination. Jiang et al. revealed that smoke can stimulate SIBLING expression and contribute to mesenchymal stem cell (MSC)-mediated lung cancer metastasis [11]. While B[a]P exposure significantly correlates with lung cancer initiation and progression, the precise molecular mechanisms and signaling cascades have yet to be fully elucidated.

Epigenetic modifications are closely associated with tumorigenesis and progression [12]. Methylation modifications of RNA are a form of epigenetic regulation that post-transcriptionally modulate gene expression without changing the underlying nucleotide sequence. M6A modification, occurring at adenine (A) residues, represents the most abundant RNA epigenetic mark across eukaryotic species [13–15]. Additionally, the presence of m6A modifications, which can be found across virtually all coding and non-coding RNA species, plays a dynamic role in modulating their respective molecular processes [16]. The dysregulation of m6A regulatory mechanisms is associated with tumorigenesis and progression [17,18]. YTH domain family 1 (YTHDF1), an m6A "reader", is expressed at elevated levels in various cancers [19–22]. Numerous studies have highlighted the pivotal role of YTHDF1 in tumorigenesis. As an m6A reader protein, YTHDF1 has been shown to promote hepatocellular carcinoma cell growth, motility, invasiveness, and cell cycle progression by activating the PI3K/AKT/mTOR signaling pathway [23]. Studies have revealed that YTHDF1 expression correlates with disease advancement in hypopharyngeal squamous cell carcinoma [24]. Additionally, YTHDF1 may promote gastric carcinogenesis by regulating the translation of FDZ7 [25]. The exact molecular mechanisms through which YTHDF1, acting as an m6A reader, regulates lung cancer initiation and progression have yet to be fully elucidated. Therefore, investigating the regulatory mechanisms of YTHDF1 in lung cancer is clinically significant.

This research explored how YTHDF1 regulates both malignantly transformed bronchial epithelial cells and A549 lung cancer cells. We first established B[a]P-induced bronchial epithelial malignant transformed cells (HBE-P35), detected the changes in YTHDF1 and m6A levels in lung cancer and malignant transformed cells, and then used proteomics, MeRIP, and RIP to probe the upstream and downstream regulatory proteins of YTHDF1. We expected to find potential therapeutic targets for lung cancer through the above studies.

2. Materials and Methods

2.1. Datasets

Tissue mRNA and miRNA sequencing data from a total of 521 LUAD patients and 504 LUSC patients was obtained from the TCGA database (http://cancergenome.nih.gov/publications/publicationguidelines/, accessed on 12 February 2017), along with their basic information. Following the application of this study's inclusion and exclusion criteria, the final analysis incorporated data from 465 LUAD patients and 429 LUSC patients. The mRNA and miRNA sequencing data in the TCGA database were level 3 visual data, which could be analyzed directly without the need for normalization or standardization. The results of all publicly available sequencing data analyses and survival analyses for LUAD in the TCGA and GEO databases were obtained from the LUADEXPRESS website (http://www.bioinfo-zs.com/luadexpress/, accessed on 15 March 2021).

2.2. Tissue Microarray and Immunohistochemistry Analysis

Tissue microarrays were sourced from Aifang Biotechnology Company (Changsha, China). These microarrays comprised 160 lung tissue samples. Following standard pathological protocols, the specimens underwent sequential processing, including 4% paraformaldehyde fixation, pruning, dehydration, embedding, sectioning, and staining, before microscopic examination and sealing.

2.3. Reverse-Transcription Quantitative (RT-q)PCR

RNA was extracted using Trizol Reagent (Invitrogen, Carlsbad, CA, USA) following the manufacturer's protocol. RNA was then reverse transcribed using HiScript-II Q RT SuperMix (Vazyme, Nanjing, China), followed by quantitative PCR analysis with 2 × ChamQ SYBR Color qPCR Master Mix. The primers used for gene amplification are listed in Table S1.

2.4. Constructing Bronchial Epithelial Malignant Transformed Cells HBE-P35

B[a]P was initially dissolved in DMSO to prepare a stock solution at a concentration of 40 μmol/mL. This stock was then diluted with RPMI-1640 culture medium to achieve a final concentration of 80 μmol/L. For B[a]P exposure, HBE cells at 80% confluence were exposed to B[a]P (80 μmol/L) or the solvent control (DMSO) for 24 h, once per passage. Next, the medium was replaced with standard RPMI-1640 complete medium, and the cells were cultured until they reached the next passage, with this process being repeated 35 times, up to passage 35 (P35). P35 cells served as the experimental cells for this study and were designated as HBE-P35, while normally cultured 16HBE cells were used as the normal control and designated as HBE. The HBE cells (CVCL_3695) we used were purchased from the Typical Culture Preservation Committee cell bank of the Chinese Academy of Sciences, and the A549 cells (CVCL_0023) were purchased from the Typical Culture Preservation Committee cell bank of the Chinese Academy of Sciences.

2.5. Cell Cycle Assay

The cells were washed with PBS and then digested with trypsin. Following the PBS wash and centrifugation, the supernatant was discarded. Next, 500 μL of 70% ethanol was added to 1×10^6 cells at 4 °C to fix the cells overnight. The fixed cells were washed with PBS to remove the fixative, then centrifuged again as previously described. Following this, 500 μL of PI/RNase A staining solution (9:1 ratio) was added to each 1×10^6 cells. The cells were incubated at room temperature, protected from light, for 30 to 60 min before being analyzed using a flow cytometer (Thermo, Waltham, MI, USA). Red fluorescence was detected at an excitation wavelength of 488 nm. Three parallel samples were prepared for each cell type, and each sample was analyzed in triplicate with the flow cytometer.

2.6. Cell Transfection

Nanjing Corex Biologicals (Nanjing, China) provided the sh-YTHDF1 lentiviral vector and its negative control, utilizing lentiviral interfering shuttle vectors with puromycin (Puro) resistance and GFP tags. The lentiviral sequence and titer information are presented in Table S1. Cells were plated in 6-well plates at a density of 3×10^5 cells per well, and lentivirus was transduced at a multiplicity of infection (MOI) of 30, corresponding to 50–60% cell confluence. An appropriate amount of polybrene was added to each well, gently mixed, and then the plates were placed in the incubator. The cells were gently washed with PBS, and fresh medium was added. They were then incubated for another 48 h, until fluorescence was observed in the cells. Successfully transduced cells were maintained in complete RPMI-1640 containing puromycin. A high concentration of puromycin (8–10 μg/mL) may be used at the onset of the screening, and as the screening progresses, the concentration is gradually reduced to 2 μg/mL and then maintained for continued culture.

Three siRNA sequences were designed for the transient knockdown of YTHDF1 expression (refer to Table S1 for sequence details). Cells were collected and plated into the appropriate well plates 12 h before transfection, reaching approximately 50% confluence. The siRNA sequences were delivered into the cells using the riboFECT CP Transfection Kit (Guangzhou Ruibo biological Technology Co., Ltd., Guangzhou, China), in a medium without penicillin–streptomycin or serum. Gene expression was observed between 24 and 72 h post transfection.

The miRNA-139/145-5p mimic and inhibitor were provided by Reebok Bio (Guangzhou, China), and the sequences of the mimic and inhibitor are kept confidential by the company. The transfection method utilized is identical to that of YTHDF1.

Six siRNA sequences were designed for the transient knockdown of CDK6 and MAP3K6 expression (refer to Table S1 for sequence details). The transfection method utilized is identical to that of YTHDF1.

2.7. *Proteomic Sample Preparation Followed by LC-MS/MS*

The proteins were labeled according to the protocol provided with Thermo's TMT labeling kit (Thermo, Waltham, MI, USA). Reversed-phase (RP) and strong cation exchange (SCX) fractionation were performed on equally mixed labeled peptides from each group. The flow rate of the HPLC system was 300 nL/min. Buffer A (0.1% formic acid aqueous) and Buffer B (0.1% formic acid acetonitrile) were used. The linear elution gradient was as follows: 6% Buffer B for 5 min, 6–30% Buffer B for 60 min, 30–40% Buffer B for 10 min, 40–100% Buffer B for 5 min, and 100% buffer B for 5 min. Separation was performed using a Thermo Scientific EASY column. The analysis was carried out using a Q-Exactive mass spectrometer (Thermo Fisher Scientific, Waltham, MI, USA). The parent ion scanning range was 300–1800 m/z, the primary mass spectrometry resolution was 70,000 (200 m/z), the AGC (automatic gain control) was 10^6, and the maximum IT was 50 ms. The dynamic exclusion time was 60.0 s. The mass charge ratio was collected according to the following methods: After each full scan, 20 fragments were collected. The HCD isolation window was 2 m/z, the secondary mass spectrometry resolution was 17,500 (200 m/z), and the normalized collision energy was 30 eV. Underfill was 0.1%. For TMT quantitative proteomic sequencing, differentially expressed proteins were identified based on fold changes (FC) > 1.2 or FC < 0.83 and $p < 0.05$.

2.8. *Cell Proliferation*

Cell viability was assessed using the CCK8 (Cell Counting Kit-8, CELLCOOK, Guangzhou, China) assay. HBE, HBE-P35, and A549 cells were plated into a 96-well plate at a density of 2000–3000 cells per well. The CCK8 reagent was then added to the wells and incubated at 37 °C for 2 h. Optical density (OD) values were recorded at a wavelength of 450 nm using a Multiskan SkyHigh (Thermo Fisher Scientific, USA).

2.9. *Luciferase Reporter Assay*

Luciferase reporter gene assays were performed using the Dual-Luciferase Reporter Assay System (Yeasen, Shanghai, China), following the manufacturer's guidelines.

2.10. Determination of Total m6A

Experiments were performed using the EpiQuikTM m6A RNA Methylation Quantification Kit (Amyjet, Wuhan, China).

2.11. Methylated RNA Immunoprecipitation Sequencing and RIP Assay

The EZ-Magna RIP RNA-Binding Protein Immunoprecipitation Kit (Merck, Darmstadt, Germany) was utilized to perform the assay. First, cells were lysed using a custom-formulated RIP lysis buffer, and the cell extracts were subsequently incubated with IgG and antibodies at 4 °C overnight. RNA was purified from the complexes, and cDNA was synthesized before being subjected to RT-qPCR.

2.12. Transwell Assay

For cell migration assays, cells were plated into the upper chamber. In total, 600 μL of medium supplemented with 20% fetal bovine serum was added to the lower chamber. Cells were fixed with paraformaldehyde and stained with violet after 24 h. Samples were examined under a microscope, and a field of view was selected for cell counting. For the invasion assay, 50 μL of a matrigel and serum-free medium mixture (1:8 ratio) was added to the upper chamber and incubated at 37 °C for 30 min. The remaining steps are identical to those of the cell migration assays.

2.13. Wound Healing Assay

A single layer of cells was scratched with the tip of a sterile 1 mL pipette to simulate a wound. Two milliliters of serum-free medium were added, and the cells were incubated. The wound was examined and analyzed under a microscope after incubation for 0, 6, 12, 24, 48, and 72 h. The scratch area was quantified using the ImageJ software (https://ij.imjoy.io/ accessed on 21 March 2023), and the healing ability of the cells was subsequently analyzed.

2.14. Western Blot Analysis

The gel was prepared by mixing liquid A and liquid B of the PAGE gel in a 1:1 ratio, and then equivalent quantities of total protein were subjected to electrophoretic separation. The separated proteins underwent electrotransfer to a PVDF membrane, followed by a single TBST rinse. The membrane was then subjected to a blocking step using 5% skim milk in TBST for 2 h. Following blocking, the PVDF membrane was incubated with primary antibody overnight at 4 °C. Subsequently, three 15 min washes with TBST were performed at room temperature. The PVDF membrane was incubated with the secondary antibody for 1 h, washed with TBST 3 times for 15 min, and then the chemiluminescence assay was performed using ECL substrate (Amersham Biosciences, Amersham, UK). The gray values were quantified using ImageJ for statistical data analysis.

2.15. Statistical Analysis

SPSS 26.0 software was used to conduct statistical analyses. Significant differences are denoted by asterisks (*) in the figures. Statistical comparisons between two groups were conducted using independent samples *t*-tests, and one-way ANOVA was utilized for multi-group data analysis. A statistical comparison of survival between the two groups was conducted using the Log-rank test, with statistical significance defined at $p < 0.05$. Statistical graphs were created using GraphPad Prism 7.0.

3. Results

3.1. Constructing HBE Cell Malignant Transformation Model Through B[a]P Exposure

The malignant phenotype of HBE-P35 cells was characterized by evaluating their proliferative capacity and metastatic potential through migration and invasion assays. The results demonstrated that after 35 generations of chronic exposure to the chemical B[a]P, the proliferative capacity of HBE-P35 gradually increased compared to normal bronchial epithelial cells (HBE) (Figure 1A). Cells chronically exposed to B[a]P demonstrated a stronger wound healing ability compared to unexposed HBE cells (Figure 1B). The results of the cell invasion and metastasis experiments further demonstrated that HBE cells exhibited a malignant phenotype following prolonged exposure to B[a]P (Figure 1C). These findings imply that B[a]P can induce the malignant transformation of HBE cells and promote tumor development in vitro.

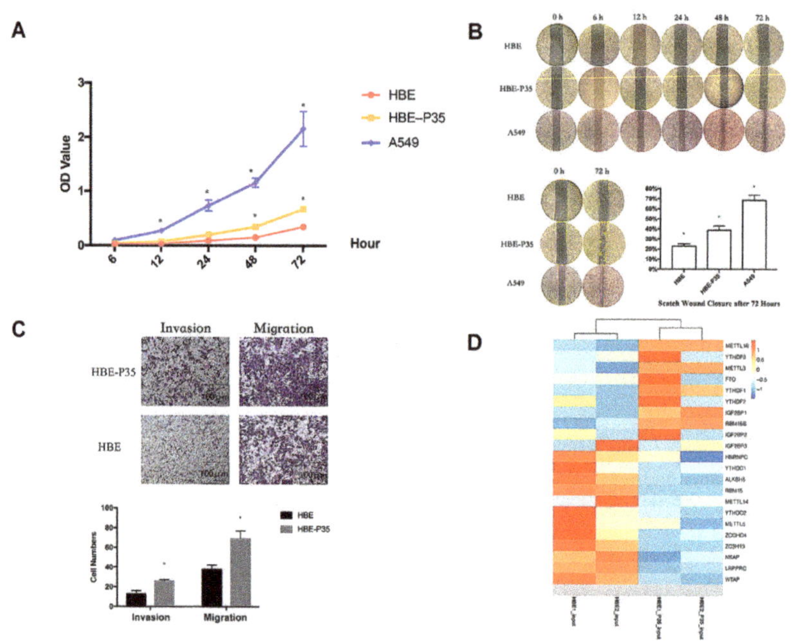

Figure 1. Long-term B[a]P exposure leads to a malignant phenotype in HBE cells. (**A**) Long-term B[a]P exposure enhances the proliferative capacity of HBE-P35 cells; (**B**) scratch assay of HBE and A549 cells with long-term B[a]P exposure; (**C**) long-term B[a]P exposure promoted HBE-P35 cell invasion and metastasis; (**D**) expression of m6A-related genes in transcriptome sequencing results of HBE and HBE-P35 cells. Values are presented as the mean ± SD. * $p < 0.05$, compared with passage-matched control HBE cells.

3.2. m6A Modification Is Implicated in the Malignant Transformation Process Induced by B[a]P Exposure

Transcriptome sequencing and MeRIP sequencing were employed to detect transcriptional and epigenetic changes in the malignant transformed HBE-P35 cells. To determine whether the level of m6A modification changes during lung cancer development, the total expression levels of m6A modification in HBE-P35 cells and lung cancer cells were examined. The results revealed that the level of m6A modification was elevated in HBE-P35 and lung adenocarcinoma cell line A549 compared to normal HBE cells (Figure S1A). To understand the impact of B[a]P exposure on the transcriptome and gene expression of HBE cells, next-generation sequencing (NGS) transcriptome sequencing was conducted on HBE and HBE-P35 cells. The results indicated that after continuous exposure to B[a]P, there are many differentially expressed transcripts and genes in HBE-P35 cells (Figure S1B–D). GO and KEGG enrichment analyses indicated that B[a]P exposure activated numerous classical pathways closely related to cancer occurrence and development, such as the PI3K signaling pathway, p53 signaling pathway, and ECM receptor (Figure S2A,B). Further analysis of the expression of m6A-related genes indicated that YTHDF1 was upregulated in HBE-P35 cells, suggesting that B[a]P exposure could promote the level of m6A modification and related protein expression to a certain extent (Figure 1D). MeRIP-Seq results indicated that there are lots of m6A-modified genes affected by B[a]P exposure (Figure S1E,F). This is not only fundamentally consistent with the results of whole-transcriptome sequencing but also indicates that m6A modification is indeed affected by B[a]P exposure and is involved in the carcinogenic and promoting processes associated with B[a]P.

3.3. YTHDF1 Regulates the Proliferation, Migration, and Invasion

YTHDF1 expression may be linked to the prognosis of lung cancer, as indicated by data from the TCGA and GEO databases (Figure S3). PCR and Western blot experiments on HBE, HBE-P35, and A549 cells demonstrated that the expression of YTHDF1 was higher in malignant transformed and lung cancer cells compared to HBE cells (Figure 2A). siRNAs and shRNAs targeting YTHDF1 were utilized to knock down YTHDF1 expression in HBE-P35 and A549 cells (Table S1). Subsequently, the cell assay confirmed that the viability of HBE-P35 and A549 cells with YTHDF1 knockdown was inhibited (Figure 2B). The migration and invasion capabilities of YTHDF1 was inhibited (Figure 2C). The wound healing further indicated that YTHDF1 promoted the migration of HBE-P35 and A549 cells (Figure 2D). Cell cycle experiments indicated that YTHDF1 knockdown caused S-phase blockade in HBE-P35 and A549 cells (Figure 2E). Collectively, the above functional experiments demonstrate that YTHDF1 regulates the proliferation, migration, and invasion of lung cancer cells. Therefore, a comprehensive investigation of YTHDF1 is essential for understanding the pathogenesis of the disease.

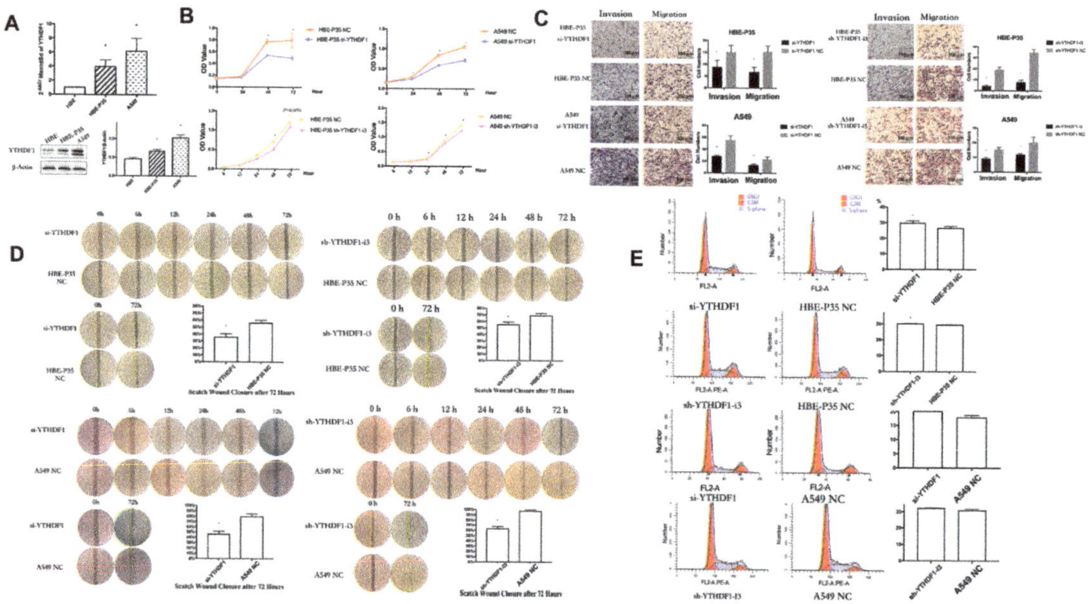

Figure 2. Knocking down YTHDF1 inhibits the growth, migration, and wound healing ability of HBE-P35 and A549 cells. (**A**) qPCR and WB analysis for YTHDF1 in HBE, HBE-P35, and A549. (**B**) CCK8 assays in A549 and HBE-P35 cells. (**C**) Transwell experiments showed that knocking down YTHDF1 reduced the invasion and migration ability of A549 cells and HBE-P35 cells. (**D**) Wound healing experiments showed that a low expression of YTHDF1 reduced the wound migration ability of cells. (**E**) Cell cycle experiments showed that the knockdown of YTHDF1 caused S-phase arrest of cells. Data are shown as means ± S.D.; * $p < 0.05$.

3.4. YTHDF1 Regulates Lung Carcinogenesis and Progression by Modulating CDK6 and MAP3K6

TMT labeling-based proteomic analysis of HBE-P35 and HBE-P35 cells was conducted with YTHDF1 knocked out (Figure S4). MAP3K6, CDK6, and PARD6β were found to be not only downregulated in YTHDF1 knockdown cells (Table S2) but also associated with cell cycle (Table S3). Therefore, we focused on these three proteins in our subsequent studies.

YTHDF1 regulates the expression levels of CDK6 and MAP3K6 proteins through m6A modification. We examined the expression of YTHDF1, CDK6, MAP3K6, and PARD-6β in clinical tissues using immunohistochemical staining (IHC) with tissue microarrays. The experimental data indicated that YTHDF1, MAP3K6, and CDK6 were significantly over-expressed in lung cancer compared to adjacent normal tissues ($p < 0.05$) (Figure 3A). Additionally, a positive correlation was observed between the expression levels of YTHDF1, MAP3K6, and CDK6 (Figure 3B). Moreover, the analysis revealed that CDK6 expression could significantly distinguish between LUAD and LUSC patients (Table S4). Unfortunately, no clear difference in PARD-6β expression was observed between paracancerous and lung cancer tissues. Moreover, no notable correlation was found between the expression levels of YTHDF1 and PARD-6β. Therefore, subsequent studies targeting downstream regulatory proteins of YTHDF1 will primarily focus on CDK6 and MAP3K6. Furthermore, the expression of CDK6 and MAP3K6 in HBE, HBE-P35, and A549 cells indicated that protein levels were significantly elevated in A549 and HBE-P35 compared to HBE ($p < 0.05$) (Figure 3C). This indicates that the expression of CDK6 and MAP3K6 was elevated during the transformation of normal cells into lung cancer cells. We further found that the expression of CDK6 and MAP3K6 proteins was also decreased in cells that knocked down YTHDF1, indicating a certain positive correlation between YTRHDF1 and CDK6 and MAP3K6 (Figure 3D,E). We subsequently examined the m6A modification status of CDK6 mRNA and MAP3K6 mRNA in HBE-P35 and A549 cells using a MeRIP-qPCR assay, confirming the presence of m6A modification sites on both CDK6 and MAP3K6 mRNA; furthermore, both were shown to bind to the YTHDF1 protein (Figure 3F). To investigate whether YTHDF1 regulates CDK6 and MAP3K6 through m6A-dependent regulation (Figure S5E), HBE-P35 and A549 cells were transfected with YTHDF1-mut (YTHDF1 with FLAG tagging in the YTH structural domain, introducing the K395A and Y397A mutation sites) and YTHDF1-wt (wild-type YTHDF1). Subsequent RIP-qPCR experiments validated the interaction between YTHDF1 and both CDK6 and MAP3K6 in HBE-P35 and A549 cells (Figure 3G). RIP analysis using an anti-FLAG antibody followed by quantitative PCR (qPCR) demonstrated efficient immunoprecipitation of CDK6 and MAP3K6 mRNA in cells transfected with YTHDF1-wt. In contrast, cells transfected with the YTHDF1-mut variant showed the significantly reduced immunoprecipitation of both CDK6 and MAP3K6 mRNA. This suggests that YTHDF1 regulates CDK6 and MAP3K6 mRNA through m6A modification.

3.5. CDK6 and MAP3K6 Regulate Proliferation, Cell Cycle, and Invasion

Cell growth, wound healing, cell cycle progression, migration, and invasion were carried out to explore the roles of CDK6 and MAP3K6. The results indicated that A549 and HBE-P35 cells with CDK6 knockdown exhibited inhibited growth (Figure 4A), wound healing (Figure 4C), and invasion (Figure 4B). Notably, S-phase blockade occurred in cells with CDK6 knockdown (Figure 4D). However, CDK6 knockdown had a limited effect on the number of cell migrations across the membrane, suggesting that CDK6 protein still possesses the ability to promote cell migration. As a cyclin, migration may not be the primary cellular function of CDK6. The knockdown of MAP3K6 inhibited the proliferation and invasion of both HBE-P35 and A549 cells (Figure 4A,B). MAP3K6 knockdown had no significant effect on wound healing and cell migration, indicating that MAP3K6 does not promote cell migration (Figure 4B,C). The S-phase arrest observed in A549 cells, but not in HBE-P35 cells, was attributed to MAP3K6 knockdown, possibly because HBE-P35 cells did not undergo sufficient malignant transformation, and MAP3K6 primarily promoted the cell cycle in cancer cells (Figure 4D). In summary, these results suggest that CDK6 and MAP3K6 function to promote lung carcinogenesis.

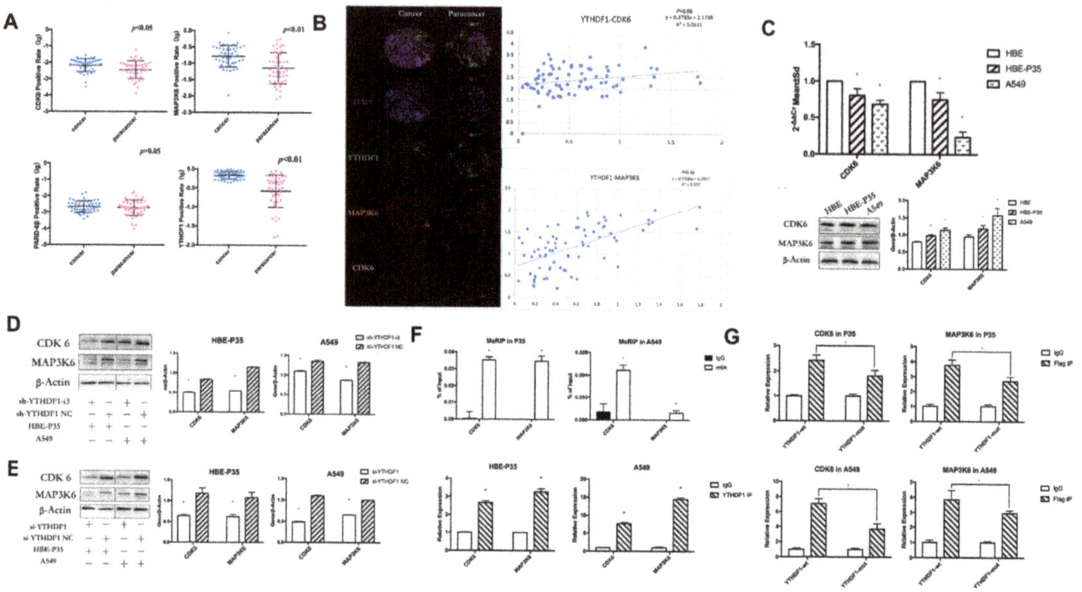

Figure 3. YTHDF1 regulates CDK6 and MAP3K6 mRNA expression through m6A. (**A**) The expression of YTHDF1, CDK6, MAP3K6, and PARD-6β in clinical lung cancer tissues by immunohistochemical staining (IHC) using tissue microarrays. (**B**) Relationship between CDK6 and MAP3K6 as well as YTHDF1 in clinical lung cancer tissues. (**C**) qPCR and WB of CDK6 and MAP3K6 in A549, HBE, and HBE-P35 cells. (**D**,**E**) After YTHDF1 knockdown, CDK6 and MAP3K6 protein expression levels. (**F**) Top: m6A Me-RIP followed by RT-qPCR. Bottom, YTHDF1 RIP followed by RT-qPCR. (**G**) RT-qPCR in A549 and HBE-P35 cells. Data are shown as means ± S.D.; * $p < 0.05$.

3.6. miR-139/145-5p Are Upstream Regulators of YTHDF1 in the Progression of Lung Cancer

Differential analysis of paired lung cancer tissue samples from TCGA revealed that the expression levels of 122 miRNAs were significantly regulated in lung cancer tissues ($p < 0.05$, | log2FC | > 1). Among these, 34 miRNAs were significantly under-expressed, while 88 miRNAs were significantly over-expressed (Figure S6A,B). The miRWalk and starBase databases were further applied to predict the upstream miRNAs of YTHDF1, while intersections were taken with the above differential miRNAs. The results showed that among the 11 miRNAs in the intersection, miR-184, miR-139-5p, and miR-145-5p were under-expressed in lung cancer tissues, which were inversely proportional to the expression of YTHDF1 and might be the key miRNAs regulating YTHDF1 (Figure S6C). Analysis of the GEO database showed that only miR-139-5p and miR-145-5p were specifically under-expressed in lung cancer patients ($p < 0.05$, | log2FC | > 1), and the expression of miR-184 was inconsistent and did not match the predicted results (Table S5). PCR reveals the expression of hsa-miR-139/145-5p decreased in HBE-P35 cells, and A549 cells compared to HBE cells (Figure S6D). Therefore, we now focus on the mechanism of miR-139-5p and miR-145-5p in lung cancer.

The regulatory relationships between miRNAs and YTHDF1 were investigated. First, the experimental results indicated that the expression of YTHDF1 was downregulated in HBE-P35 and A549 cells over-expressing miR-139/145-5p (Figure 5A,B). The proteins levels of CDK6 and MAP3K6 changed significantly, while the mRNA levels did not change (Figure 5A,B). These results showed that miR-139-5p/miR-145-5p were negatively correlated withYTHDF1 expression. Furthermore, the regulatory relationship between miR-

139-5p/miR-145-5p and the downstream genes CDK6 and MAP3K6 mirrored the effect of YTHDF1 on these two genes.

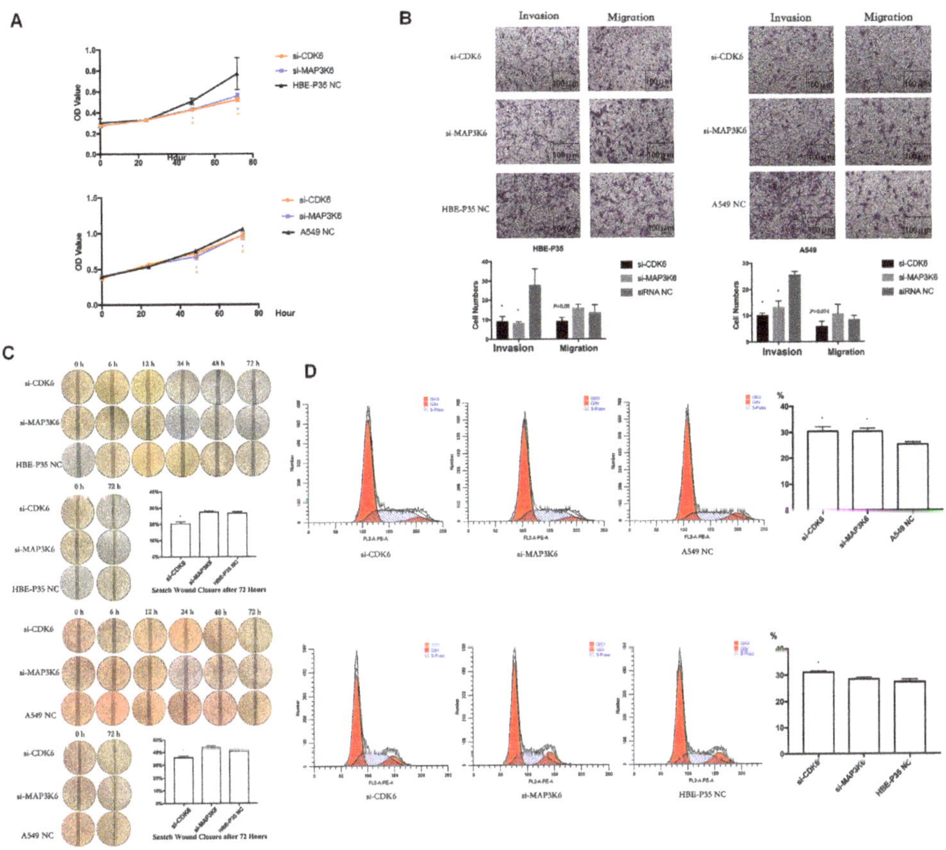

Figure 4. (**A**) CCK8 assays in A549 and HBE-P35 cells. (**B**) Transwell experiments showed that knocking down CDK6 and MAP3K6 reduced the invasion ability of A549 cells and HBE-P35 cells. (**C**) Wound healing experiments showed that a low expression of CDK6 reduced the wound migration ability of cells. (**D**) Cell cycle experiments showed that the knockdown of CDK6 caused S-phase arrest of A549cells and HBE-P35 cells. Data are shown as means ± S.D.; * $p < 0.05$.

When HBE-P35 and A549 cells were treated with miR-139-5p inhibitors (Figure 5C,D), both YTHDF1 mRNA and protein expression were elevated with statistical significance in HBE-P35 and A549 cells ($p < 0.05$). The protein expression of CDK6 and MAP3K6 was also elevated; conversely, the reduction in miR-139-5p expression promoted CDK6 mRNA elevation and had no effect on MAP3K6 mRNA. In HBE-P35, when miR-145-5p expression was suppressed, it still had a negative regulatory relationship on the expression of YTHDF1, CDK6, and MAP3K6 protein and had no effect on CDK6 and MAP3K6 mRNA. However, it showed the inhibition of the proteins of YTHDF1, CDK6, and MAP3K6 in A549 cells. In conclusion, miR-139-5p was negatively correlated with YTHDF1 expression in both HBE-P35 and A549 cells, and it increased the protein expression of both CDK6 and MAP3K6. In this regulatory process, the inhibition of miR-139-5p expression exerted a negative regulatory effect on CDK6 mRNA. This finding suggests that miR-139-5p, as an upstream regulator, may modulate CDK6 through multiple regulatory axes and mechanisms. While the regulatory relationship of miR-145-5p on YTHDF1, CDK6, and MAP3K6 showed diametrically opposite results in HBE-P35 and A549 cells, which needs to be supplemented by subsequent experiments.

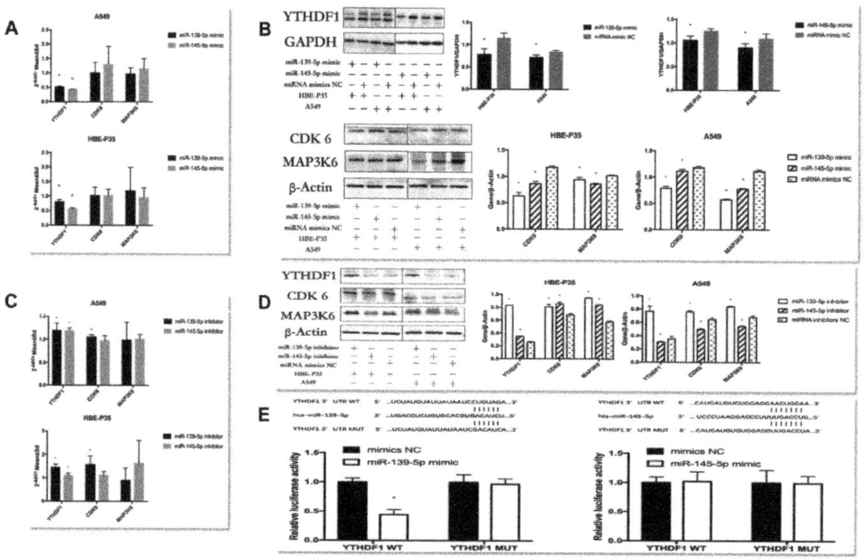

Figure 5. Explore the regulatory role between YTHDF1 and hsa-miR-139/145-5p. (**A**,**B**) RT-qPCR and Western blot explore the expression of YTHDF1, CDK6, and MAP3K6 in hsa-miR-139/145-5p over-expressed in A549 cells and HBE-P3 cells. (**C**,**D**) The expression of YTHDF1, CDK6, and MAP3K6 in A549 cells and HBE-P35 cells with low expression of hsa-miR-139/145-5p was detected by RT-qPCR and Western blot. (**E**) Luciferase reporter genes reveal that miR-139 could reduce cellular luciferase activity. Data are shown as means ± S.D.; * $p < 0.05$.

To verify whether hsa-miR-139/145-5p directly targets YTHDF1 in HBE-P35 and A549 cells, we cloned YTHDF1 mRNA (designated as YTHDF1 WT) along with two mutants (designated as YTHDF1 MUT). After the co-transfection of YTHDF1 wild-type/mutant plasmids with miR-139-5p NC/mimic, only the fluorescence intensity of PmirGLO YTHDF1-3′UTR-WT in the miR-139-5p mimic group was significantly lower compared to that of the other three groups (Figure 5E). This result indicates an miR-139-5p-YTHDF1 mRNA binding interaction, with the binding site being the one predicted with TargetScan (http://www.targetscan.org/); after the co-transfection of YTHDF1 wild-type/mutant plasmid and miR-145-5p NC/mimic, there was no difference in the fluorescence intensity of all four groups (Figure 5E), indicating that miR-145-5p and YTHDF1 mRNA do not bind through the binding site predicted by TargetScan and do not bind to each other. These results indicate that YTHDF1 mRNA is a target of miR-139-5p and is directly regulated by it. By contrast, miR-145-5p does not appear to directly regulate YTHDF1.

3.7. miR-139/145-5P Regulate the Proliferation, Cell Cycle, Migration, and Invasion of Lung Cancer Cells

To analyze the biological function of hsa-miR-139/145-5p, two types of mimics were used to enhance the expression of hsa-miR-139/145-5p in A549 and HBE-P35 cells (Figure S5). CCK8 assays indicated that the proliferation of HBE-P35 and A549 cells was inhibited with an enhanced expression of hsa-miR-139/145-5p (Figure 6A). Transwell assays further demonstrated that the enhanced expression of hsa-miR-139/145-5p inhibited the migration and invasion capabilities of HBE-P35 and A549 cells (Figure 6B). The wound healing assay further demonstrated that hsa-miR-139/145-5p inhibited the migration of lung cancer cells (Figure 6C). Cell cycle experiments indicated that the knockdown of miR-139/145-5p in A549 cells resulted in S-phase arrest, suggesting that these two miRNAs promote cell cycle progression (Figure 6D). However, the knockdown of miR-139/145-5p in HBE-P35 cells did not lead to S-phase arrest, possibly because the malignancy of HBE-P35 cells is lower than that of lung cancer A549 cells. These results suggest that hsa-miR-139/145-5p plays a role in the development of lung cancer.

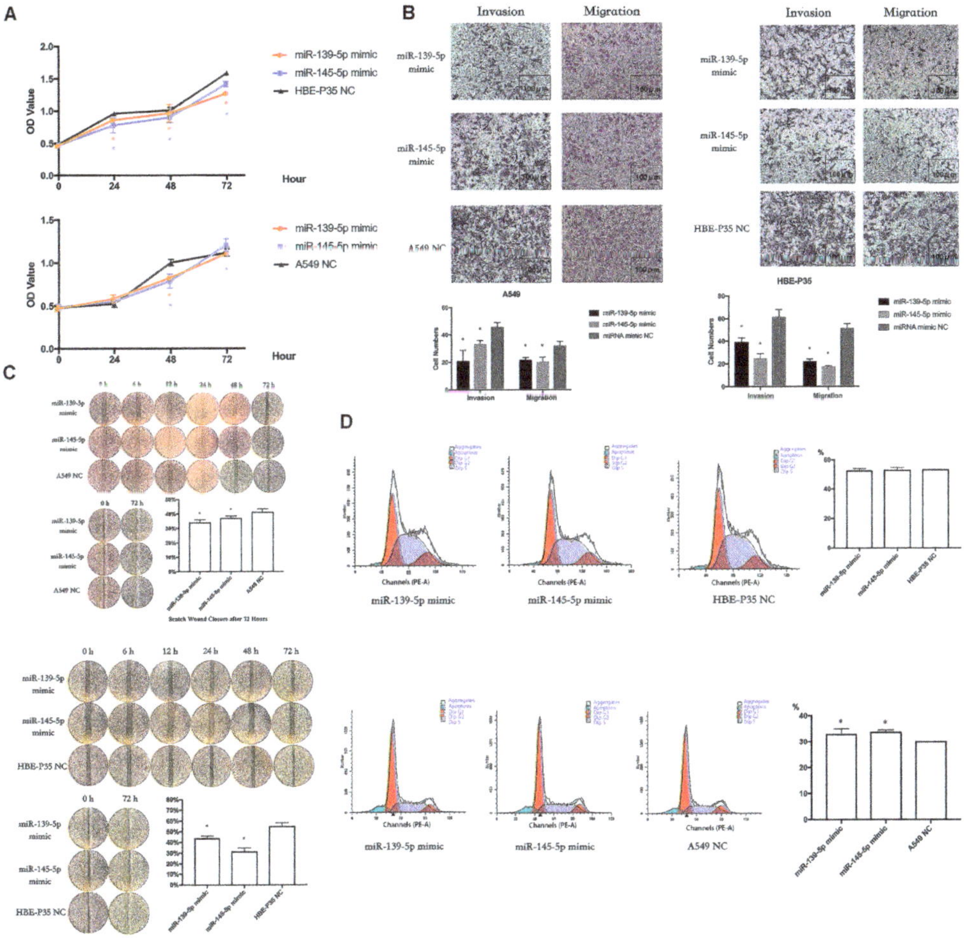

Figure 6. miR-139/145-5P regulates the proliferation, cell cycle, migration, and invasion of lung cancer cells. (**A**) CCK8 assays in A549 and HBE-P35 cells with hsa-miR-139/145-5p over-expressed. (**B**) Transwell experiments showed that over-expression of hsa-miR-139/145-5p inhibited the invasion and migration of cells. (**C**) Wound healing experiments showed that over-expression of hsa-miR-139/145-5p inhibited cell migration. (**D**) Cell cycle experiments showed that over-expression of hsa-miR-139/145-5p caused S-phase arrest of A549 cells. Data are shown as means ± SD; * $p < 0.05$.

4. Discussion

An altered expression of m6A is strongly linked to the development of various tumors [26]. Our study showed that m6A expression was elevated in B[a]P-induced HBE-P35 and A549 cells compared to HBE cells. Tumor growth and invasion are regulated by m6A-associated genes, including "writers", "readers", and "erasers", highlighting the importance of exploring the expression and interactions between m6A and its associated genes in tumors [27,28]. Although some studies have investigated the pathogenic mechanism of YTHDF1 in lung cancer [29–31], the progression of lung cancer results from the mutual regulation of multiple factors, with fewer studies conducted to investigate the regulatory axis of YTHDF1. Our study revealed that the YTHDF1 gene was upregulated in NSCLC within the TCGA cohorts. Subsequent experiments involving the immunohistochemical staining of clinical lung cancer tissue microarrays and detection of YTHDF1 expression levels in HBE-P35 and A549 cells further confirmed this trend. Notably, analysis of GEO survival data revealed that elevated YTHDF1 expression was associated with overall survival, suggesting that YTHDF1 mRNA expression could serve as a prognostic marker for overall survival in NSCLC. The loss-of-function experiment results showed that YTHDF1 in HBE-P35 and A549 cells promoted cell growth, wound healing, and the invasion and migration of cells. Further cell cycle experiments indicated that S-phase arrest occurred in YTHDF1 knockdown cells, suggesting that YTHDF1 functions to drive the cell cycle forward. Thus, YTHDF1 plays a crucial role in the onset and progression of NSCLC.

YTHDF1 regulates the expression of CDK6 and MAP3K6 proteins through m6A modification. To further investigate the mechanism of YTHDF1 in lung cancer, TMT labeling-based proteomic analysis was performed using cells with YTHDF1 knockdown. The results revealed a reduction in CDK6 and MAP3K6 in YTHDF1 knockdown cells. Previous studies have demonstrated that CDK6 promotes lung cancer cell proliferation by advancing the cell cycle, and that CDK6 expression is linked to overall survival in lung cancer patients [32,33]. The MAP3K family is also implicated in cancer progression [34]. Therefore, by combining TMT labeling-based proteomic analysis with previous findings, we explored the roles of CDK6 and MAP3K6 in lung cancer development and the relationship between YTHDF1, CDK6, and MAP3K6. Immunohistochemical staining (IHC) experiments on clinical lung cancer tissues using tissue microarrays demonstrated a positive correlation between YTHDF1 and its downstream proteins, CDK6 and MAP3K6. MeRIP-qPCR experiments indicated that the m6A expression of CDK6 and MAP3K6 were elevated in HBE-P35 and A549 cells. Two subsequent RIP-qPCR experiments further indicated that YTHDF1 regulates the expression levels of CDK6 and MAP3K6 proteins through m6A-dependent regulation. Our experiments also indicated that CDK6 and MAP3K6 are involved in regulating cancer cell proliferation, invasion, migration, wound healing, and cell cycle progression.

miR-139/145-5p act as upstream regulators of YTHDF1 in the development of lung cancer. A recent study suggested that environmental exposures may affect the health of the organism by influencing the expression of non-coding RNAs [35]. Analysis of the TCGA database, online resources, and our cellular experiments revealed that miR-139-5p was lowly expressed in HBE-P35 and A549 cells. Moreover, it has been shown that miR-139-5p inhibits the development of lung cancer [36,37]. Our experimental results were consistent with these findings. Furthermore, it has been shown that miR-145-5p regulates tumor development [38,39]. Our analysis also revealed that miR-145-5p was lowly expressed in lung cancer tissues and cells. Therefore, studying the function of hsa-miR-139/145-5p in non-small-cell lung cancer (NSCLC) is important.

miR-139/145-5p tended to decrease the protein levels of YTHDF1 in HBE-P35 and A549 cells. An opposite trend of YTHDF1 was observed in HBE-P35 cells with suppressed miR-139/145-5p expression. However, in A549 cells, as miR-145-5p expression decreased, YTHDF1 also exhibited a trend of downregulation, suggesting a more complex regulatory mechanism between miR-145-5p and YTHDF1 in NSCLC. The luciferase reporter assay further demonstrated that YTHDF1 mRNA was directly regulated by miR-139-5p but not by miR-145-5p. Our experimental results are consistent with those of a previous report, which indicated that miR-145-5p could directly target YTHDF2 [38]. Cellular function experiments demonstrated that miR-139-5p regulates cell proliferation, wound healing, invasion, and migration, and drives the cell cycle. In conclusion, miR-139-5p promotes lung cancer cell growth through the direct regulation of YTHDF1 mRNA.

In conclusion, B[a]P exposure can facilitate the progression of non-small-cell lung cancer (NSCLC) by altering m6A expression. miR-139-5p promotes the growth of HBE-P35 and A549 cells through the direct regulation of YTHDF1 mRNA. YTHDF1 regulates CDK6 and MAP3K6 expression through m6A in B[a]P-induced HBE-P35 and A549 cells. Since our study lacks epidemiological studies on specific populations, as well as in vivo animal studies, we will later study the toxic effects of BaP through m6A in more depth from these two aspects. In conclusion, our study presents a potential target for the diagnosis and treatment of lung cancer.

Supplementary Materials: The following supporting information can be downloaded at https://www.mdpi.com/article/10.3390/toxics13040280/s1. Figure S1: B[a]P-induced changes of m6A expression level in HBE-P35 cells; Figure S2: Long-term B[a]P exposure leads to a malignant phenotype in HBE cells; Figure S3: Expression of m6A and YTHDF1 in lung cancer and relationship between YTHDF1 and overall survival time; Figure S4: TMT labelling-based proteomic analysis was performed on YTHDF1 knockdown lung cancer cells and controls; Figure S5: Transfection efficiency; Figure S6: The expression of hsa-miR-139/145-5p. Table S1: Sequence of YTHDF1, CDK6, MAP3K6; Table S2: The expression of differentially expressed proteins in YTHDF1 knockdown cells; Table S3: MAP3K6, CDK6 and PARD6β localization signaling pathways; Table S4: Clinical information and gene expression analysis of tissue microarray; Table S5: Expression analysis of key microRNAs in the GEO database lung cancer population sequencing dataset.

Author Contributions: Conceptualization, S.X.; data curation, S.X. and J.L.; funding acquisition, G.L.; investigation, S.X. and J.L.; validation, S.X. and J.L.; visualization, S.X., J.L. and S.Y.; writing—original draft, S.X. and J.L.; writing—review and editing, S.Y., P.Y., Y.N., Y.G. and G.L. All authors have read and agreed to the published version of the manuscript.

Funding: This research was funded by the National Natural Science Foundation of China, grant numbers 81972998, 82173478.

Institutional Review Board Statement: The study was conducted in accordance with the Declaration of Helsinki. The cancer tissue microarrays were provided by Ai Hunan Hunan Bio-technology Co., Ltd. (Changsha, China), and local ethical approval was obtained by the company.

Informed Consent Statement: Informed consent was obtained from all subjects involved in the study.

Data Availability Statement: The datasets generated and analyzed during the current study are available from the TCGA database (http://cancergenome.nih.gov/publications/publicationguidelines/, accessed on 12 February 2017) and GEO databases (http://www.bioinfo-zs.com/luadexpress/, accessed on 15 March 2021). Data will be made available on request.

Conflicts of Interest: The authors declare no conflicts of interest.

References

1. Sung, H.; Ferlay, J.; Siegel, R.L.; Laversanne, M.; Soerjomataram, I.; Jemal, A.; Bray, F. Global Cancer Statistics 2020: GLOBOCAN Estimates of Incidence and Mortality Worldwide for 36 Cancers in 185 Countries. *CA Cancer J. Clin.* **2021**, *71*, 209–249. [PubMed]
2. Miller, K.D.; Nogueira, L.; Mariotto, A.B.; Rowland, J.H.; Yabroff, K.R.; Alfano, C.M.; Jemal, A.; Kramer, J.L.; Siegel, R.L. Cancer treatment and survivorship statistics, 2019. *CA Cancer J. Clin.* **2019**, *69*, 363–385. [CrossRef] [PubMed]
3. Montano, L.; Baldini, G.M.; Piscopo, M.; Liguori, G.; Lombardi, R.; Ricciardi, M.; Esposito, G.; Pinto, G.; Fontanarosa, C.; Spinelli, M.; et al. Polycyclic Aromatic Hydrocarbons (PAHs) in the Environment: Occupational Exposure, Health Risks and Fertility Implications. *Toxics* **2025**, *13*, 151. [CrossRef]
4. Menck, H.R.; Casagrande, J.T.; Henderson, B.E. Industrial air pollution: Possible effect on lung cancer. *Science* **1974**, *183*, 210.
5. Meng, H.; Li, G.; Wei, W.; Bai, Y.; Feng, Y.; Fu, M.; Guan, X.; Li, M.; Li, H.; Wang, C.; et al. Epigenome-wide DNA methylation signature of benzo[a]pyrene exposure and their mediation roles in benzo[a]pyrene-associated lung cancer development. *J. Hazard. Mater.* **2021**, *416*, 125839. [PubMed]
6. Hu, X.; Geetha, R.V.; Surapaneni, K.M.; Veeraraghavan, V.P.; Chinnathambi, A.; Alahmadi, T.A.; Manikandan, V.; Manokaran, K. Lung cancer induced by Benzo(A)Pyrene: ChemoProtective effect of sinapic acid in swiss albino mice. *Saudi J. Biol. Sci.* **2021**, *28*, 7125–7133. [CrossRef]
7. Kasala, E.R.; Bodduluru, L.N.; Barua, C.C.; Sriram, C.S.; Gogoi, R. Benzo(a)pyrene induced lung cancer: Role of dietary phytochemicals in chemoprevention. *Pharmacol. Rep.* **2015**, *67*, 996–1009.
8. Friedberg, E.C. DNA damage and repair. *Nature* **2003**, *421*, 436–440. [CrossRef]
9. Friedberg, E.C.; McDaniel, L.D.; Schultz, R.A. The role of endogenous and exogenous DNA damage and mutagenesis. *Curr. Opin. Genet. Dev.* **2004**, *14*, 5–10.
10. Denissenko, M.F.; Pao, A.; Tang, M.S.; Pfeifer, G.P. Preferential formation of benzo[a]pyrene adducts at lung cancer mutational hotspots in P53. *Science* **1996**, *274*, 430–432.
11. Jiang, Y.J.; Chao, C.C.; Chang, A.C.; Chen, P.C.; Cheng, F.J.; Liu, J.F.; Liu, P.I.; Huang, C.L.; Guo, J.H.; Huang, W.C.; et al. Cigarette smoke-promoted increases in osteopontin expression attract mesenchymal stem cell recruitment and facilitate lung cancer metastasis. *J. Adv. Res.* **2022**, *41*, 77–87. [PubMed]
12. Adams, J.M.; Cory, S. Modified nucleosides and bizarre 5′-termini in mouse myeloma mRNA. *Nature* **1975**, *255*, 28–33.
13. Oerum, S.; Meynier, V.; Catala, M.; Tisné, C. A comprehensive review of m6A/m6Am RNA methyltransferase structures. *Nucleic Acids Res.* **2021**, *49*, 7239–7255. [PubMed]
14. Dominissini, D.; Moshitch-Moshkovitz, S.; Schwartz, S.; Salmon-Divon, M.; Ungar, L.; Osenberg, S.; Cesarkas, K.; Jacob-Hirsch, J.; Amariglio, N.; Kupiec, M.; et al. Topology of the human and mouse m6A RNA methylomes revealed by m6A-seq. *Nature* **2012**, *485*, 201–206. [PubMed]
15. Zhang, H.; Shi, X.; Huang, T.; Zhao, X.; Chen, W.; Gu, N.; Zhang, R. Dynamic landscape and evolution of m6A methylation in human. *Nucleic Acids Res.* **2020**, *48*, 6251–6264.
16. Gu, C.; Shi, X.; Dai, C.; Shen, F.; Rocco, G.; Chen, J.; Huang, Z.; Chen, C.; He, C.; Huang, T.; et al. RNA m(6)A Modification in Cancers: Molecular Mechanisms and Potential Clinical Applications. *Innovation* **2020**, *1*, 100066.
17. Wang, T.; Kong, S.; Tao, M.; Ju, S. The potential role of RNA N6-methyladenosine in Cancer progression. *Mol. Cancer* **2020**, *19*, 88.
18. Hao, J.; Yu, X.; Gao, W.; Wei, J.; Qi, M.; Han, L.; Shi, S.; Lin, C.; Wang, D. The perturbed expression of m6A in parthenogenetic mouse embryos. *Genet. Mol. Biol.* **2019**, *42*, 666–670.
19. Wang, X.; Zhao, B.S.; Roundtree, I.A.; Lu, Z.; Han, D.; Ma, H.; Weng, X.; Chen, K.; Shi, H.; He, C. N(6)-methyladenosine Modulates Messenger RNA Translation Efficiency. *Cell* **2015**, *161*, 1388–1399.
20. Shi, Y.; Fan, S.; Wu, M.; Zuo, Z.; Li, X.; Jiang, L.; Shen, Q.; Xu, P.; Zeng, L.; Zhou, Y.; et al. YTHDF1 links hypoxia adaptation and non-small cell lung cancer progression. *Nat. Commun.* **2019**, *10*, 4892.
21. Bai, Y.; Yang, C.; Wu, R.; Huang, L.; Song, S.; Li, W.; Yan, P.; Lin, C.; Li, D.; Zhang, Y. YTHDF1 Regulates Tumorigenicity and Cancer Stem Cell-Like Activity in Human Colorectal Carcinoma. *Front. Oncol.* **2019**, *9*, 332. [CrossRef] [PubMed]
22. Zhao, X.; Chen, Y.; Mao, Q.; Jiang, X.; Jiang, W.; Chen, J.; Xu, W.; Zhong, L.; Sun, X. Overexpression of YTHDF1 is associated with poor prognosis in patients with hepatocellular carcinoma. *Cancer Biomark.* **2018**, *21*, 859–868. [CrossRef]
23. Luo, X.; Cao, M.; Gao, F.; He, X. YTHDF1 promotes hepatocellular carcinoma progression via activating PI3K/AKT/mTOR signaling pathway and inducing epithelial-mesenchymal transition. *Exp. Hematol. Oncol.* **2021**, *10*, 35. [CrossRef]
24. Ye, J.; Wang, Z.; Chen, X.; Jiang, X.; Dong, Z.; Hu, S.; Li, W.; Liu, Y.; Liao, B.; Han, W.; et al. YTHDF1-enhanced iron metabolism depends on TFRC m(6)A methylation. *Theranostics* **2020**, *10*, 12072–12089. [CrossRef] [PubMed]
25. Pi, J.; Wang, W.; Ji, M.; Wang, X.; Wei, X.; Jin, J.; Liu, T.; Qiang, J.; Qi, Z.; Li, F.; et al. YTHDF1 Promotes Gastric Carcinogenesis by Controlling Translation of FZD7. *Cancer Res.* **2021**, *81*, 2651–2665. [CrossRef] [PubMed]

26. Duruisseaux, M.; Esteller, M. Lung cancer epigenetics: From knowledge to applications. *Semin. Cancer Biol.* **2018**, *51*, 116–128. [CrossRef]
27. Ma, J.Z.; Yang, F.; Zhou, C.C.; Liu, F.; Yuan, J.H.; Wang, F.; Wang, T.T.; Xu, Q.G.; Zhou, W.P.; Sun, S. METTL14 suppresses the metastatic potential of hepatocellular carcinoma by modulating N(6) -methyladenosine-dependent primary MicroRNA processing. *Hepatology* **2017**, *65*, 529–543. [CrossRef]
28. Cheng, M.; Sheng, L.; Gao, Q.; Xiong, Q.; Zhang, H.; Wu, M.; Liang, Y.; Zhu, F.; Zhang, Y.; Zhang, X.; et al. The m(6)A methyltransferase METTL3 promotes bladder cancer progression via AFF4/NF-κB/MYC signaling network. *Oncogene* **2019**, *38*, 3667–3680. [CrossRef]
29. Tsuchiya, K.; Yoshimura, K.; Inoue, Y.; Iwashita, Y.; Yamada, H.; Kawase, A.; Watanabe, T.; Tanahashi, M.; Ogawa, H.; Funai, K.; et al. YTHDF1 and YTHDF2 are associated with better patient survival and an inflamed tumor-immune microenvironment in non-small-cell lung cancer. *Oncoimmunology* **2021**, *10*, 1962656. [CrossRef]
30. Diao, H.; Tan, H.; Hu, Y.; Wang, R.; Cai, P.; Huang, B.; Shao, X.; Yan, M.; Yin, C.; Zhang, Y. The m(6)A Reader YTHDF1 Promotes Lung Carcinoma Progression via Regulating Ferritin Mediate Ferroptosis in an m(6)A-Dependent Manner. *Pharmaceuticals* **2023**, *16*, 185. [CrossRef]
31. Zhang, R.N.; Wu, D.M.; Wu, L.P.; Gao, G.W. LncRNA LINC00337 sponges mir-1285-3p to promote proliferation and metastasis of lung adenocarcinoma cells by upregulating YTHDF1. *Cancer Cell Int.* **2021**, *21*, 550.
32. Mu, R.; Liu, H.; Luo, S.; Patz, E.F., Jr.; Glass, C.; Su, L.; Du, M.; Christiani, D.C.; Jin, L.; Wei, Q. Genetic variants of CHEK1, PRIM2 and CDK6 in the mitotic phase-related pathway are associated with nonsmall cell lung cancer survival. *Int. J. Cancer* **2021**, *149*, 1302–1312. [PubMed]
33. Yin, M.; Cheng, M.; Liu, C.; Wu, K.; Xiong, W.; Fang, J.; Li, Y.; Zhang, B. HNRNPA2B1 as a trigger of RNA switch modulates the miRNA-mediated regulation of CDK6. *Iscience* **2021**, *24*, 103345. [PubMed]
34. Ferrero, G.; Festa, R.; Follia, L.; Lettieri, G.; Tarallo, S.; Notari, T.; Giarra, A.; Marinaro, C.; Pardini, B.; Marano, A.; et al. Small noncoding RNAs and sperm nuclear basic proteins reflect the environmental impact on germ cells. *Mol. Med.* **2024**, *30*, 12.
35. Cheung, A.H.; Wong, K.Y.; Liu, X.; Ji, F.; Hui, C.H.L.; Zhang, Y.; Kwan, J.S.H.; Chen, B.; Dong, Y.; Lung, R.W.M.; et al. MLK4 promotes glucose metabolism in lung adenocarcinoma through CREB-mediated activation of phosphoenolpyruvate carboxykinase and is regulated by KLF5. *Oncogenesis* **2023**, *12*, 35.
36. Zhang, M.; Lin, B.; Liu, Y.; Huang, T.; Chen, M.; Lian, D.; Deng, S.; Zhuang, C. LINC00324 affects non-small cell lung cancer cell proliferation and invasion through regulation of the miR-139-5p/IGF1R axis. *Mol. Cell Biochem.* **2020**, *473*, 193–202.
37. Yan, Y.; Jin, X.; Sun, H.; Pang, S.; Kong, X.; Bu, J.; Xu, S. MiR-139-5p Targetedly Regulates YAF2 and Mediates the AKT/P38 MAPK Signaling Pathway to Alleviate the Metastasis of Non-Small Cell Lung Cancer Cells and Their Resistance Against Cisplatin. *Cancer Manag. Res.* **2021**, *13*, 3639–3650.
38. Yang, Z.; Li, J.; Feng, G.; Gao, S.; Wang, Y.; Zhang, S.; Liu, Y.; Ye, L.; Li, Y.; Zhang, X. MicroRNA-145 Modulates N(6)-Methyladenosine Levels by Targeting the 3′-Untranslated mRNA Region of the N(6)-Methyladenosine Binding YTH Domain Family 2 Protein. *J. Biol. Chem.* **2017**, *292*, 3614–3623.
39. Li, J.; Baila, B.; Xu, T.X.; Song, J.; Rina, S.; Wu, J.; Wang, T. Effects of hsa-mir-145-5p on the Regulation of msln Expression in Colorectal Adenocarcinoma. *Anal. Cell Pathol.* **2022**, *2022*, 5587084.

toxics

MDPI

Article

Internal Bisphenol Analogue Exposure in an Elderly Chinese Population: Knowledge from Dietary Exposure

Xinjie Duan [1,†], Mengyuan Liang [2,†], Beibei Wei [1,3], Jie Gu [2], Qian Zhao [4], Guixiang Ji [2], Shengyang Jin [5,*] and Huanhuan Chen [1,*]

1 Department of Endocrinology, The First Affiliated Hospital of Nanjing Medical University, No. 300, Guangzhou Road, Gulou District, Nanjing 210029, China; duanxinjie0307@163.com (X.D.); 18914712609@163.com (B.W.)
2 Nanjing Institute of Environmental Science, Ministry of Ecology and Environment, No. 8, Jiangwangmiao Street, Xuanwu District, Nanjing 210042, China; liangmengyuan@nies.org (M.L.); gujie@nies.org (J.G.); jgx@nies.org (G.J.)
3 Department of Endocrinology, Nanjing Lishui People's Hospital, No. 86, Chongwen Road, Lishui District, Nanjing 211200, China
4 Department of Endocrinology, Nanjing Liuhe District People's Hospital, No. 28, Yanan Road, Liuhe District, Nanjing 211500, China; zq_19871011@163.com
5 Development Area Branch of Lianyungang Municipal Bureau of Ecology and Environment, No. 601, Huaguoshan Road, Lianyungang Economic & Technological Development Area, Lianyungang 222069, China
* Correspondence: jsyhn@126.com (S.J.); drchenhuanhuan@njmu.edu.cn (H.C.)
† These authors contributed equally to this work.

Abstract: Due to its endocrine-disrupting effects and neurotoxicity, Bisphenol A (BPA) has been banned from some products and some countries; therefore, alternatives are increasingly being used. Studies have been performed to evaluate internal Bisphenol analogue (BP) exposure in children, adolescents and adults; however, little information on elderly age groups is available. In this study, a cohort of 161 senior residents aged 60–70 years, from a coastal residential district in Jiangsu Province of China, was selected, and blood samples were collected from these individuals to evaluate internal BP exposure. The serum concentrations of eleven BPs (BPA, BPB, BPC, BPE, BPF, BPS, BPZ, BPP, BPAF, BPAP and TBBPA) were quantitatively determined by HPLC-MS/MS. In parallel, demographic and dietary surveys were conducted, and the potential association between BP levels and dietary habits was analyzed. Noteworthily, the detection rate of 10 BPs in serum samples exceeded 78%. Of all the BPs, BPA displayed the highest level, followed by BPAF, BPB, and BPS. Interestingly, the levels of most types of BPs in males were higher than those in females, and individuals above 65 years of age exhibited significantly higher BPA levels. Dietary analysis indicated a significant correlation between meat consumption and BP levels, implying that this is an important source of BP exposure. The current study uncovers previously unknown aspects of BPs exposure, characterized by high internal BP levels in the elderly, and risk factors such as gender and meat consumption. This offers valuable insights for preventing region-specific BP exposure in the elderly.

Keywords: bisphenol analogues; internal exposure; influencing factors; exposure assessment

1. Introduction

Environmental endocrine-disrupting chemicals (EDCs) are a class of exogenous substances that can cause endocrine toxicity, as well as developmental and reproductive toxicity [1]. Bisphenol A (BPA), a typical EDC, has been widely used in the production of polycarbonate (PC), epoxy resins, paints, food packaging and food containers since 1957 [2]. BPA has the ability to bind with both estrogen receptors, namely ERα and ERβ. While it exhibits a greater affinity for ERβ, its overall binding affinity to these receptors is considerably lower compared to that of 17β-estradiol [3]. Its ubiquitous presence in the environment has raised significant health concerns, due to its potential linkage to obesity, diabetes, eclampsia, hyperlipidemia, neoplasms, cardiovascular disease, chronic kidney disease, infertility, polycystic ovary syndrome, etc. [2,4–8]. Therefore, the European Union banned BPA-containing plastic baby bottles in 2011 [9]. Therefore, alternatives to BPA are increasingly being used, such as bisphenol F (BPF), bisphenol AF (BPAF) and bisphenol S (BPS). For example, BPS has found applications in the manufacturing of food packaging, baby bottles and thermal paper; BPF is predominantly utilized in epoxy resins, coatings and structural adhesives; and BPAF serves as a cross-linking agent in the electronics and fibre optics industries [10].

Since the usage of BPs has gradually increased, their exposure level urgently needs to be evaluated. Studies have revealed that humans are exposed to bisphenol analogues through a wide spectrum of media, such as air, food, drinking water and indoor dust [11]. For safety, the U.S. Environmental Protection Agency (U.S.EPA) set the maximum daily intake (MDI) of BPA at 0.05 mg/kg·bw/d in 1993, Health Canada set an MDI of BPA at 0.025 mg/kg·bw/d in 2008, and the European Food Safety Authority (EFSA) set an MDI of BPA at 0.05 mg/kg·bw/d in 2006, which was readjusted in 2015 to 0.004 mg/kg·bw/d [12]. Recently, an increasing number of studies have focused on measuring BP levels in humans [13–16]. For example, the median concentrations of BPA and BPS in urine samples from Guangdong, China, were 31.07 and 7.37 ng/mL, respectively [13]. Intriguingly, BPA and BPS levels were significantly higher in males than in females [13]. In a study examining the relationship between BPA and hyperlipidemia among the elderly population in Hubei, China, the median BPA concentration was determined to be 3.09 ng/mL, with a range extending from 0.08 to 8.14 ng/ml [14]. This study also identified several other Bisphenol analogues, with the following geometric mean (GM) concentrations: BPF (0.228 ng/mL), BPAF (0.018 ng/mL) and BPS (0.029 ng/mL) [14].

Nonetheless, the vast majority of studies on the issue of BP exposure are focused on BPA in the urine of children, adolescents and adults; information on its substitutes in blood (serum), as well as its risk factors, are still unknown. The purpose of this study was to evaluate the internal BP exposure in an elderly Chinese population; moreover, the underlying risk factors are also discussed in the present work.

2. Materials and Methods

2.1. Chemicals and Reagents

BPA, BPB, BPC, BPE, BPF, BPS, BPZ, BPP, BPAF and BPAP standards with purity $\geq$ 98% were purchased from J&K Scientific (Shanghai, China). Isotope internal standards, such as BPA-d6, BPS-d8, BPAF-d4, were purchased from Accustandard, Inc. (Market Street, New Haven, CT, USA).

HPLC-grade methanol, hexane and dichloromethane were purchased from Merck KGaA (Darmstadt, Germany). Deionized water was prepared by the Milli-Q® Water Purification System (Billerica, MA, USA). Formic acid (HPLC-grade) was bought from Sigma-Aldrich (Saint Louis, MO, USA). A Hydrophilic–Lipophilic Balance (HLB) cartridge (500 mg, 6 mL) was bought from Waters Corporation (Milford, MA, USA).

2.2. Participant Sample Collection

This study employed a cross-sectional design to assess BP exposure and associated risk factors in an elderly population in a city on the eastern coast of Jiangsu Province. A total of 161 permanent residents aged 60–70 years were randomly selected from a residential community. Participants were included if they had resided in the community for at least 5 years. Blood samples (5 mL) were collected from the population; a self-designed questionnaire containing questions on age, gender and environmental and occupational risk factors was used to investigate the selected participants. Moreover, a dietary survey was carried out on the survey population. We distributed dietary questionnaires to the subjects of the survey, which included questions on daily dietary habits, types of food, food weight, etc., and required the respondents to carefully recall and fill in the information truthfully. Data were reviewed for completeness and plausibility. The study was reviewed and approved by the Ethics Committee of the First Affiliated Hospital of Nanjing Medical University (Jiangsu Provincial People's Hospital) (Luncheon Review: No. 2023-SR-234). All study subjects signed an informed consent form.

2.3. Blood Sample Preparation

Samples were thawed at 4 °C, vortexed and mixed. To precipitate proteins, 400 μL of serum was pipetted into an Ep tube, and 800 μL of methanol solution containing 0.2% formic acid was added. Methanol was used to precipitate proteins from the serum samples, and formic acid (0.2%) was added to the methanol solution to improve the ionization of BPs during Liquid Chromatography–Tandem Mass Spectrometry (LC-MS/MS) analysis. The mixture was vortexed to precipitate the protein, transferred to a low-temperature centrifuge and centrifuged at 8000 rpm for 10 min. The supernatant was then transferred to a new cuvette, and 20 mL of purified water was added and mixed. The mixture was left to be purified.

A solid-phase extraction (SPE) column was pre-conditioned with sequential rinses of 5 mL of hexane, 5 mL of dichloromethane, 10 mL of methanol and 10 mL of laboratory-grade water to make it better integrated with the target. Following this preparation, the sample was then passed through the SPE column at a flow rate of 3 mL to 5 mL per minute, for adsorption of the targets. After this, the column was rinsed with 5 mL of 10% methanol aqueous solution to wash away non-specific/unwanted compounds. Then, the column was dried under a stream of nitrogen gas. The retained compounds were then eluted using 5 mL of methanol and 10 mL of dichloromethane. The collected eluate was concentrated under nitrogen to a final volume of less than 1 mL. The solvent was exchanged, and the sample was brought up to a fixed volume of 50 μL with methanol; subsequently, it was allowed to stand before proceeding to analysis. The serum samples were purified using solid-phase extraction (SPE), according to the method described by Maknun L et al. [17].

2.4. Instrumental Analysis

In this study, a liquid chromatography–tandem triple quadrupole mass spectrometer (AB SCIEX 5500, Framingham, MA, USA) was used, which was equipped with an electrospray ion source (ESI). The mobile phase for the column's A phase consisted of a 0.05% aqueous ammonia solution, while phase B was acetonitrile. We injected a 5 μL sample at a column temperature of 35 °C and a flow rate of 0.3 mL/min. The gradient elution programme was as follows: phase B started at 10% for the initial minute (0–1 min), then increased to 50% over the next 0.5 min (1–1.5 min), and subsequently ramped up to 100% by 6 min, where it was maintained for 3 min. During the final stage, from 9 to 9.1 min, the proportion of phase B was reduced back to 10% and held for an additional minute.

The mass spectrometer was operated in negative ion mode with multi-stage reaction monitoring (MRM). The ion source temperature was set at 350 °C. The spray voltage was established at −4000 V, with the atomization temperature and nebulizing gas pressure set at 550 °C and 45 psi, respectively. The auxiliary gas pressure was maintained at 60 psi.

2.5. Method Validation

Each of the 20 samples were inserted to analyze one full procedure blank, one solvent blank and one matrix spiked sample; BPA and BPAF were detected in the full procedure blank, which were below the detection limit. The concentration range of the standard curve was 0.5 ng/mL–200 ng/mL, and the linearity of the standard curve was ≥0.995. The recoveries of the target spiked with the spiked concentration of 10 ng/mL were in the range of 68.4–112%, and the RSDs were in the range of 3.3–18%. To ensure accuracy and minimize potential drift, calibration standards were run at the beginning, middle and end of each analytical batch [18]. Furthermore, a quality control (QC) sample at a known concentration was analyzed every 10 samples to monitor instrument performance throughout the run. The measured values for the QC samples were consistently within the acceptable range (±15% of the nominal value).

2.6. Statistical Analysis

Descriptive statistics were used to describe demographic characteristics, food intake and levels of BPs in blood samples. Since the data collected in this study did not demonstrate normal distribution, the total score was thus expressed as the median M and interquartile spacing Q_U-Q_L, in which Q_U stands for the upper quartile (Q3) and Q_L stands for the lower quartile (Q1), and the rank sum test was used for between-group comparisons. Subsequently, correlations between BPs and food were tested by Spearman correlation analysis. Finally, because dietary levels were skewed, we therefore did not transform the BP data, but rather graded them by quartiles (Q1/Q2/Q3/Q4), and then assessed the effect of diet on the detection of BPs using ordered logistic regression analysis. All statistical methods were performed using SPSS 26.0, and $p < 0.05$ was statistically significant.

3. Results

3.1. Basic Information of Survey Population

A total of 161 elderly permanent residents in a community in Lianyungang were investigated, of which 104 were females, accounting for 64.6%; the average age of the respondents was 67.48 ± 5.06 years old, with the youngest being 57 years old and the oldest being 80 years old. The age distribution was as follows: 67 individuals were 65 years old or younger, while 94 were 65 years old and above. For body mass index (BMI), the normal population was 33.5%, the underweight population was 0.6%, the overweight population was 44.7% and the obese population was 21.1%. The study population had a normal diet, excluding those with a history of diabetes mellitus or intentional dieting. Most of the study population denied a history of smoking and alcohol consumption. Detailed information is shown in Table 1.

Table 1. Demographic characteristics of elderly people in a community in Lianyungang (n = 161).

Characteristics	*n*	Proportion (%)
Gender		
Male	57	35.4
Female	104	64.6
Age		

Table 1. *Cont.*

Characteristics	*n*	Proportion (%)
≤65	67	41.6
>65	94	58.4
Education level		
None	46	28.6
Elementary school (did not graduate)	9	5.6
Elementary school	24	14.9
Middle school	51	31.7
High school/middle school/technical school	28	17.4
Junior college	3	1.8
BMI		
Underweight	1	0.6
Normal weight	54	33.5
Overweight	72	44.7
Obese	34	21.1
High blood pressure		
Yes	60	39.5
No	101	60.5
Diabetes		
Yes	0	0.0
No	161	100.0
Smoking		
Never	120	74.5
Quit	12	7.5
Remain	27	16.8
Deficiencies	2	1.2
Drinking		
Regular	18	11.2
Sometimes	18	11.2
Never	123	76.4
Quit	2	1.2

3.2. *BP Internal Exposure in the Elderly*

The BP levels in the serum of the investigated population were investigated, including BPA, BPB, BPC, BPE, BPF, BPAP, BPS, BPZ and BPP. It was found that BPA levels in the investigated population were significantly higher than the levels of other bisphenol compounds, with a range of 0.07–104.35 ng/mL and a median of 6 ng/mL.

For other BPA substitutes, the median concentrations of BPB, BPAF and BPS reached 2.01, 3.68 and 1.44 ng/mL, with ranges of 0.14–116.25, 0–30.55 and 0–23.1 ng/mL, respectively (Table 2 and Figure 1).

Table 2. The levels of bisphenol analogues in the serum of elderly people in a community in Lianyungang, China (n = 161, ng/mL).

BPs	LOD	Detection Frequency (%)	Median	Min	P25	P75	Max
BPA	0.070	100	6.000	0.070	4.350	9.750	104.35
BPB	0.050	97.5	2.010	<LOD	0.570	3.380	30.55
BPC	0.200	78.9	0.560	<LOD	0.360	0.820	15.35
BPE	0.050	98.1	0.640	<LOD	0.500	0.750	13.8
BPF	0.060	99.3	0.600	<LOD	0.340	1.150	41.2
BPAP	0.007	96.4	0.160	<LOD	0.120	0.240	3.45
BPAF	0.003	100	3.680	0.140	1.710	6.170	116.25
BPS	0.010	98.8	1.440	<LOD	1.090	2.050	23.1
BPZ	0.040	96.3	0.880	<LOD	0.530	3.320	359.45
BPP	0.040	98.1	0.200	<LOD	0.100	0.410	3.41
TBBPA	0.100	24.2	< LOD	<LOD	<LOD	<LOD	1.54

LOD: limit of detection; SD: standard deviation; Min: minimum; Max: maximum; P25: percentile of 25; P75: percentile of 75.

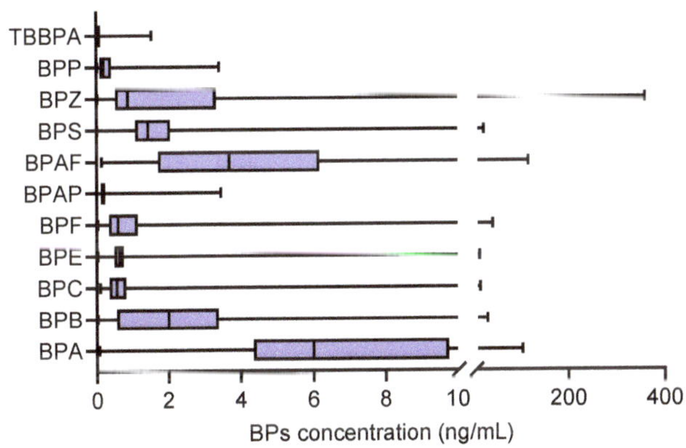

Figure 1. The levels of bisphenol analogues in the serum of elderly people in a community in Lianyungang, China (n = 161, ng/mL).

3.3. Associations Between Serum BP Levels and Gender and Age

Having determined the internal levels of BPs, we then grouped the survey population according to gender and age. The total scores were expressed using the median M and interquartile spacing Q_U–Q_L, and the rank sum test was used for between-group comparisons. It showed that almost all types of BPs were higher in the male group than in females. In addition, almost all types of BPs were higher in the elderly population aged > 65 years than in those aged $\leq$ 65 years (Table 3).

Table 3. Analysis of differences in BP concentrations among different genders and age groups (M, QU–QL) (ng/mL).

BPs	Gender		Z-Value	*p*-Value	Age		Z-Value	*p*-Value
	Male (Median, Range)	Female (Median, Range)			≤65	>65		
BPA	6.43, 4.76–11.10	5.76, 4.08–8.83	−1.649	0.099	5.32, 4.06–7.28	7.08, 4.72–10.80	−2.445	0.014 *
BPB	2.13, 0.59–3.49	1.97, 0.56–3.36	−0.375	0.708	1.81, 0.53–3.10	2.24, 0.77–3.50	−1.320	0.187
BPC	0.57, 0.37–0.93	0.55, 0.33–0.74	−0.416	0.678	0.56, 0.41–0.73	0.56, 0.25–0.87	−0.190	0.850
BPE	0.63, 0.52–0.78	0.66, 0.50–0.75	−1.011	0.312	0.63, 0.50–0.72	0.67, 0.50–0.79	−1.087	0.277
BPF	0.64, 0.35–1.60	0.58, 0.34–1.09	−0.456	0.648	0.72, 0.40–1.31	0.56, 0.32–1.00	−1.595	0.111
BPAP	0.18, 0.12–0.25	0.15, 0.11–0.24	−0.969	0.333	0.16, 0.11–0.24	0.16, 0.12–0.24	−0.400	0.689
BPAF	3.75, 1.82–6.68	3.52, 1.64–5.95	−0.979	0.327	3.65, 1.70–6.94	3.70, 1.76–6.05	−0.322	0.747
BPS	1.43, 1.07–2.11	1.44, 1.09–2.02	−0.064	0.949	1.37, 1.12–1.98	0.50, 1.08–2.12	−0.333	0.739
BPZ	0.93, 0.57–7.95	0.89, 0.52–3.42	−0.636	0.525	0.88, 0.50–3.47	0.90, 0.61–3.87	−0.410	0.682
BPP	0.20, 0.11–0.46	0.20, 0.10–0.41	−0.937	0.349	0.21, 0.09–0.38	0.19, 0.11–0.44	−0.837	0.403

Note: * $p < 0.05$.

Considering that BPs are widely found in a variety of consumer products, including polycarbonate and other forms of plastics, food and beverage container linings, thermal printing paper and dental materials, people are therefore usually exposed to multiple BPs, and different BPs may have similar sources or routes of exposure. Also, BPS, BPF, BPB, etc., are inherently substitutes for BPA, so there are a variety of complex interactions. Therefore, we performed correlation analyses of different BPs, and these showed that there were significant correlations between almost all of the BPs. For example, there was a significant positive correlation between BPA and BPS (r = 0.571, $p < 0.01$) (Figure 2 and Table S2).

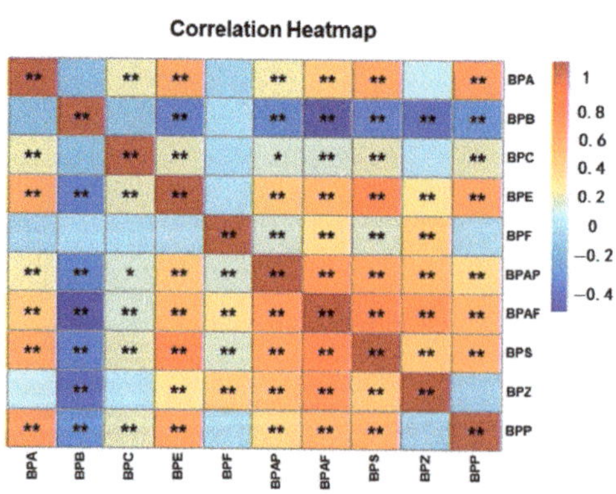

Figure 2. Heatmap of Spearman correlation analyses: associations among BPs. (** $p < 0.01$; * $p < 0.05$).

3.4. Relationship Between Serum BP Levels and Diet

Diet is the main route of exposure to BPs, so we collected data on the diet of the above-mentioned surveyed population, and a correlation analysis was performed between serum BPs and diet. Through the questionnaire survey, we found that the elderly population in the region mainly consumed staple foods such as rice. In addition to this, the intake of other foods, such as meat, vegetables and fruits, was balanced. The analysis found that almost all of the BPs showed a significant correlation with meat, except for BPC and BPAP, and the levels of BPA, BPE, BPF, BPAF, BPS, BPZ and BPP were all significantly and positively correlated with meat intake, which is presumed to be related to the lipophilicity of the BPs. In addition, a positive correlation was found between BPZ levels and rice intake. In addition, both BPAP and BPZ levels were negatively correlated with aquatic products (Table 4 and Figure 3). These results indicate that differences in lifestyle and dietary habits may contribute to regional differences in exposure to BPs.

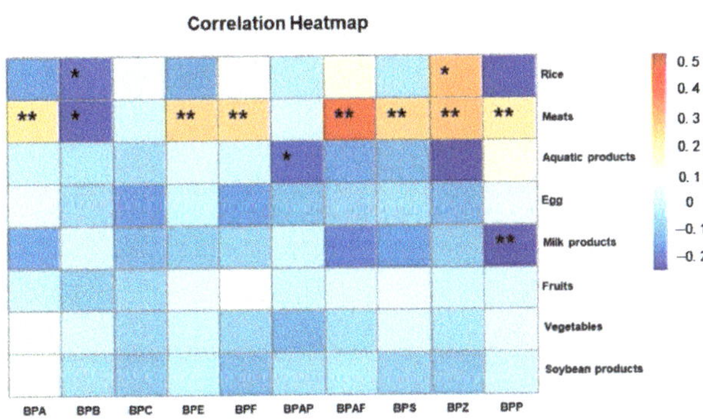

Figure 3. Heatmap of Spearman correlation analyses: associations among BPs and dietary situation. (** $p < 0.01$; * $p < 0.05$).

Table 4. Spearman correlation analyses of serum concentration of BPs and dietary situation.

	BPA	BPB	BPC	BPE	BPF	BPAP	BPAF	BPS	BPZ	BPP
Rice	−0.109	−0.167 *	0.094	−0.093	0.107	0.008	0.128	−0.003	0.289 **	−0.179
Meats	0.218 **	−0.179 *	0.035	0.251 **	0.248 **	0.053	0.452 **	0.254 **	0.285 **	0.204 **
Aquatic products	0.020	−0.006	−0.025	0.052	0.040	−0.164 *	−0.101	−0.075	−0.211 **	0.132
Egg	0.070	−0.024	−0.120	0.021	−0.111	−0.059	−0.036	−0.020	−0.077	0.075
Milk products	−0.107	0.042	−0.074	−0.045	−0.034	0.028	−0.139	−0.113	−0.047	−0.226 **
Fruits	0.022	−0.050	−0.032	0.073	0.108	0.029	0.061	0.078	0.035	0.041
Vegetables	0.100	0.047	−0.031	0.030	−0.031	−0.079	−0.021	0.053	−0.016	0.066
Soybean products	0.105	−0.023	−0.054	0.013	−0.068	−0.018	−0.006	−0.039	−0.056	0.033

* $p < 0.05$; ** $p < 0.01$ (2-tailed).

4. Discussion

Our study revealed the serum BPS levels in older adults in coastal areas, and some similar studies have been conducted around the world. One report on an elderly population in Hubei, China, indicated that the median serum concentration of BPA was 3.09 ng/mL, with a range of 0.08–8.14 ng/mL [14]; and a study in a Malaysian population showed that the serum BPA levels ranged from 0.81 to 3.65 ng/mL [19]; while in a Thai population, the mean serum BPA level was 0.34 ng/mL, with a range of 0.071–0.746 ng/mL [20]. In Western countries, a study performed on a Swedish elderly population revealed that the median serum BPA concentration was 3.76 ng/mL, with a range of 2.02–6.52 ng/mL [21]. In a Chinese population study with 81 samples, it was found that the plasma concentrations of total BPs in adults ranged from 0 to 6.56 ng/mL, and the mean plasma concentrations (range) of BPA, BPS and BPAF were 0.40 (0–5.0) ng/mL, 0.15 (0–62.0) ng/mL and 0.073 (0–44.6) ng/mL, respectively. In serum samples collected from an elderly population living near e-waste recycling facilities in China, the concentrations of BPA, BPAF and BPF were 3.2, 0.0074 and 0.062 ng/mL, respectively [13], which were lower than those found in the coastal areas in this study. These results collectively indicate that BPA remains the prominent BP distributed globally. In the current study, slightly higher BPA levels, with a wider range of fluctuation, were observed, which may be presumed to be related to geographic location and population factors. Other studies are provided in Supplementary Table S2.

We found that serum BP levels were higher in most men than women, and higher in the elderly population aged > 65 years than in those aged ≤ 65 years. In support of this, Wang et al. [13] reported that men had significantly higher urinary levels of BPA and BPS than women, which may be ascribed to smoking, alcohol consumption, dietary habits and high blood levels of androgens [19,22]. Research shows that serum elevated BPF and BPS exposure have negative associations with estrogen (E2) levels and E2/T (total testosterone) ratio, which may affect fertility [23]. In women with PCOS, serum BPS concentrations were found to be significantly higher compared to those in control subjects [7]. In 181 serum samples from pregnant Chinese women, ten BPs were positively identified and quantified by 0–144 ng/mL, of which TBBPS and BPS reached 0.593 and 0.113 ng/mL, respectively [24]. Some studies have found a gradual decrease in BPA concentrations with age, with significantly higher BPA levels in children than in adults, especially in those younger than 30 years of age [13,19,22,25], which may be associated with more frequent exposure to boxed lunches, beverages and other dietary habits. Free BPA is active and can be metabolized after ingestion, mainly by glucuronidation (BPA-G) and sulphation (BPA-S). The majority of BPA is metabolized in the liver through the production of BPA-G by the uridine 5′-bisphosphate glucuronide transferase (UDP-glycosyltransferase (UGT)) system, and is excreted by the kidneys [26]. In human hepatocytes, the contributions of glucuronidation and sulfation were found to be 94.04% and 5.96%, respectively [27]. Furthermore, it was shown that BPA had the highest intrinsic clearance, followed by BPF and then BPS [27]. With age, the activity of various enzymes in the body decreases, which we hypothesized to be one of the reasons for the higher levels of BPs in the elderly in the present study [28].

However, the concentration of BPs in residents near an electronics factory [29] was lower than that found in the coastal areas in this study; we speculated that this might be related to regional differences, so we investigated the eating habits of the study population, trying to determine the relationship between BPs and food.

The relationship between meat intake and higher serum BP levels may be due to the following reasons. Firstly, BPs in fresh meat may have been produced through environmental sources before slaughter. Animal feeds may contain BPs; Di et al. [30] selected feeds from different farms for detection, and found that most of the feed contained BPA, ranging from 1.0 ng/g to 50.0 ng/g. Meanwhile, samples from two farms were contaminated with BPA at concentrations ranging from 50.0 ng/g to 100.0 ng/g, and in one farm, BPA was found at levels even higher than 100.0 ng/g. In addition, BPA has been detected in feeds stored in woven bags, e.g., 0.52 μg/kg in cereals and 1.36 μg/kg in oilseeds, because the inner layer of a woven bag is polyethylene (PE) film [31]. BPA has also been detected in the feces or urine of livestock (e.g., cattle, pigs, sheep) and poultry (e.g., chickens, ducks and geese) [32]. Secondly, food conveyor belts, cutting boards, etc., are often used in processing and production, and these tools are usually made of PE, which is obviously contaminated with BPs [33]. Thirdly, different habits may also be one of the influencing factors of BP exposure. People who buy meat often directly use plastic bags, plastic boxes or cartons with plastic film, which are usually made of High-Density Polyethylene (HDPE) or Polypropylene (PP) [34], and there is a certain level of BP migration from the plastic bag to the meat [35]. In addition, more than 20 BPs, including BPA, BPS and BPAF, have been detected in takeaway containers made from Polystyrene (PS) plastic [36]. Finally, many households often use polycarbonate (PC) plastic containers to heat food, and after 9 min in a microwave oven, the average BPA concentration in hot pork cooked in PC containers increased to 14 ppb [37].

5. Conclusions

In this study, we selected 161 elderly permanent residents in an eastern coastal area of China as the research subjects, measured the concentrations of various BPs in their serum, and analyzed the differences in serum levels of various BPs among different genders and age groups. BPA levels were observed to be notably higher compared to the levels of other bisphenol compounds. Additionally, exposure levels of alternative compounds, such as BPB, BPAF and BPS, were also found to be elevated in human serum. It is important to note that BP concentrations tended to be generally higher in males as compared to females. Furthermore, examining the relationship between BP exposure and dietary habits uncovered a significant correlation between the consumption of meat products and the levels of most BPs. This finding offers novel insights and potential targets for interventions aimed at reducing BP exposure. Our dietary analysis revealed a significant correlation between meat consumption and serum BP levels, suggesting that meat is a major contributor to BP exposure in this population. Therefore, targeted interventions focused on reducing BP contamination in meat products could be effective in lowering overall BP exposure in elderly individuals. To the best of our knowledge, this is the first study of BP levels in a population-based serological sample in this region, filling a gap in the field.

Supplementary Materials: The following supporting information can be downloaded at https://www.mdpi.com/article/10.3390/toxics13040259/s1: Table S1: Levels of BPA and other BPs in populations in different studies; Table S2: Results of Spearman correlation analyses: associations among BPs. Refs. [38,39] are cited in Supplementary Materials.

Author Contributions: Conceptualization, G.J., S.J. and H.C.; data curation, J.G.; formal analysis, X.D.; funding acquisition, G.J. and H.C.; investigation, B.W.; methodology, X.D. and M.L.; project administration, G.J.; resources, Q.Z.; software, X.D. and M.L.; supervision, S.J. and H.C.; validation, X.D. and M.L.; visualization, M.L.; writing—original draft, X.D.; writing—review and editing, X.D., G.J. and H.C. All authors have read and agreed to the published version of the manuscript.

Funding: This research received no external funding.

Institutional Review Board Statement: The study was conducted in accordance with the guidelines of the Declaration of Helsinki, and approved by the Ethics Committee of the First Affiliated Hospital of Nanjing Medical University (Jiangsu Provincial People's Hospital) (Luncheon Review: No. 2023-SR-234).

Informed Consent Statement: Informed consent was obtained from all subjects involved in the study. Written informed consent has been obtained from the patients to publish this paper.

Data Availability Statement: The original contributions presented in the study are included in the article and Supplementary Materials; further inquiries can be directed to the corresponding authors.

Acknowledgments: This work was supported by the Jiangsu Province Ecological Environment Research Project (2022014), and the Central Scientific Research Projects for Public Welfare Research Institutes. This work was also supported by Jiangsu Provincial Key Medical Discipline (ZDXK202202), and by the Postgraduate Research & Practice Innovation Program of Jiangsu Province (JX10214189).

Conflicts of Interest: The authors declare no conflicts of interest.

References

1. Qiu, W.; Zhan, H.; Hu, J.; Zhang, T.; Xu, H.; Wong, M.; Xu, B.; Zheng, C. The occurrence, potential toxicity, and toxicity mechanism of bisphenol S, a substitute of bisphenol A: A critical review of recent progress. *Ecotoxicol. Environ. Saf.* **2019**, *173*, 192–202. [CrossRef] [PubMed]
2. Dagdeviren, G.; Arslan, B.; Keles, A.; Yucel Celik, O.; Arat, O.; Caglar, A.T. The evaluation of serum bisphenol A in patients with preeclampsia. *J. Obstet. Gynaecol. Res.* **2023**, *49*, 1322–1327. [CrossRef] [PubMed]
3. Gramec Skledar, D.; Peterlin Mašič, L. Bisphenol A and its analogs: Do their metabolites have endocrine activity? *Environ. Toxicol. Pharmacol.* **2016**, *47*, 182–199. [CrossRef] [PubMed]
4. Pivonello, C.; Muscogiuri, G.; Nardone, A.; Garifalos, F.; Provvisiero, D.P.; Verde, N.; de Angelis, C.; Conforti, A.; Piscopo, M.; Auriemma, R.S.; et al. Bisphenol A: An emerging threat to female fertility. *Reprod. Biol. Endocrinol.* **2020**, *18*, 22. [CrossRef]
5. Hong, X.; Wang, G.; Liu, X.; Wu, M.; Zhang, X.; Hua, X.; Jiang, P.; Wang, S.; Tang, S.; Shi, X.; et al. Lipidomic biomarkers: Potential mediators of associations between urinary bisphenol A exposure and colorectal cancer. *J. Hazard. Mater.* **2022**, *427*, 127863. [CrossRef]
6. Nie, H.; Wang, F.; Zhang, Y.; Zhang, S.; Han, X.; Zhang, X.; Guo, H.; He, M. Associations of serum bisphenol A levels with incident chronic kidney disease risk. *Sci. Total. Environ.* **2021**, *771*, 145401. [CrossRef]
7. Jurewicz, J.; Majewska, J.; Berg, A.; Owczarek, K.; Zajdel, R.; Kaleta, D.; Wasik, A.; Rachon, D. Serum bisphenol A analogues in women diagnosed with the polycystic ovary syndrome—Is there an association? *Environ. Pollut.* **2021**, *272*, 115962. [CrossRef]
8. Oliviero, F.; Marmugi, A.; Viguie, C.; Gayrard, V.; Picard-Hagen, N.; Mselli-Lakhal, L. Are BPA Substitutes as Obesogenic as BPA? *Int. J. Mol. Sci.* **2022**, *23*, 4238. [CrossRef]
9. European Parliament and Council. Directive 2011/8/EU of the European Parliament and of the Council of 25 January 2011 amending Directive 2008/122/EC as regards the use of bisphenol A in plastic infant feeding bottles. *Off. J. Eur. Union* **2011**, *2011*, 11–12. Available online: https://eur-lex.europa.eu/eli/dir/2011/8/oj/eng (accessed on 28 January 2024).
10. Moreman, J.; Lee, O.; Trznadel, M.; David, A.; Kudoh, T.; Tyler, C.R. Acute Toxicity, Teratogenic, and Estrogenic Effects of Bisphenol A and Its Alternative Replacements Bisphenol S, Bisphenol F, and Bisphenol AF in Zebrafish Embryo-Larvae. *Environ. Sci. Technol.* **2017**, *51*, 12796–12805. [CrossRef]
11. Michalowicz, J. Bisphenol A—Sources, toxicity and biotransformation. *Environ. Toxicol. Pharmacol.* **2014**, *37*, 738–758. [CrossRef] [PubMed]
12. Chen, W.-Y.; Shen, Y.-P.; Chen, S.-C. Assessing bisphenol A (BPA) exposure risk from long-term dietary intakes in Taiwan. *Sci. Total. Environ.* **2016**, *543*, 140–146. [CrossRef] [PubMed]
13. Wang, H.; Gao, R.; Liang, W.; Wei, S.; Zhou, Y.; Zeng, F. Assessment of BPA and BPS exposure in the general population in Guangzhou, China—Estimation of daily intakes based on urinary metabolites. *Environ. Pollut.* **2022**, *315*, 120375. [CrossRef]
14. Yao, J.; Wang, F.; Zhang, Y.; Zhang, Z.; Bi, J.; He, J.; Li, P.; Han, X.; Wei, Y.; Zhang, X.; et al. Association of serum BPA levels with changes in lipid levels and dyslipidemia risk in middle-aged and elderly Chinese. *Ecotoxicol. Environ. Saf.* **2022**, *241*, 113819. [CrossRef]
15. Liang, J.; Xu, C.; Xu, J.; Yang, C.; Kong, W.; Xiao, Z.; Chen, X.; Liu, Q.; Weng, Z.; Wang, J.; et al. PPARα Senses Bisphenol S to Trigger EP300-Mediated Autophagy Blockage and Hepatic Steatosis. *Environ. Sci. Technol.* **2023**, *57*, 21581–21592. [CrossRef]
16. Fu, Z.; Jin, H.; Mao, W.; Hu, Z. Conjugated bisphenol S metabolites in human serum and whole blood. *Chemosphere* **2024**, *357*, 142082. [CrossRef] [PubMed]
17. Maknun, L.; Kińska, K.; González-Álvarez, I.; Ouerdane, L.; Lauga, B.; Siripinyanond, A.; Szpunar, J.; Lobinski, R. Quantitative Determination of Iron-Siderophore Complexes in Peat by Isotope-Exchange Size-Exclusion UPLC-Electrospray Ionization High-Resolution Accurate Mass (HRAM) Mass Spectrometry. *Anal. Chem.* **2023**, *95*, 9182–9190. [CrossRef]
18. Gervais, A.; Dirksen, E.H.C.; Pohl, T.; Bechtold-Peters, K.; Burkitt, W.; D'Alessio, V.; Greven, S.; Lennard, A.; Li, X.; Lössner, C.; et al. Compliance and regulatory considerations for the implementation of the multi-attribute-method by mass spectrometry in a quality control laboratory. *Eur. J. Pharm. Biopharm.* **2023**, *191*, 57–67. [CrossRef]
19. Santhi, V.A.; Sakai, N.; Ahmad, E.D.; Mustafa, A.M. Occurrence of bisphenol A in surface water, drinking water and plasma from Malaysia with exposure assessment from consumption of drinking water. *Sci. Total. Environ.* **2012**, *427–428*, 332–338. [CrossRef]

20. Aekplakorn, W.; Chailurkit, L.O.; Ongphiphadhanakul, B. Relationship of serum bisphenol A with diabetes in the Thai population, National Health Examination Survey IV, 2009. *J. Diabetes* **2015**, *7*, 240–249. [CrossRef]
21. Olsen, L.; Lampa, E.; Birkholz, D.A.; Lind, L.; Lind, P.M. Circulating levels of bisphenol A (BPA) and phthalates in an elderly population in Sweden, based on the Prospective Investigation of the Vasculature in Uppsala Seniors (PIVUS). *Ecotoxicol. Environ. Saf.* **2012**, *75*, 242–248. [CrossRef]
22. He, Y.; Miao, M.; Herrinton, L.J.; Wu, C.; Yuan, W.; Zhou, Z.; Li, D.-K. Bisphenol A levels in blood and urine in a Chinese population and the personal factors affecting the levels. *Environ. Res.* **2009**, *109*, 629–633. [CrossRef] [PubMed]
23. Zeng, J.-Y.; Chen, P.-P.; Liu, C.; Deng, Y.-L.; Miao, Y.; Zhang, M.; Cui, F.-P.; Lu, T.-T.; Shi, T.; Yang, K.-D.; et al. Bisphenol A analogues in associations with serum hormone levels among reproductive-aged Chinese men. *Environ. Int.* **2022**, *167*, 107446. [CrossRef] [PubMed]
24. Li, A.; Zhuang, T.; Shi, W.; Liang, Y.; Liao, C.; Song, M.; Jiang, G. Serum concentration of bisphenol analogues in pregnant women in China. *Sci. Total Environ.* **2020**, *707*, 136100. [CrossRef] [PubMed]
25. Jin, H.; Zhu, J.; Chen, Z.; Hong, Y.; Cai, Z. Occurrence and Partitioning of Bisphenol Analogues in Adults' Blood from China. *Environ. Sci. Technol.* **2018**, *52*, 812–820. [CrossRef]
26. Rolfo, A.; Nuzzo, A.M.; De Amicis, R.; Moretti, L.; Bertoli, S.; Leone, A. Fetal-Maternal Exposure to Endocrine Disruptors: Correlation with Diet Intake and Pregnancy Outcomes. *Nutrients* **2020**, *12*, 1744. [CrossRef]
27. Durcik, M.; Gramec Skledar, D.; Tomasic, T.; Trontelj, J.; Peterlin Masic, L. Last piece in the puzzle of bisphenols BPA, BPS and BPF metabolism: Kinetics of the in vitro sulfation reaction. *Chemosphere* **2022**, *303*, 135133. [CrossRef]
28. Kim, D.; Yoo, S.H.; Yeon, G.-B.; Oh, S.S.; Shin, W.-H.; Kang, H.-C.; Lee, C.-K.; Kim, H.W.; Kim, D.-S. Senescent Astrocytes Derived from Human Pluripotent Stem Cells Reveal Age-Related Changes and Implications for Neurodegeneration. *Aging Dis.* **2024**, *15*, 1–17. [CrossRef]
29. Song, S.; Duan, Y.; Zhang, T.; Zhang, B.; Zhao, Z.; Bai, X.; Xie, L.; He, Y.; Ouyang, J.-P.; Huang, X.; et al. Serum concentrations of bisphenol A and its alternatives in elderly population living around e-waste recycling facilities in China: Associations with fasting blood glucose. *Ecotoxicol. Environ. Saf.* **2019**, *169*, 822–828. [CrossRef]
30. Di Marco Pisciottano, I.; Guadagnuolo, G.; Busico, F.; Alessandroni, L.; Neri, B.; Vecchio, D.; Di Vuolo, G.; Cappelli, G.; Martucciello, A.; Gallo, P. Determination of 20 Endocrine-Disrupting Compounds in the Buffalo Milk Production Chain and Commercial Bovine Milk by UHPLC-MS/MS and HPLC-FLD. *Animals* **2022**, *12*, 410. [CrossRef]
31. Wang, R.; Huang, Y.; Dong, S.; Wang, P.; Su, X. The occurrence of bisphenol compounds in animal feed plastic packaging and migration into feed. *Chemosphere* **2021**, *265*, 129022. [CrossRef] [PubMed]
32. Xu, P.; Zhou, X.; Xu, D.; Xiang, Y.; Ling, W.; Chen, M. Contamination and Risk Assessment of Estrogens in Livestock Manure: A Case Study in Jiangsu Province, China. *Int. J. Environ. Res. Public Health* **2018**, *15*, 125. [CrossRef] [PubMed]
33. Aliyu, A.B.; Saleha, A.A.; Jalila, A.; Zunita, Z. Risk factors and spatial distribution of extended spectrum β-lactamase-producing-Escherichia coli at retail poultry meat markets in Malaysia: A cross-sectional study. *BMC Public Health* **2016**, *16*, 699. [CrossRef]
34. Musavian, H.S.; Butt, T.M.; Larsen, A.B.; Krebs, N. Combined steam-ultrasound treatment of 2 seconds achieves significant high aerobic count and Enterobacteriaceae reduction on naturally contaminated food boxes, crates, conveyor belts, and meat knives. *J. Food Prot.* **2015**, *78*, 430–435. [CrossRef]
35. Wang, X.; Nag, R.; Brunton, N.P.; Siddique, M.A.B.; Harrison, S.M.; Monahan, F.J.; Cummins, E. A probabilistic approach to model bisphenol A (BPA) migration from packaging to meat products. *Sci. Total Environ.* **2023**, *854*, 158815. [CrossRef]
36. Zhao, N.; Zhu, J.; Zhao, M.; Jin, H. Twenty bisphenol analogues in take-out polystyrene-made food containers: Concentration levels, simulated migration, and risk evaluation. *Environ. Sci. Pollut. Res.* **2023**, *30*, 10516–10526. [CrossRef]
37. Lim, D.S.; Kwack, S.J.; Kim, K.-B.; Kim, H.S.; Lee, B.M. Potential risk of bisphenol A migration from polycarbonate containers after heating, boiling, and microwaving. *J. Toxicol. Environ. Health Part A* **2009**, *72*, 1285–1291. [CrossRef]
38. Liao, C.; Liu, F.; Guo, Y.; Moon, H.B.; Nakata, H.; Wu, Q.; Kannan, K. Occurrence of eight bisphenol analogues in indoor dust from the United States and several Asian countries: Implications for human exposure. *Environ. Sci. Technol.* **2012**, *46*, 9138–9145. [CrossRef]
39. Yang, Y.; Guan, J.; Yin, J.; Shao, B.; Li, H. Urinary levels of bisphenol analogues in residents living near a manufacturing plant in south China. *Chemosphere* **2014**, *112*, 481–486. [CrossRef]

toxics

MDPI

Article

Lead Causes Lipid Droplet Accumulation by Impairing Lysosomal Function and Autophagic Flux in Testicular Sertoli Cells

Chengwei Guo [1], Lingqiao Wang [1], Ke Cui [1], Guowei Zhang [1], Yao Tan [1], Weiyan Chen [1], Yiqi Wang [1], Jijun Liu [2], Wenbin Liu [1], Guanghui Zhang [1] and Ziyuan Zhou [1,*]

[1] Department of Environmental Health, College of Preventive Medicine, Third Military Medical University (Army Medical University), Chongqing 400038, China; 15123001480@163.com (C.G.); mamababa520qq@163.com (L.W.); cuike@tmmu.edu.cn (K.C.); zhangguowei@tmmu.edu.cn (G.Z.); xiaoyue7122@tmmu.edu.cn (Y.T.); weiyanchen@tmmu.edu.cn (W.C.); wangyiqi@tmmu.edu.cn (Y.W.); liuwenbin@tmmu.edu.cn (W.L.); zhgh221@tmmu.edu.cn (G.Z.)

[2] Chongqing Center for Disease Control and Prevention, Chongqing 400707, China; cqliujijun2007@163.com

* Correspondence: ziyuanzhou@tmmu.edu.cn

Abstract: Lead (Pb) is one of the most common environmental pollutants that negatively impacts male reproductive health. Thus far, the underlying molecular mechanisms of Pb-induced reproductive toxicity are still not well understood. In this study, 64 male ICR mice were given drinking water with Pb (0, 100, 200, and 300 mg/L) for 90 days. We found that exposure to 300 mg/L Pb resulted in reduced sperm quality and elevated autophagy-related protein levels in the mouse testes. Our findings indicate that the Pb hindered the autophagic clearance by impairing the lysosomes' function and then obstructing the fusion of lysosomes and autophagosomes. The autophagy cycle obstruction prevented the lipid droplets from breakdown and led to their accumulation in the Sertoli cells. In turn, the ccytotoxic effects that resulted from the interruption of the autophagy maturation stage, instead of the elongation phase, could be alleviated by either Chloroquine or Bafilomycin A1. Furthermore, exposure to 400 μM Pb initiated the TFE3 nuclear translocation and caused the increased expression of its target genes. Then, the knockdown of TFE3 reduced the formation of the autophagosome. In addition, the use of the antioxidant NAC notably enhanced the autophagic activity and reduced the occurrence of lipid droplets in the Sertoli cells. This study demonstrated that Pb disrupted the autophagic flow, which caused lipid droplet accumulation in the TM4 cells. Consequently, focusing on the maturation stage of autophagy might offer a potential therapeutic approach to alleviate male reproductive toxicity caused by Pb exposure.

Keywords: autophagy; lead; male reproduction; TFE3; ROS

1. Introduction

Lead (Pb) is widely used as an industrial raw material in metallurgy, batteries, printing, and the chemical and other industries, causing considerable pollution to the natural environment and human diet [1]. Additionally, Pb toxicity is amplified by its prolonged half-life. The general population exposure to Pb mainly occurs through contaminated food, drinking water, leaded gasoline, and dust [2]. Considering the amplified toxicity derived from Pb's non-degradability and long biological half-life in both the environment and organisms, there has been growing concern that occupational or environmental Pb exposure may affect male reproductive function. Pb is recognized to possess male reproductive toxicity linking to growth retardation, pubertal maturation delay, and semen quality decline [3]. Further research also demonstrated that Pb has harmful impacts on male reproductive health by disrupting hormone regulation and spermatogenesis [4,5]. However, the mechanisms underlying Pb-induced reproductive toxicity still remain unclear.

Sertoli cells, which serve as a physical barrier and supply nutrients to developing germ cells, are the primary targets of Pb toxicity. Studies have reported that Pb induces pyroptosis in Sertoli cells, which, in turn, leads to testicular fibrosis [6]. Earlier research demonstrated that exposure to 10 μM Pb for 24 h resulted in a significant increase in reactive oxygen species [7]. Sertoli cells absorb glucose from the extracellular environment and transform it into lactate, supplying energy to germ cells [8]. In this metabolic scenario, the oxidation of fatty acids stored in lipid droplets generates the ATP required by the Sertoli cells [9]. It is reported that a 1 μM Pb treatment for 24 h can affect lactate production and transportation in Sertoli cells [10]. In addition, lipid droplets are formed when Sertoli cells engulf and metabolize dead germ cells [11]. The dysfunction of lysosomes and the buildup of lipids have been documented in the testicular tissue of individuals suffering from late onset hypogonadism [12]. After rats were treated with Pb water at a dose of 25 mg/kg b.w. for 90 days, an increased lysosome content and phagocytosis of apoptotic bodies were also observed in the Sertoli cells [13]. The above research demonstrated that Pb could negatively influence the lysosomal activity of support cells, leading to irregularities in lipid metabolism and phagocytic processes.

Autophagy refers to a mechanism through which eukaryotic cells utilize lysosomes to break down their own cytoplasmic proteins and deteriorated organelles, which is regulated by genes associated with autophagy [14]. This mechanism can control the levels of lipids within the cell by decomposing lipid droplets, which is known as a process of lipophagy [15]. Autophagy plays an important role in the normal growth and development of male reproductive organs but also in male reproductive physiological processes, including blood–testis barrier integrity maintenance, testosterone synthesis, spermatogenesis, testosterone synthesis, and the stability of the blood–testis barrier [16,17]. In male reproductive toxicity caused by environmental endocrine-disrupting chemicals (EDCs), autophagy is also two-sided, with both protective and damaging effects [18,19]. Nevertheless, the function of autophagy in Pb-induced toxicity affecting testicular organs is still unclear, necessitating further investigation into its mechanisms. The protein TFE3, which contains a bHLH-leucine zipper domain, has been recognized as a key regulator for gene expression associated with autophagy and the formation of lysosomes [20]. Thus, in each stage of autophagy, TFE3 is involved through promoting the formation of the autophagosome and aiding its fusion with lysosomes, as well as maintaining the degradation function of lysosomes. However, more details still need to be elucidated to what extent does abnormal autophagy contribute to Pb-induced male reproductive toxicity and how autophagy is regulated by TFE3.

In the current research, we explored the effects of a 90-day Pb exposure on sperm quality and testicular autophagy-related proteins in mice. Furthermore, we investigated the particular elements of the impact of autophagy on the Pb-triggered cytotoxicity and its underlying upstream mechanism in TM4 cells. To explain the relationship between the observed impairment of sperm motility in mice and the markedly increased expression of autophagy-related proteins in the testes, we further evaluated the effects of Pb on various stages of autophagy and the role of TFE3 in regulating the Pb-triggered autophagy. To our knowledge, this research first demonstrated that Pb exposure led to lipid droplet accumulation in Sertoli cells, and antioxidant NAC significantly mitigated this process.

2. Materials and Methods

2.1. Animals and Treatment

A total of 64 five-week-old male SPF ICR mice (Vital River Laboratory Animal Technology Co., Beijing, China) were housed with ad libitum access to water and food, with five per cage. A regular light and dark cycle was maintained for 12 h each. The male mice were randomly divided into four groups according to body weight and given distilled water with lead acetate Pb $(AC)_2$ concentrations of 0, 100, 200, and 300 (mg/L, as Pb^{2+}). The Pb treatments were administered for a duration of 90 days. All animal procedures complied with the National Institute of Health's ethical guidelines for laboratory animals and were approved by the Laboratory Animal Welfare and Ethics Committee of the Army Medical University (AMUWEC 20230252).

2.2. Semen Quality Analysis

The computer-assisted sperm analysis system (CASA; Microptic S.L., Barcelona, Spain) was employed to evaluate the parameters of sperm quality, including sperm concentration, total count, progressive mobility, and total motility.

2.3. Histological Analysis and Immunofluorescent Labeling in Murine Testicular Tissue

Mice were sacrificed after anesthesia with pentobarbital and testes were fixed in 4% paraformaldehyde overnight. For the HE staining, we embedded the testes in paraffin according to standard protocols [21]. A 5 μm thick tissue section was prepared from the central region, stained with hematoxylin–eosin, and examined using a light microscope. For immunofluorescence, the paraffin sections were fixed, permeabilized, and subjected to blocking using standardized protocols. The slides were incubated at 4 °C overnight with rabbit anti-LC3 (1:500, CST, 43566S, Danvers, MA, USA) and rabbit anti-P62 (1:500, CST, D6M5X) anti-bodies in immunostaining dilution buffer, then incubated with Donkey Anti-Rabbit IgG (H+L) conjugated with Alexa Fluor 555 (Beyotime, Shanghai, China) at a 1:200 dilution for one hour at 37 °C, ensuring protection from light. The nucleus was stained for 5 min with DAPI staining solution (Beyotime, China) to identify the labels. The stained specimens were analyzed with a Lecia confocal laser scanning microscope (Lecia, Stellaris 5).

2.4. Cell Culture and Treatment

A Sertoli cell line from mouse testicles (TM4) was purchased from Pricella (Wuhan, China) and was originally sourced from the American Type Culture Collection (ATCC). The cells were cultured in DMEM/F12 medium (Thermo Scientific, MA, USA) supplemented with 10% fetal calf serum and 1% penicillin/streptomycin in a 37 °C humidified incubator with a 5% CO_2 atmosphere. When the cells reached about 70% confluence, they were exposed to various concentrations (0, 25, 100, and 400 μM) of Pb for either 24 h or 48 h. Lead acetate (Sigma, 32307, St. Louis, MS, USA) was dissolved in ultrapure water and diluted in DMEM/F12 medium.

2.5. Cell Viability

Rapamycin (TargetMol, T1537, Boston, MA, USA), 3-Methyladenine (TargetMol, T1879), chloroquine (TargetMol, T8689), and bafilomycin A1 (TargetMol, T6740) were dissolved in DMSO, and N-Acetylcysteine (TargetMol, T0875) was dissolved in ultrapure water. The TM4 cells were exposed to rapamycin (R, 200 nM), 3-Methyladenine (3-MA, 2 mM), chloroquine (CQ, 20 μM), bafilomycin A1 (Baf, 10 nM), or N-Acetylcysteine (NAC, 2 mM), either alone or in combination with Pb (400 μM), for a duration of 24 h. The working concentrations of these reagents were derived from previous reports [22]. The cell viability was measured by the MTT kit (Solarbio, M1020, Beijing, China) to assess the cytotoxic effects of Pb on the TM4 cell lines [23]. In brief, 5000 cells were inoculated into a 96-well plate and cultured for 24 h. After 24 h of Pb treatment, 10 μL of MTT solution was added to each well and incubated for 4 h. The absorbance at 490 nm was measured by an enzyme labeling instrument (Molecular Devices, M3, San Jose, CA, USA). The viability of the cells was represented as the ratio of absorbance from treated cultures in comparison with control cultures.

2.6. Transmission Electron Microscopy

In order to investigate the autophagy triggered by Pb on the TM4 cells, the treated cells underwent washing with a Hanks buffer (Beyotime, C0218) and were subsequently fixed using 4% glutaraldehyde (Sigma, G5882). Autophagic vacuoles were quantified using a JEM-1400Plus electron microscope (JEOL, Tokyo, Japan) to examine the cells.

2.7. Oil Red O (ORO) Staining

Oil Red O (ORO) (Beyotime, C0157S) is a dye used for lipid staining in histology and biological research. Lipid accumulation in the TM4 cells was assessed using ORO staining. The TM4 cells were washed with Hanks buffer (Beyotime, C0218), then stained with Oil Red O for 20 min. After staining, the cells were washed three times with Hanks buffer and immediately imaged under an Olympus CKX41 microscope (Olympus, Tokyo, Japan).

2.8. Measurement of ROS

2′,7′-Dichlorodihydrofluorescein diacetate (DCFH-DA) is a cell-permeable fluorescent probe used to detect the production of reactive oxygen species (ROS) within cells. The DCFH-DA (Beyotime, S0033S) stock solution was diluted 1000 times in DMEM/F12 medium to become the working solution (20 μM). The TM4 cells were washed with Hanks buffer (Beyotime, C0218), then stained with DCFH-DA for 30 min. After staining, the cells were washed three times with Hanks buffer and immediately photographed using a Leica Stellaris 5 confocal laser scanning microscope (Leica, Wetzlar, Germany).

2.9. Measurement of Lysosomal pH

LysoSensor Green DND-189 is a fluorescent dye that is primarily used to measure the pH of acidic organelles, such as lysosomes within cells. The LysoSensor Green DND-189 (Meilunbio, MB6043, Dalian, China) stock solution was diluted 1000 times in DMEM/F12 medium to become the working solution (1 μM). The TM4 cells were washed with Hanks buffer (Beyotime, C0218), then stained with LysoSensor Green DND-189 for 1 h. After staining, the cells were washed three times with Hanks buffer and immediately photographed by a Leica Stellaris 5 confocal laser scanning microscope (Leica, Wetzlar, Germany).

2.10. Acridine Orange (AO) Staining

Acridine orange (AO) is a cell-permeable nucleic-acid-selective fluorescent dye, mainly used for observing the permeability of lysosomal membranes. The AO (Beyotime, C0233S) stock solution was diluted 1000 times in DMEM/F12 medium to become the working solution (30 μM). The TM4 cells were washed with Hanks buffer (Beyotime, C0218), then stained with AO for 20 min. After staining, the cells were washed three times with Hanks buffer and immediately photographed by a Leica Stellaris 5 confocal laser scanning microscope (Leica, Wetzlar, Germany).

2.11. LysoTracker Red Staining

LysoTracker Red is a lysosomal red fluorescent probe that is commonly used for the specific fluorescent staining of lysosomes in live cells. The LysoTracker Red (Beyotime,

C0218) stock solution was diluted 10,000 times in DMEM/F12 medium to become the working solution (50 nM). The TM4 cells were washed with Hanks buffer (Beyotime, C0218), then stained with LysoTracker Red for 30 min. After staining, the cells were washed three times with Hanks buffer and immediately photographed by a Leica Stellaris 5 confocal laser scanning microscope (Leica, Wetzlar, Germany).

2.12. Apoptosis Assay

Annexin V-FITC (FITC) and Propidium Iodide (PI) are two fluorescent dyes commonly used in apoptosis assays. FITC (BD Pharmingen, 559763, San Diego, CA, USA) and PI (BD Pharmingen, 559763) can effectively distinguish cells in different apoptotic states. The TM4 cells were washed with Hanks buffer (Beyotime, C0218), then stained with annexin FITC and PI for 15 min. After staining, 1×10^4 cells were collected by flow cytometry (BD, Accuri C6) and the proportion of Annexin V-positive cells was analyzed. All groups of cells were examined by flow cytometry within 1 h to ensure the signal strength and data accuracy. The experimental data were evaluated with the help of FlowJo V10 software.

2.13. Transfection

A small interfering RNA (siRNA) that targets TFE3 and a control siRNA were provided by Tsingke Biotech (Beijing, China). The siRNA was dissolved in ultrapure water as the stock solution (100 μM). Lipo8000™ Transfection Reagent (Beyotime, C0533) is a high-efficiency nanomaterial-based cell transfection reagent. Prior to transfection, 1 μL of siRNA solution and 1 μL of Lipo8000 transfection reagent were mixed in 1 mL of Opti-MEM medium (Gibco, 31985062, Waltham, MA, USA) for 15 min. Following this, the TM4 cells underwent a 6 h treatment with combined transfection reagents, followed by a transfer to a fresh medium for 24 h to prepare for further experiments.

2.14. Immunocytochemical Analysis

Immunofluorescence was conducted following established protocols. Briefly, cells developed to the appropriate density on a circular glass slide situated within a 24-well plate were fixed in 4% paraformaldehyde (Beyotime, P0099) for 30 min, followed by 0.25% Triton X-100 (Beyotime, P0096) permeabilizing for 10 min. Thereafter, cells were blocked with Immunol Staining Blocking Buffer (Beyotime, P0260) for 30 min, and then were incubated at 4 °C overnight in immunostaining buffers with diluted antibodies: rabbit anti-TFEB (1:500, ABclonal, A21657, Wuhan, China), rabbit anti-TFE3 (1:500, ELK Biotechnology, ES7376, Wuhan, China), rabbit anti-LC3 (1:500, CST, 43566S), and rat anti-LAMP-1 (1:250, Invitrogen, LY1C6, Carlsbad, CA, USA). The cells were washed three times using a Western wash buffer (Beyotime, P0023C). Either Donkey Anti-Rabbit IgG (H+L) with Alexa Fluor 555 or Goat Anti-Mouse IgG (H+L) with Alexa Fluor 488 (both from Beyotime, China) were incubated for one hour at 37 °C, diluted 1:200, while shielded from light. The nucleus was stained for 5 min with DAPI staining solution (Beyotime, C1005) to identify the labels, followed by three washes with 5% TBST after the staining procedure. Ultimately, the circular cell-climbing tablets were inverted onto a glass slide and preserved in the Anti-fade Mounting Medium (Solarbio, China) at 4 degrees Celsius while shielded from light. The cell slides were imaged and examined promptly by a Lecia confocal laser scanning microscope (Lecia, Stellaris 5).

2.15. Real-Time PCR Analysis

The cells were lysed with Trizol (Beyotime, R0016) and then total RNA was extracted. A total of 1 μg total RNA of each sample was reverse transcribed using a cDNA synthesis kit (ABclonal, RM21400). The RT product was amplified with SYBR Master Mix (ABclonal, RM21203), data were generated by a TFX-96 Real-Time PCR Detection System (Bio-Rad,

Hercules, CA, USA), and the relative expression was calculated by the $2^{-\Delta\Delta CT}$ method. The levels of beta-actin gene expression served as the internal standard. The primer sequences for the genes relevant to this study are presented in Table 1.

Table 1. Primer used in the current study.

	Forward Sequence (5′–3′)	Reverse Sequence (5′–3′)
Becn1	ATGGAGGGGTCTAAGGCGTC	TGGGCTGTGGTAAGTAATGGA
Atg5	TGTGCTTCGAGATGTGTGGTT	ACCAACGTCAAATAGCTGACTC
Atg12	CGGAAGATTCAGAGGTTGTGCT	CAGCCTTCAGCAGGATGTCAA
Ulk1	AAGTTCGAGTTCTCTCGCAAG	ACCTCCAGGTCGTGCTTCT
Pik3c3	GGGCTATACCAAGAGACATGC	CGCCTTGTAGGATGTTCTGACT
Map1lc3b	TTATAGAGCGATACAAGGGGGAG	CGCCGTCTGATTATCTTGATGAG
Lamp1	CAGCACTCTTTGAGGTGAAAAAC	CCATTCGCAGTCTCGTAGGTG
Lamp2	TGTATTTGGCTAATGGCTCAGC	TATGGGCACAAGGAAGTTGTC
Clcn7	GACAACAGCGAGAATCAGCTC	CCAATGAGGGCACAGATAACC
Ctsb	CAGGCTGGACGCAACTTCTAC	TCACCGAACGCAACCCTTC
Ctsd	CGATTATCAGAATCCCTCTGCG	GGTCTTAGGCGATGACTGCAT
Gba	GTATGGCCTAAGATTCTGGGC	CTAGGTCACGGGAAATGAAGTC
Atp6v1g1	CCCAGGCTGAAATTGAACAGT	TTCTGGAGGACGGTCATCTTC

2.16. Western Blot Analysis

The cells were harvested after PBS washing. The cells were lysed with a Western blotting and immunoprecipitation cell lysis buffer (Beyotime, P0013) that contained protease inhibitors (Beyotime, ST506) and incubated on ice for 30 min. The sodium dodecyl sulfate-polyacrylamide gel (Beyotime, P0012A) was then used to separate the protein mixture. Following this, the proteins were moved onto PVDF membranes, which were then incubated with a Blocking Buffer for Western Blotting (Beyotime, P0220) for a duration of 20 min. The membranes were incubated with specific antibodies against LC3 (1:1000, CST, E7X4S), P62 (1:1000, CST, D6M5X), TFEB (1:1000, ABclonal, A21657), TFE3 (1:500, ELK Biotechnology, ES7376), ACTB (1:50,000, ABclonal, AC026), and GAPDH (1:50,000, ABclonal, A19056) at 4 °C overnight. After three TBST washes, the membrane was incubated with HRP-conjugated Goat Anti-Rabbit IgG (Beyotime, A0208) at room temperature for 1 h. The membrane was washed thrice with TBST and then incubated in a chemiluminescent solution for development, and protein bands were obtained. Glyceraldehyde-3-phosphate dehydrogenase (GAPDH) and β-actin (ACTB) were used as internal control proteins.

2.17. Statistical Analysis

The results are presented as the mean ± SEM. All quantitative measurements were collected from at least three independent experiments, each carried out in triplicate. The statistical analysis and evaluation of the experimental data were conducted utilizing SPSS 25.0 software. The means of two experimental data sets were compared by unpaired Student's *t*-tests, while the means of three or more groups were compared by one-way ANOVA, followed by Tukey's post hoc test. A p-value < 0.05 was thought to have statistical significance.

3. Results

3.1. Lead Exposure Resulted in Reduced Sperm Quality and Increased Autophagy in Mouse Testes

The sperm density of the three Pb exposure groups (100, 200, and 300 mg/L) were 18.37×10^6/L, 15.3×10^6/L, and 11.15×10^6/L, respectively, and showed no significant reduction when compared with the 14.37×10^6/L of sperm density in the control group (Figure 1A). The proportions of immobile sperm (IM) increased in all three Pb exposure groups (25.94%, 29.13%, and 40.63%), but only the 300 mg/L group exhibited a significantly greater IM proportion compared with the control group (22.06%, $p < 0.05$) (Figure 1B). As shown in Figure 1C, the progressively mobile sperm (PM) in the control group comprised 61.94%, and except for the 100 mg/L group (55.44%), both the 200 mg/L and 300 mg/L groups showed significant decreases in their PMs to 49.5% and 38%, respectively ($p < 0.05$). The structure of the seminiferous tubules showed no obvious variation when comparing the control group with the three experimental groups (Figure 1D). As previously reported, pathological changes in mouse testicles only occurred when the exposure dose reached 1000 mg/L of Pb [24]. Immunofluorescence analysis revealed elevated LC3 and P62 expressions in the testes across all experimental groups, indicating a blockage in the autophagy flow (Figure 1E,F).

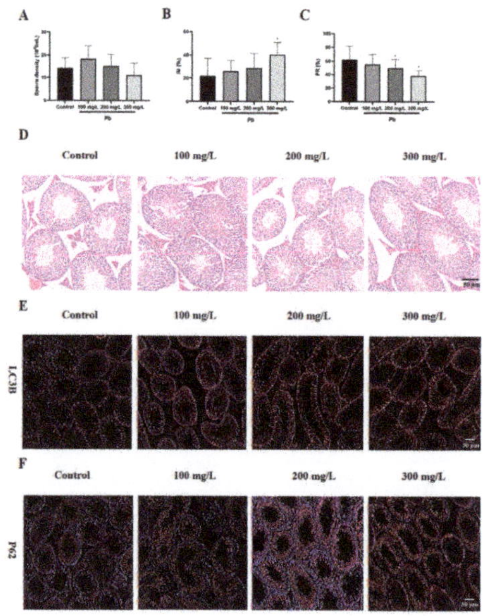

Figure 1. The impact of Pb on sperm movement and the structure of the testicles was investigated. The male mice were exposed to 0, 100, 200, and 300 mg/L Pb for 90 days. (**A**) Sperm density, (**B**) percentage of immotile sperm, and (**C**) percentage of progressive sperm in male mice. (**D**) HE staining of testicular tissue. Immunofluorescence analysis of (**E**) LC3B expression and (**F**) P62 expression. The results are presented as the mean ± SEM and were analyzed via one-way ANOVA. A significance level of * $p < 0.05$ when compared with the control group ($n = 16$).

3.2. *Pb Blocked Autophagy Flux in TM4 Cells*

This study examined the 24 h survival rate of the TM4 cells exposed to different Pb concentrations using the MTT assay. The exposure of cells to 25, 100, and 400 μM of Pb led to reductions in the cell viability by approximately 21%, 23%, and 29%, respectively (Figure 2A). The examination of autophagy activation in the TM4 cells implicated that the block of autophagy flux possibly contributed to the observed cellular damage induced by Pb exposure. Of the core genes related to autophagosome formation, including *Becn1*, *Atg5*, *Atg12*, *Ulk1*, *Pik3c3*, and *Map1lc3b*, their mRNA levels exhibited a marked elevation following exposure to Pb, particularly in the 400 μM group, where all the genes showed dramatically increased mRNA expression (Figure 2B). As a common marker for tracking the autophagy flux and measuring the autophagy activity, LC3-II and P62 both had significantly increased protein levels after the Pb treatment, especially the LC3-II level elevated in a time- and dose-dependent manner, which was comparable with the changes in its mRNA expression pattern (Figure 2C,D). Assays for autophagic flux were performed to ascertain whether LC3-II accumulation was due to autophagy induction or a subsequent process blockage. The increased P62 levels after Pb treatment implied the inhibition of autophagic degradation (Figure 2C,D). In addition, transmission electron microscopy revealed a significant rise in the quantity of autophagosomes and lipid droplets within the TM4 cells (Figure 2E) and the oil red test also confirmed the increased lipid accumulation in the TM4 cells in the Pb-treated group (Figure 2F). The results mentioned above indicate that Pb-induced autophagy may manage intracellular lipid concentrations by degrading the lipid droplets, a process referred to as lipophagy, in TM4 cells.

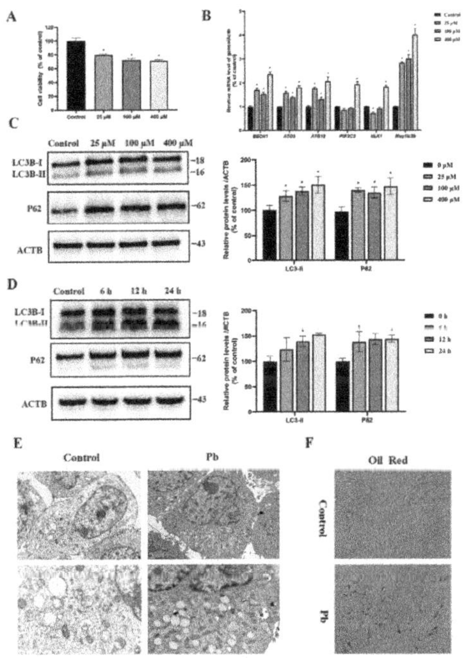

Figure 2. Pb induced the accumulation of autophagosomes and lipid droplets in the TM4 cells. After being exposed to 0, 25, 200, or 400 μM of Pb for 24 h, (**A**) cell viability assessed by an MTT assay, (**B**) mRNA expression levels of autophagy-related genes evaluated by RT-qPCR, (**C**) protein levels of LC3 and P62 subjected to varying concentrations of Pb (from 0 to 400 μM) over a duration of 24 h, and (**D**) 400 μM Pb for different time intervals (from 0 to 24 h). ACTB served as the internal standard. (**E**) TM4 cells were treated with Pb (400 μM) for 24 h, where electron microscopy demonstrated a higher quantity of autophagic vesicles (AVs) and lipid droplets; the lower panels display enlarged sections of the upper panels. The red arrows indicate lipid droplets; yellow arrows indicate autophagosomes. (**F**) Images of oil red staining for cells in the control and Pb (400 μM) treatment groups. The results are presented as the mean ± SEM and were analyzed via one-way ANOVA. A significance level of * $p < 0.05$ when compared with the control group ($n = 3$).

3.3. Preventing the Fusion of Autophagosomes with Lysosomes Reduced Pb-Induced Cell Damage

To assess autophagy's role in Pb-induced cell death, rapamycin, 3MA, CQ, and Baf were used to treat the cells exposed to Pb to modulate the autophagy levels. 3MA and rapamycin act as inhibitors and activators respectively in the initiation stage of autophagy; both CQ and Baf had the ability to disrupt lysosomal acidification and prevent the merging of autophagosomes with lysosomes. Neither 3-MA nor rapamycin influenced the cytotoxic effects induced by Pb (Figure 3A,B). These results suggest that both the inhibition and promotion of autophagosome formation failed to safeguard the cells against Pb-induced cell death. In contrast, CQ and Baf significantly increased the survival of the Pb-treated cells, indicating that the Pb-induced damage was restrained by controlling the autophagy maturation stage (Figure 3C,D). To further validate this finding, the impact of CQ on the apoptosis of the TM4 cells exposed to Pb was subsequently assessed. Since our previous experimental results show that there was no obvious apoptosis after 24 h of Pb treatment, we extended the treatment time to 48 h. Consistent with our assumptions, the CQ treatment significantly reduced the apoptosis induced by Pb (Figure 3E). Immunoblotting results confirmed that rapamycin reduced the p62 expression after Pb exposure, indicating that rapamycin restored the autophagic flux (Figure 3G). The presence of CQ did not significantly enhance LC3-II accumulation induced by Pb, supporting the hypothesis that Pb disrupts autophagosome–lysosome fusion (Figure 3F).

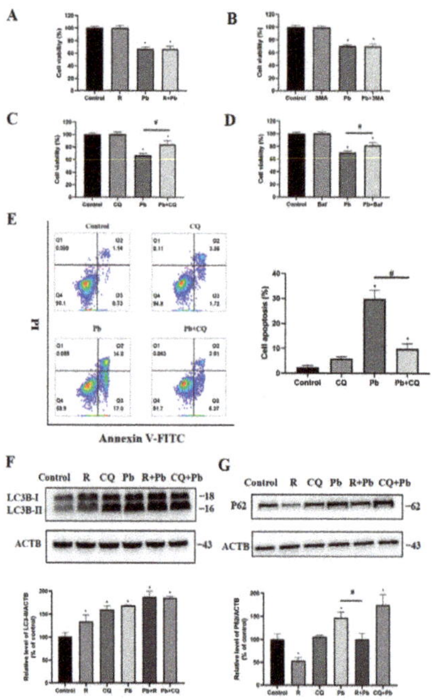

Figure 3. Chloroquine reduces Pb-induced cytotoxicity by inhibiting the autophagosome–lysosome fusion in the TM4 cells. After the treatment with Pb (400 μM) for 24 h, the MTT assay was used to access the cell viability both in the absence and presence of (**A**) rapamycin (R, 200 nM), (**B**) 3-MA (2 mM), (**C**) bafilomycin A1 (Baf, 10 nM), and (**D**) chloroquine (CQ, 20 μM). After the treatment with Pb (400μM) for 48 h, flow cytometry was used to detect the (**E**) apoptosis in the TM4 cells with or without chloroquine (CQ, 20 μM). An analysis that involved immunoblotting and quantification was conducted for (**F**) LC3-II and (**G**) P62 after treating TM4 cells with Pb (400 μM) for 24 h, either with or without the presence of rapamycin (R, 200 nM) or chloroquine (CQ, 20 μM). ACTB served as the internal standard. The results are presented as the mean ± SEM and were analyzed via one-way ANOVA. * $p < 0.05$ when compared with the control group; # $p < 0.05$ when compared with the Pb (400 μM) group ($n = 3$).

3.4. The Autophagosomes–Lysosomes Fusion and Lysosomal Function in the TM4 Cells Were Disrupted by Pb

The autophagosomes, which contain cellular waste material, must first fuse with lysosomes in order to be degraded and recycled by the cell. The immunostaining for LC3 and LAMP1 was performed to assess the process of autophagosome–lysosome fusion under Pb exposure; as shown in Figure 4A, the LC3-positive autophagosome (red) were not co-localized well with the LAMP1-positive lysosome (green). Given that red fluorescence means acridine orange (AO) accumulation in lysosomes, AO staining was performed to determine whether LMP (lysosomal membrane permeabilization) is affected by Pb exposure, and the cell images with significantly decreased red fluorescence may implicate the reduction of AO accumulation in lysosomes (Figure 4B). In addition, by using LysoTracker Red staining to trace the morphological change of lysosomes, an increased number of lysosomes that swelled into large vacuoles was found (Figure 4C), which implicates that the Pb caused lysosome morphological changes and impaired the function of the lysosomes. Sequentially, the lysosome pH was tested and an increased pH value of lysosomes in the Pb-treated group was observed that also indicated the impaired function of lysosomes (Figure 4D). Based on these data, the Pb blocked the merging of autophagosomes with autolysosomes, disrupted lysosomal function, and consequently resulted in the buildup of LC3 positive autophagosomes.

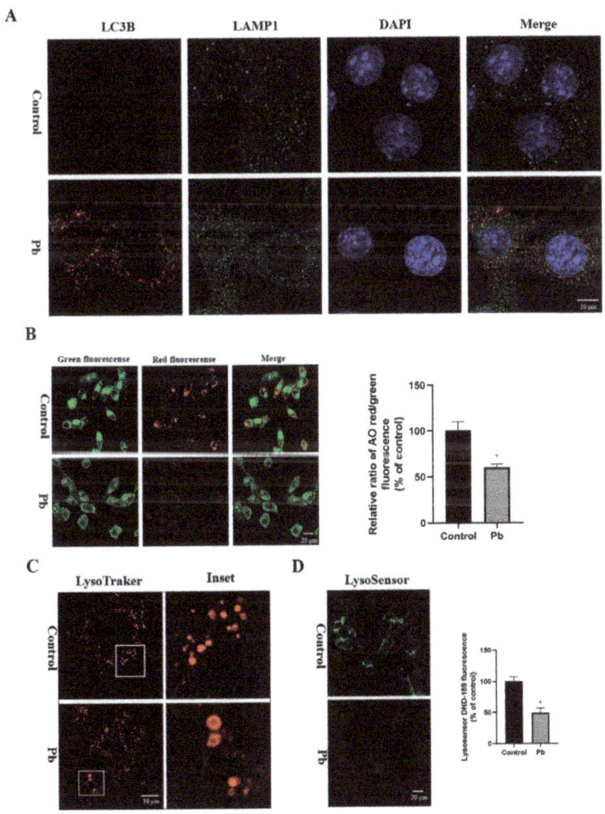

Figure 4. Pb disrupted the autophagosome–lysosome fusion and lysosomal function. The TM4 cells were treated with Pb (400 μM) for 24 h. (**A**) Immunofluorescence staining was used to label LC3 and LAMP1. (**B**) Acridine orange fluorescence was employed to study the LMP (lysosomal membrane permeabilization) through confocal microscopy. (**C**) LysoTracker Red fluorescence served to assess the morphology of lysosomes using confocal microscopy. (**D**) LysoSensor Green DND-189 fluorescence served to assess the lysosome pH using confocal microscopy. The results are presented as the mean ± SEM and were analyzed via one-way ANOVA. A significance level of * $p < 0.05$ when compared with the control group ($n = 3$).

3.5. Pb Treatment Caused Nuclear Translocation of TFE3 Protein

Since the MiT/TFE family members TFEB and TFE3 can interact with CLEAR elements and then regulate the expression of relative autophagic and lysosomal genes, we further explored whether TFEB and TFE3 were involved and their potential roles in the Pb-induced autophagy in TM4 cells. Immunoblot analysis indicated that the TFEB and TFE3 expression levels remained unchanged in TM4 cells exposed to Pb (Figure 5A,B), but the TFE3 protein translocation into the nucleus was observed after the Pb exposure (Figure 5C,D). As expected, treatment with Pb resulted in a notable enhancement of mRNA levels for genes associated with lysosomal biogenesis, including lysosomal transmembrane proteins (*Lamp1*, *Lamp2*, and *Clcn7*), lysosomalhydrolases (*Ctsb*, *Ctsd*, and *Gba*), and lysosomal V-ATPase (*Atp6v1g1*) (Figure 5E). Taken together, our results imply that the elevated expression of TFE3 response genes was very likely associated with Pb-induced TFE3 protein nuclear translocation.

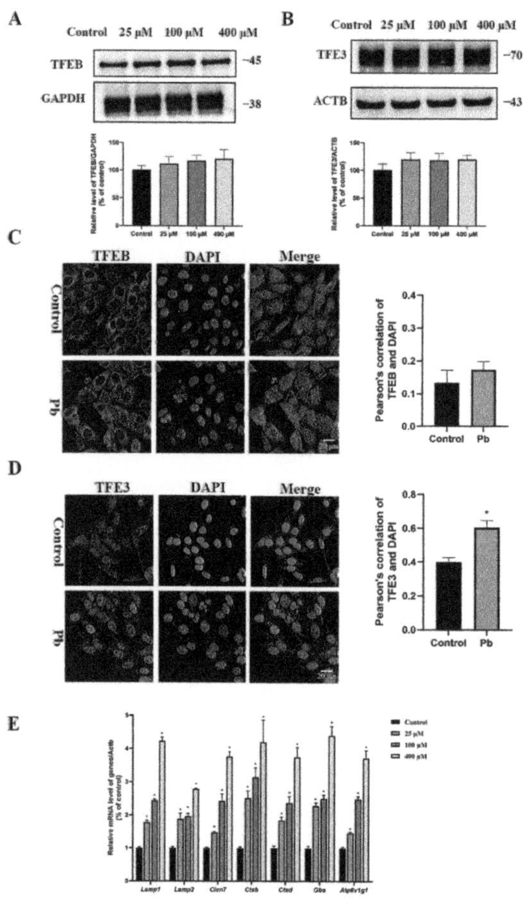

Figure 5. Pb induced the nuclear translocation of TFE3 in the TM4 cells. After exposure to 0, 25, 100, or 400 μM of Pb for 24 h, immunoblotting and quantification were used to assess the protein levels of (**A**) TFEB and (**B**) TFE3. GAPDH and ACTB served as the internal standard. Immunofluorescence analysis of the 400 μM Pb group for 24 h using the (**C**) anti-TFEB antibody and (**D**) anti-TFE3 antibody. (**E**) mRNA expression levels of the TFE3 target genes, including *Lamp1*, *Lamp2*, *Clcn7*, Ctsb, *Ctcd*, *Gba*, and *Atp6v1g1*. The results are presented as the mean ± SEM and were analyzed via one-way ANOVA. A significance level of * $p < 0.05$ when compared with control group ($n = 3$).

3.6. TFE3 Mediated Pb-Induced Autophagy in TM4 Cells

To evaluate the TFE3 function of the TFE3 in the Pb-triggered autophagy, RNAi-mediated silencing of the TFE3 was performed. Analysis through immunoblotting revealed that the administration of TFE3 siRNA decreased the levels of TFE3 and LC3-II following the exposure to Pb, while it did not influence the expression of p62 (Figure 6B). The immunofluorescence analysis indicated that TFE3 siRNA notably diminished the nuclear translocation of TFE3 (Figure 6C). Our results demonstrated that TFE3 siRNA reduced the level of Pb-induced autophagy. However, TFE3 knockdown did not restore the autophagic flux in Pb-induced cells, nor did it restore the cell viability (Figure 6A). In summary, the TFE3 played a role in the Pb-induced autophagosome formation phase.

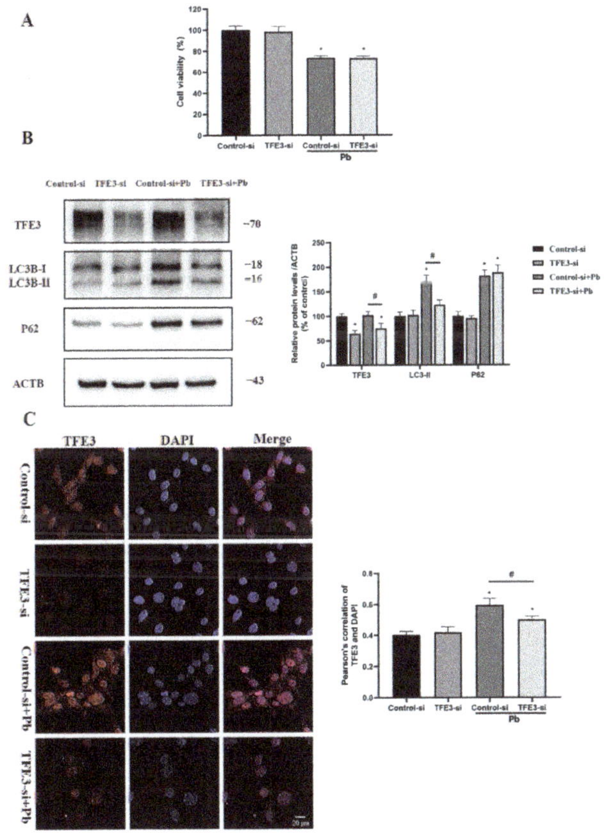

Figure 6. Pb activated the TFE3-mediated autophagy pathway. The TM4 cells were transfected with 100 nM TFE3 siRNA or control siRNA and then treated with 400 μM Pb for 24 h. (**A**) Viability of TM4 cells. (**B**) The immunoblot and quantification analysis of TFE3, LC3-II, and P62 in TM4 cells. ACTB served as the internal standard. (**C**) The immunofluorescence analysis was conducted on the TM4 cells using anti-TFE3 antibody and DAPI. The results are presented as the mean ± SEM and were analyzed via one-way ANOVA. * $p < 0.05$ when compared with the control group; # $p < 0.05$ when compared with the Pb (400 μM) group ($n = 3$).

3.7. Inhibition of ROS Partially Restored Autophagic Flux and Reduced Lipid Droplet Accumulation

Considering the essential role of ROS in autophagy, it is vital to examine its involvement in autophagy and the cytotoxic effects triggered by Pb. As shown in Figure 7, the antioxidant NAC had no protective effect on the viability of cells exposed to Pb (Figure 7A), though the elevated levels of ROS after Pb exposure was significantly mitigated by the NAC treatment (Figure 7B). These results suggest that ROS may not be a key contributor in Pb-induced toxicity. Concomitantly, LC3-II and P62 protein levels were found to be significantly reduced by the NAC treatment (Figure 7C), which indicates that ROS played a critical role in autophagy. Notably, cells in the NAC- and Pb-treated groups showed only a small accumulation of lipid droplets (Figure 7D), suggesting that restoring autophagic flux can effectively decompose lipid droplets.

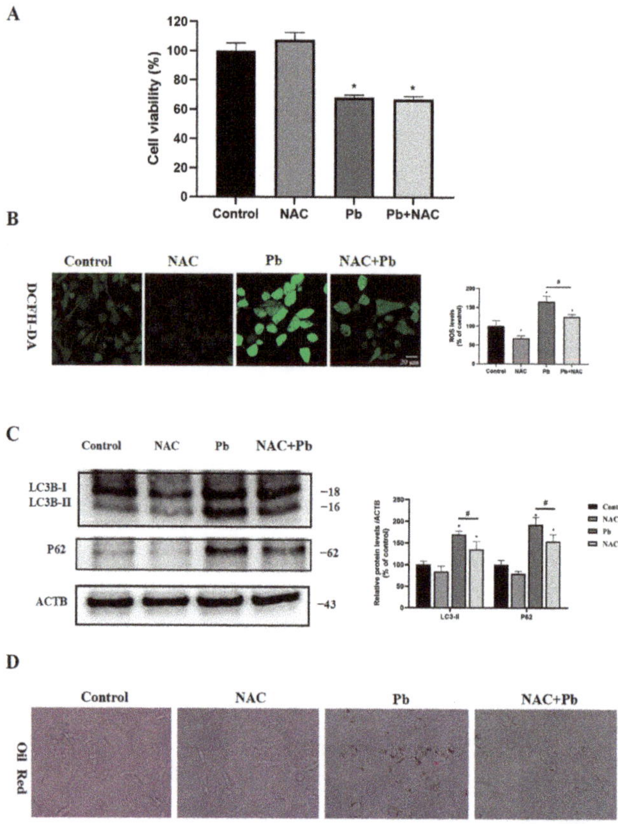

Figure 7. In the TM4 cells, the ROS acted as the upstream signaling molecule that triggered the Pb-induced autophagy. The TM4 cells were treated with 400 μM Pb, with or without NAC (2 mM), for 24 h. (**A**) Viability of the TM4 cells. (**B**) ROS levels of the TM4 cells. (**C**) A representative immunoblot and quantification analysis of LC3-II and P62 in the TM4 cells were performed. ACTB served as the internal standard. (**D**) Microscope image of the TM4 cells stained with oil red. The results are presented as the mean ± SEM and were evaluated using one-way ANOVA. * $p < 0.05$ when compared with the control group; # $p < 0.05$ when compared with the Pb (400 μM) group ($n = 3$).

4. Discussion

Pb is a widespread environmental pollutant known to cause male reproductive toxicity. Pb-induced toxic effects on Sertoli cells, one of the most important functional cells in testes, have been reported [25,26]; however, whether autophagy plays a role and the underlying mechanisms remain unclear. Autophagy, a process of membrane trafficking that has been conserved throughout evolution, is essential for preserving intracellular metabolism and energy balance by breaking down damaged organelles and cytoplasmic proteins [27]. In many instances, autophagy is regarded as a protective mechanism for cells. However, when autophagy is overactivated or dysfunctional, causing damage to organelles, it can be harmful to cells. Recently, multiple research investigations indicated a link between autophagy impairment and the decline in Sertoli cell functionality. The autophagy pathway is essential for maintaining Sertoli cell polarity and enhancing male fertility by removing SCIN and HDAC6, which negatively impact F-actin cytoskeleton organization [28]. Apoptotic cells are cleared from the system through the phagocytosis and autophagy of Sertoli cells, providing a normal environment for sperm maturation [29]. An investigation into the expression profiles of microRNAs and their functional networks within mouse testes following Pb exposure showed that the pathways that are associated with lysosomes and autophagy were the most affected pathways [30]. An electron microscopic observation of Pb-exposed rats showed that the lysosome content increased in Sertoli cells [13]. Clarifying the mechanisms of autophagy and lysosomal pathways in Pb-induced Sertoli cell death is crucial.

This research demonstrated that Pb toxicity is associated with alterations in the autophagy levels. In fact, we found that some autophagy-related key genes, such as *Becn1*, *Atg5*, *Atg12*, *Ulk1*, *Pik3c3*, and *Map1lc3b*, were upregulated after the Pb exposure, and the Pb-induced increase in the LC3-II and P62 levels suggests an obstruction of autophagic degradation within lysosomes. In the meantime, immunofluorescence also showed low levels of colocalization of LC3 and Lamp1, which implies that the autophagosome–lysosome merging was inhibited. Our research showed that Pb caused lysosomal membrane permeabilization, lysosome expansion into large vacuoles, and the elevation of pH in lysosome. The results support that Pb disrupts autophagic flow in TM4 cells by impeding autophagosome–lysosome fusion and reducing lysosomal activity. The function of autophagy concerning lead toxicity continues to be a debated issue. Earlier research has indicated that cell death through autophagy is associated with the impairment of learning and memory that results from Pb exposure [31,32]. In contrast, autophagy functions as a protective factor in the death of osteoblasts following Pb treatment [33]. Our research indicates that blocking the formation of autophagosomes failed to safeguard the cells from injury caused by Pb, suggesting it was not autophagic cell death. In addition, restored autophagic flux also failed to improve the cell survival. Surprisingly, the inhibition of autophagosome–lysosome fusion significantly improved the cell viability, suggesting that targeting the autophagy maturation stage could be a potential strategy for mitigating the cytotoxic effects of Pb.

With regard to TFE3, this is a member of the MiT/TFE helix–loop–helix subfamily that is linked to autophagy and lysosomal function [34]. Notably, the MiT/TFE family exists in an inactive form in the cytoplasm and enters the nucleus after activation. Nuclear translocation of the MiT/TFE family modulates lysosomal function and crucial phases of autophagy, including autophagosome formation, their fusion with lysosomes, and substrate degradation [35]. The capacity of TFE3 to carry out two contrasting cellular outcomes is influenced by the type of cell and the specific stimulus. For example, TFE3 overexpression maintains the lysosome–mitochondria axis and subsequently protected neurons from cadmium-induced apoptosis [36]. When autophagy is harmful to cells, the activation of TFE3 might trigger excessive autophagy and possibly cause cell death [37]. Given the fact that the nuclear translocation of TFE3 may upregulate the transcription of its target genes, TFE3 is likely activated in the compensatory role after Pb-induced impairment of autophagic flux. The use of TFE3 siRNA to inhibit autophagy activation indicates TFE3's role in regulating the prolonged phase of autophagy. However, the knockdown of TFE3 had no effect on cell viability, demonstrating that the cytotoxicity by Pb is not restrained by the aggregation of autophagosomes. Further investigation is required to determine whether TFE3 overexpression protects against Pb-induced injury.

Reactive oxygen species (ROS) are involved in cellular processes like apoptosis, necrosis, and autophagy. The generation of ROS due to drug metabolism and environmental contaminants can lead to significant harm to macromolecules and organelles within cells. In some reports, pretreatment with N-acetylcysteine (NAC) demonstrates a notable beneficial impact on the ROS generated by Pb exposure, as well as on DNA damage and programmed cell death [38]. After the Pb treatment, the ROS levels in the TM4 cells were significantly increased, which was inhibited by NAC. We found that the antioxidant NAC restored the autophagic flux and significantly reduced the accumulation of lipid droplets. In fact, therapeutic approaches to reduce lipid droplet accumulation by increasing autophagy have been used in hepatic steatosis. TFE3 overexpression alleviates hepatic steatosis by activating autophagy and PGC-1α-mediated fatty acid metabolism [39]. These data indicate that Pb induces multiple signaling pathways for autophagy in TM4 cells. Indeed, the suppression of ROS does not safeguard TM4 cells against cell death induced by Pb, indicating that oxidative stress may not be a critical target of lead cytotoxicity.

Overall, our study filled a gap in comprehending the fundamental mechanisms associated with Pb-induced reproductive toxicity, offering insights into the function of autophagy in the molecular events triggered by Pb. Notably, blocking autophagosome–lysosome fusion could present a novel approach for addressing reproductive toxicity caused by Pb exposure, such as mitochondrial generation and energy metabolism.

Author Contributions: Conceptualization, C.G. and L.W.; Methodology, K.C. and W.C.; Investigation, W.L. and Y.T.; Formal analysis, G.Z., (Guowei Zhang), Y.W. and J.L.; Writing—original draft preparation, C.G.; Writing—review and editing, G.Z. (Guanghui Zhang) and Z.Z.; Project administration, G.Z. (Guanghui Zhang) and Z.Z.; Funding acquisition, Z.Z. All authors read and agreed to the published version of this manuscript.

Funding: This research was funded by the National Key Research and Development Program of China (No. 2022YFC2702902), the Key Joint Project of the National Natural Science Foundation of China (U23A20494), the Natural Science Foundation of Chongqing (CSTB2024NSCQLZX0142), and the National Natural Science Foundation of China (82273663).

Institutional Review Board Statement: This research received approval from the Laboratory Animal Welfare and Ethics Committee of the Army Medical University (approval no. AMUWEC 20230252).

Informed Consent Statement: Not applicable.

Data Availability Statement: The supporting data for the findings of this research can be obtained from the corresponding author upon a reasonable request.

Acknowledgments: We thank Liting Wang for their help and guidance in the use of laser confocal microscopy.

Conflicts of Interest: There are no conflicts of interest.

References

1. Han, L.; Gao, B.; Hao, H.; Zhou, H.; Lu, J.; Sun, K. Lead contamination in sediments in the past 20 years: A challenge for China. *Sci. Total Environ.* **2018**, *640–641*, 746–756. [CrossRef] [PubMed]
2. Jonasson, M.E.; Afshari, R. Historical documentation of lead toxicity prior to the 20th century in English literature. *Hum. Exp. Toxicol.* **2018**, *37*, 775–788. [CrossRef] [PubMed]
3. Williams, P.L.; Mínguez-Alarcón, L.; Korrick, S.A.; Lee, M.M.; Plaku-Alakbarova, B.; Burns, J.S.; Smigulina, L.; Dikov, Y.; Abou Ghayda, R.; Hauser, R.; et al. Association of peripubertal blood lead levels with reproductive hormones and semen parameters in a longitudinal cohort of Russian men. *Hum. Reprod.* **2022**, *37*, 848–858. [CrossRef] [PubMed]
4. Calogero, A.E.; Fiore, M.; Giacone, F.; Altomare, M.; Asero, P.; Ledda, C.; Romeo, G.; Mongioi, L.M.; Copat, C.; Giuffrida, M.; et al. Exposure to multiple metals/metalloids and human semen quality: A cross-sectional study. *Ecotoxicol. Environ. Saf.* **2021**, *215*, 112165. [CrossRef] [PubMed]

5. Xie, J.; Yu, J.; Fan, Y.; Zhao, X.; Su, J.; Meng, Y.; Wu, Y.; Uddin, M.B.; Wang, C.; Wang, Z. Low dose lead exposure at the onset of puberty disrupts spermatogenesis-related gene expression and causes abnormal spermatogenesis in mouse. *Toxicol. Appl. Pharmacol.* **2020**, *393*, 114942. [CrossRef] [PubMed]
6. Zheng, X.; Guo, C.; Lv, Z.; Jiang, H.; Li, S.; Yu, L.; Zhang, Z. From animal to cell model: Pyroptosis targeted-fibrosis is a novel mechanism of lead-induced testicular toxicity. *Food Chem. Toxicol.* **2023**, *178*, 113886. [CrossRef]
7. Li, Z.; Liu, X.; Wang, L.; Wang, Y.; Du, C.; Xu, S.; Zhang, Y.; Wang, C.; Yang, C. The role of PGC-1alpha and MRP1 in lead-induced mitochondrial toxicity in testicular Sertoli cells. *Toxicology* **2016**, *355–356*, 39–48. [CrossRef] [PubMed]
8. Rato, L.; Alves, M.G.; Socorro, S.; Duarte, A.I.; Cavaco, J.E.; Oliveira, P.F. Metabolic regulation is important for spermatogenesis. *Nat. Rev. Urol.* **2012**, *9*, 330–338. [CrossRef]
9. Gorga, A.; Rindone, G.M.; Regueira, M.; Pellizzari, E.H.; Camberos, M.C.; Cigorraga, S.B.; Riera, M.F.; Galardo, M.N.; Meroni, S.B. PPARgamma activation regulates lipid droplet formation and lactate production in rat Sertoli cells. *Cell Tissue Res.* **2017**, *369*, 611–624. [CrossRef]
10. Yu, J.; Sun, J.; Fan, Y.; Su, J.; Xie, J.; Wu, Y.; Liu, X.; Wang, C. Exposure to Pb and Cd alters MCT4/CD147 expression and MCT4/CD147-dependent lactate transport in mice Sertoli cells cultured in vitro. *Toxicol. In Vitro* **2019**, *56*, 30–40. [CrossRef]
11. Wang, H.; Wang, H.; Xiong, W.; Chen, Y.; Ma, Q.; Ma, J.; Ge, Y.; Han, D. Evaluation on the phagocytosis of apoptotic spermatogenic cells by Sertoli cells in vitro through detecting lipid droplet formation by Oil Red O staining. *Reproduction* **2006**, *132*, 485–492. [CrossRef] [PubMed]
12. Deng, Z.; Zhao, L.; Li, S.; Chen, X.; Ling, X.; Zheng, J.; Yu, K.; Xu, J.; Yao, C.; Han, S.; et al. Targeting dysregulated phago-/auto-lysosomes in Sertoli cells to ameliorate late-onset hypogonadism. *Nat. Aging* **2024**, *4*, 647–663. [CrossRef] [PubMed]
13. Shafai, A.E.; Zohdy, N.; Mulla, K.E.; Hassan, M.; Morad, N. Light and electron microscopic study of the toxic effect of prolonged lead exposure on the seminiferous tubules of albino rats and the possible protective effect of ascorbic acid. *Food Chem. Toxicol.* **2011**, *49*, 734–743. [CrossRef] [PubMed]
14. Loos, B.; Engelbrecht, A.M.; Lockshin, R.A.; Klionsky, D.J.; Zakeri, Z. The variability of autophagy and cell death susceptibility: Unanswered questions. *Autophagy* **2013**, *9*, 1270–1285. [CrossRef] [PubMed]
15. Singh, R.; Kaushik, S.; Wang, Y.; Xiang, Y.; Novak, I.; Komatsu, M.; Tanaka, K.; Cuervo, A.M.; Czaja, M.J. Autophagy regulates lipid metabolism. *Nature* **2009**, *458*, 1131–1135. [CrossRef]
16. Wang, H.; Wan, H.; Li, X.; Liu, W.; Chen, Q.; Wang, Y.; Yang, L.; Tang, H.; Zhang, X.; Duan, E.; et al. Atg7 is required for acrosome biogenesis during spermatogenesis in mice. *Cell Res.* **2014**, *24*, 852–869. [CrossRef]
17. Gao, F.; Li, G.; Liu, C.; Gao, H.; Wang, H.; Liu, W.; Chen, M.; Shang, Y.; Wang, L.; Shi, J.; et al. Autophagy regulates testosterone synthesis by facilitating cholesterol uptake in Leydig cells. *J. Cell Biol.* **2018**, *217*, 2103–2119. [CrossRef] [PubMed]
18. Zhang, G.; Liu, K.; Ling, X.; Wang, Z.; Zou, P.; Wang, X.; Gao, J.; Yin, L.; Zhang, X.; Liu, J.; et al. DBP-induced endoplasmic reticulum stress in male germ cells causes autophagy, which has a cytoprotective role against apoptosis in vitro and in vivo. *Toxicol. Lett.* **2016**, *245*, 86–98. [CrossRef] [PubMed]
19. Wang, Y.; Zheng, W.; Bian, X.; Yuan, Y.; Gu, J.; Liu, X.; Liu, Z.; Bian, J. Zearalenone induces apoptosis and cytoprotective autophagy in primary Leydig cells. *Toxicol. Lett.* **2014**, *226*, 182–191. [CrossRef]
20. Martina, J.A.; Diab, H.I.; Lishu, L.; Jeong, A.L.; Patange, S.; Raben, N.; Puertollano, R. The nutrient-responsive transcription factor TFE3 promotes autophagy, lysosomal biogenesis, and clearance of cellular debris. *Sci. Signal.* **2014**, *7*, ra9. [CrossRef] [PubMed]
21. Liu, H.; Zhu, R.; Liu, C.; Ma, R.; Wang, L.; Chen, B.; Li, L.; Niu, J.; Zhao, D.; Mo, F.; et al. Evaluation of Decalcification Techniques for Rat Femurs Using HE and Immunohistochemical Staining. *Biomed Res. Int.* **2017**, *2017*, 9050754. [CrossRef] [PubMed]
22. Hao, Y.; Huang, J.; Ran, Y.; Wang, S.; Li, J.; Zhao, Y.; Ran, X.; Lu, B.; Liu, J.; Li, R. Ethylmalonic encephalopathy 1 initiates overactive autophagy in depleted uranium-induced cytotoxicity in the human embryonic kidney 293 cells. *J. Biochem. Mol. Toxicol.* **2021**, *35*, e22669. [CrossRef] [PubMed]
23. Ghasemi, M.; Turnbull, T.; Sebastian, S.; Kempson, I. The MTT Assay: Utility, Limitations, Pitfalls, and Interpretation in Bulk and Single-Cell Analysis. *Int. J. Mol. Sci.* **2021**, *22*, 12827. [CrossRef]
24. Wang, X.; Wang, M.; Dong, W.; Li, Y.; Zheng, X.; Piao, F.; Li, S. Subchronic exposure to lead acetate inhibits spermatogenesis and downregulates the expression of Ddx3y in testis of mice. *Reprod. Toxicol.* **2013**, *42*, 242–250. [CrossRef]
25. Zheng, X.; Guo, C.; Lv, Z.; Li, J.; Jiang, H.; Li, S.; Yu, L.; Zhang, Z. Novel findings from arsenic-lead combined exposure in mouse testicular TM4 Sertoli cells based on transcriptomics. *Sci. Total Environ.* **2024**, *913*, 169611. [CrossRef] [PubMed]
26. Huang, S.; Ye, J.; Yu, J.; Chen, L.; Zhou, L.; Wang, H.; Li, Z.; Wang, C. The accumulation and efflux of lead partly depend on ATP-dependent efflux pump-multidrug resistance protein 1 and glutathione in testis Sertoli cells. *Toxicol. Lett.* **2014**, *226*, 277–284. [CrossRef]
27. Mizushima, N.; Yoshimori, T.; Ohsumi, Y. The role of Atg proteins in autophagosome formation. *Annu. Rev. Cell Dev. Biol.* **2011**, *27*, 107–132. [CrossRef]

28. Wang, K.; Kong, F.; Qiu, Y.; Chen, T.; Fu, J.; Jin, X.; Su, Y.; Gu, Y.; Hu, Z.; Li, J. Autophagy regulation and protein kinase activity of PIK3C3 controls sertoli cell polarity through its negative regulation on SCIN (scinderin). *Autophagy* **2023**, *19*, 2934–2957. [CrossRef] [PubMed]
29. Yefimova, M.G.; Ravel, C.; Rolland, A.D.; Bourmeyster, N.; Jegou, B. MERTK-Mediated LC3-Associated Phagocytosis (LAP) of Apoptotic Substrates in Blood-Separated Tissues: Retina, Testis, Ovarian Follicles. *Cells* **2021**, *10*, 1443. [CrossRef] [PubMed]
30. Ma, H.; Yu, J.; Xie, J.; Liu, D.; Zhang, Z.; Wang, Z.; Wang, C. Genome-wide identification and functional analysis of long non-coding RNAs and mRNAs in male mice testes at the onset of puberty after low dose lead exposure. *Toxicol. Appl. Pharmacol.* **2021**, *422*, 115556. [CrossRef]
31. Ji, X.; Wang, B.; Paudel, Y.N.; Li, Z.; Zhang, S.; Mou, L.; Liu, K.; Jin, M. Protective Effect of Chlorogenic Acid and Its Analogues on Lead-Induced Developmental Neurotoxicity Through Modulating Oxidative Stress and Autophagy. *Front. Mol. Biosci.* **2021**, *8*, 655549. [CrossRef] [PubMed]
32. Zhang, J.; Cai, T.; Zhao, F.; Yao, T.; Chen, Y.; Liu, X.; Luo, W.; Chen, J. The Role of α-synuclein and Tau Hyperphosphorylation-Mediated Autophagy and Apoptosis in Lead-induced Learning and Memory Injury. *Int. J. Biol. Sci.* **2012**, *8*, 935–944. [CrossRef]
33. Lv, X.H.; Zhao, D.H.; Cai, S.Z.; Luo, S.Y.; You, T.; Xu, B.L.; Chen, K. Autophagy plays a protective role in cell death of osteoblasts exposure to lead chloride. *Toxicol. Lett.* **2015**, *239*, 131–140. [CrossRef]
34. Wang, H.; Wang, N.; Xu, D.; Ma, Q.; Chen, Y.; Xu, S.; Xia, Q.; Zhang, Y.; Prehn, J.H.M.; Wang, G.; et al. Oxidation of multiple MiT/TFE transcription factors links oxidative stress to transcriptional control of autophagy and lysosome biogenesis. *Autophagy* **2020**, *16*, 1683–1696. [CrossRef] [PubMed]
35. Settembre, C.; Di Malta, C.; Polito, V.A.; Garcia Arencibia, M.; Vetrini, F.; Erdin, S.; Erdin, S.U.; Huynh, T.; Medina, D.; Colella, P.; et al. TFEB links autophagy to lysosomal biogenesis. *Science* **2011**, *332*, 1429–1433. [CrossRef] [PubMed]
36. Pi, H.; Li, M.; Xie, J.; Yang, Z.; Xi, Y.; Yu, Z.; Zhou, Z. Transcription factor E3 protects against cadmium-induced apoptosis by maintaining the lysosomal-mitochondrial axis but not autophagic flux in Neuro-2a cells. *Toxicol. Lett.* **2018**, *295*, 335–350. [CrossRef]
37. Pi, H.; Li, M.; Zou, L.; Yang, M.; Deng, P.; Fan, T.; Liu, M.; Tian, L.; Tu, M.; Xie, J.; et al. AKT inhibition-mediated dephosphorylation of TFE3 promotes overactive autophagy independent of MTORC1 in cadmium-exposed bone mesenchymal stem cells. *Autophagy* **2019**, *15*, 565–582. [CrossRef]
38. Siddarth, M.; Chawla, D.; Raizada, A.; Wadhwa, N.; Banerjee, B.D.; Sikka, M. Lead-induced DNA damage and cell apoptosis in human renal proximal tubular epithelial cell: Attenuation via N-acetyl cysteine and tannic acid. *J. Biochem. Mol. Toxicol.* **2018**, *32*, e22038. [CrossRef] [PubMed]
39. Xiong, J.; Wang, K.; He, J.; Zhang, G.; Zhang, D.; Chen, F. TFE3 Alleviates Hepatic Steatosis through Autophagy-Induced Lipophagy and PGC1α-Mediated Fatty Acid β-Oxidation. *Int. J. Mol. Sci.* **2016**, *17*, 387. [CrossRef] [PubMed]

toxics

MDPI

Article

Paternal DEHP Exposure Triggers Reproductive Toxicity in Offspring via Epigenetic Modification of H3K27me3

Lu Zhang [1,2,†], Rui Yang [1,2,†], Guiyong Xu [1,2], Lingqiao Wang [2], Weiyan Chen [2], Yao Tan [2], Guowei Zhang [2], Wenbin Liu [2], Guanghui Zhang [2], Jun Li [1,*] and Ziyuan Zhou [1,2,*]

1 The Key Laboratory of Environmental Pollution Monitoring and Disease Control, School of Public Heath, Ministry of Education, Guizhou Medical University, Guiyang 561113, China; zl1332271608@163.com (L.Z.); yangr202501@163.com (R.Y.); xuguiyong73@163.com (G.X.)
2 Department of Environmental Health, College of Preventive Medicine, Third Military Medical University (Army Medical University), Chongqing 400038, China; mamababa520qq@163.com (L.W.); weiyanchen@tmmu.edu.cn (W.C.); xiaoyue7122@tmmu.edu.cn (Y.T.); zhangguowei@tmmu.edu.cn (G.Z.); liuwenbin@tmmu.edu.cn (W.L.); zhgh221@tmmu.edu.cn (G.Z.)
* Correspondence: gygwlj@163.com (J.L.); ziyuanzhou@tmmu.edu.cn (Z.Z.)
† These authors contributed equally to this work.

Abstract: Di (2-ethylhexyl) phthalate (DEHP) is an acknowledged endocrine disruptor with male reproductive toxicity; nevertheless, the transgenerational impacts on male offspring resulting from paternal exposure, along with the mechanisms involved, are not well understood. To develop a transgenerational model of DEHP paternal exposure, male C57BL/6J mice (4-week) exposed to DEHP (5, 250, and 500 mg/kg/d) for 35 days were then bred with unexposed female mice at a ratio of 1:2 to produce offspring. Findings indicate that the sperm quality and relative sex hormones were adversely affected in males of F1 and F2 generations, and pathological damage in the testes and the apoptosis of testicular cells were also observed. Interestingly, an increase in the expression levels of H3K27me3 was observed in the testicular tissues of male descendants. It was further confirmed by in vitro approach that H3K27me3 may down-regulate the expression of Bcl-2 and plays a role in regulating the initiation of apoptosis in Leydig cells triggered by MEHP (the primary metabolite of DEHP). Additionally, the down-regulation of Bcl-2 can be reversed by treatment with the H3K27me3 inhibitor GSK126. To conclude, DEHP leads to transgenerational harm to male offspring reproductive systems, with the epigenetic mechanism of H3K27me3 playing a key role in mediating these effects.

Keywords: DEHP; paternal exposure; male offspring effect; H3K27me3; apoptosis

1. Introduction

In recent years, global male semen concentrations and total sperm counts have declined by more than 50% [1]. At the same time, studies have shown that environmental pollution can cause damage to sperm, which is an early warning sentinel of human health [2]. Environmental pollution, including heavy metals [3], environmental endocrine disruptors [4], and persistent organic pollutants [5], can cause adverse effects on the male reproductive system, such as reduced sperm quality and pathologic changes in gonadal tissue, which may increase the risk of infertility. Consequently, male reproductive toxicity has already become a significant public concern. Exposure to environmental endocrine disruptors is among the most critical causes of male reproductive harm [6]. DEHP is one of these, and it is abundant in the environment because it is unstable in bonding with plastics and easily escapes into the environment [7]. Research has found that DEHP resulted in a

https://doi.org/10.3390/toxics13030172

reduction in relative testicular weight and serum testosterone levels in male mice, with sperm quality also being adversely affected, ultimately leading to decreased fertility [8]. Similarly, exposure of adolescent male mice to DEHP at doses of 500 mg/kg/d was found to down-regulate histone methylation levels and induce reproductive disorders, including germ cell apoptosis and reduced testosterone levels [9]. Furthermore, DEHP entering the mother causes hypermethylation of spermatogenesis-associated genes in the F1 generation of male mice, resulting in down-regulation of gene expression and spermatogenesis defects [10]. The experimental studies described above emphasize the risk of reproductive and developmental toxicity of DEHP in males and its potential to negatively affect offspring.

Research evidence indicates that parental lifestyle [11], diet [12], and exposure to endocrine disruptors [13] may be transmitted to offspring through epigenetic modifications, and that offspring may exhibit adverse phenotypes, including abnormal embryonic development, altered reproductive endocrinology, and changes in growth and development. DEHP is recognized as epigenotoxic [14]. DEHP-induced intergenerational and transgenerational epigenetic effects can be transmitted through epigenetic mechanisms including DNA methylation [15], small noncoding RNAs [16], or histone modifications [17], particularly through histone modifications. Histone H3K27 trimethylation, a conserved histone modification, represses gene expression and serves as an epigenetic mechanism to regulate transgenerational genetic effects in Caenorhabditis elegans [18], Drosophila melanogaster [19], and mice [20].

Given that the fetus develops within the maternal environment, it is particularly susceptible to intrauterine exposure [21], and previous research has focused on the effects of maternal DEHP exposure on pregnancy outcomes, as well as the growth and development of the offspring. Recently, it has been demonstrated that DEHP causes not only male reproductive damage but also adverse phenotypes in their offspring, but the reasons for these alterations still remain unclear [22]. Overall, in this research we aim to elucidate the adverse effects of paternal DEHP exposure on male offspring by establishing a transgenerational animal model. Furthermore, we seek to investigate the potential involvement of the histone modification H3K27me3 in the transgenerational effects induced by DEHP.

2. Materials and Methods

2.1. Animal Model

Forty C57BL/6J male mice (Beijing Vital River Laboratory Animal Technology Co., Ltd., Beijing, China), 3 weeks old and weighing 13–16 g, were housed in a standard environment and given adequate water and food. After one week, they were divided into control (corn oil) and DEHP-contaminated groups (5, 250, and 500 mg/kg/d) of 10 mice each according to the randomized numeric table method (Figure 1). Corn oil and DEHP were purchased from Sigma-Aldrich (St. Louis, MI, USA). Gavage was performed at the same time every day for 35 days (one spermatogenic cycle) based on body weight. All animal studies were authorized by the Laboratory Animal Welfare and Ethical Committee of the Army Medical University (AMUWEC20226243).

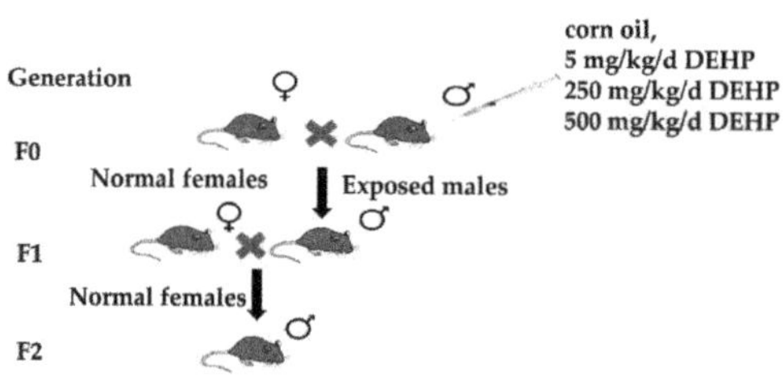

Figure 1. Schematic diagram of cross-generation model construction for paternal DEHP exposure.

2.2. Reproduction and Culture of Offspring

As shown in Figure 1, male mice were directly exposed to DEHP and mated (1:2) with DEHP-unexposed female mice to breed the F1 generation; then, male mice of the F1 generation were mated (1:2) with unexposed female mice to produce the F2 generation. The F1 generation is called intergenerational and the F2 generation is called transgenerational.

2.3. Anogenital Distance (AGD) and Prepuce Separation Test

In male offspring, at postnatal days 14, 19, and 24 (PND14, PND19, and PND24), the anogenital distance was measured using vernier calipers and their body weights were recorded [23]. Starting from PND21, male mice were observed daily for foreskin separation, and the time of foreskin separation and body weight were recorded.

2.4. Organization Sample Collection

Male mice were weighed and bled in the eyeballs and then severed and executed, and the abdomen was cut open to rapidly separate the testes and epididymis bilaterally, which were weighed and recorded (testis coefficient = bilateral testis weight/body weight × 100%; epididymis coefficient = bilateral epididymis weight/body weight × 100%). Some organs were fixed with 4% paraformaldehyde, and the rest were stored at −80 °C. Determination of reproductive hormone levels in the serum of male offspring was conducted according to the instructions of the mouse testosterone ELISA kit, mouse LH ELISA kit, mouse FSH ELISA kit, and mouse ABP ELISA kit (Weiao Biotechnology, Shanghai, China).

2.5. Sperm Quality Assessment

Semen parameters of male offspring were examined by using a computer-aided sperm analysis (CASA) system. Isolated epididymal tails were placed in 1 mL of medium containing BSA at 37 °C and incubated, immediately following the addition of 10 μL of sperm-containing culture solution on a disposable sperm counting plate, and the concentration and viability were assessed using the CASA system, with a minimum of 500 spermatozoa per mouse used for data analysis.

2.6. Testicular Pathologic Histologic Analysis

Fixed testicular tissue slides were stained with hematoxylin and eosin and photographed under light microscopy. Testicular tissue lumen area, seminiferous tubular area, epithelial height, and diameter were assessed. The black line area shown in Figure 2 indicates the cross-sectional area of the spermatogenic tubules and the red line area is the lumen area. The yellow line represents the vertical diameter of the varicocele, and the average length of the solid portion of the line represents the height of the varicocele epithelium [24]. Apoptosis in testicular paraffin sections was identified using a TUNEL staining kit (Servicebio, Wuhan, China) according to the instructions and the sections were analyzed using confocal fluorescence microscopy.

2.7. Cell Processing

Mouse testicular mesenchymal cells TM3 were purchased from Timesaver (Shanghai, China) and cultured in F12 medium (Sigam, Newbury, UK) containing 5% fetal bovine serum (FBS (fetal bovine serum), Hyclone, Logan, UT, USA). Cells treated with MEHP (100, 200, and 400 μM) were incubated at 37 °C for 24 h in an incubator with 5% CO_2.

2.8. Apoptosis Assay

Based on the experimental procedures, we employed the Annexin V-FITC kit (BD Pharmingen, Franklin Lakes, NJ, USA) to detect apoptosis. Cells treated with MEHP were incubated with Annexin V-FITC and propidium iodide (PI) for 15 min at room temperature, and protected from light. Subsequently, flow cytometry was utilized to carry out the assay. A total of 10,000 cells were collected from each sample and the apoptosis rate was calculated by flow cytometry based on the number of apoptotic cells identified by fluorescence (Apoptosis rate = number of apoptotic cells/10,000 × 100%).

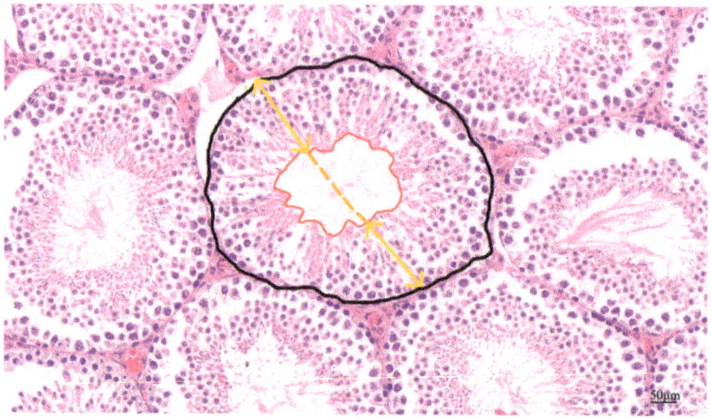

Figure 2. Schematic diagram of parameters for quantitative assessment of testicular tissue in male mice.

2.9. Protein Extraction and Western Blot

Cells were lysed on ice with RIPA buffer for 30 min; testicular tissue was homogenized for 6 min, and then centrifuged for 10 min to extract the supernatant; and protein concentration was determined by BCA Protein Assay Kit (Biotronik, Beijing, China). The protein samples were separated by SDS-PAGE electrophoresis and then transferred to PVDF membranes (Millipore, Bedford, MA, USA). The membranes were incubated with anti-β-actin (rabbit, AC026), anti-TriMethyl-Histone H3-K27 (rabbit, A22396), anti-Bax (rabbit, A19684), and anti-Histone H3 (rabbit, A17562) from ABclonal (Wuhan, China), and anti-Bcl-2 (mouse, 68103-1-Ig) from Proteintech (Wuhan, China), at 4 °C overnight. After washing three times, the membrane was incubated with HRP coupled secondary antibody (1:2000) for 1 h and then the signals were detected using enhanced chemiluminescence (ECL) solution (Millipore, USA).

2.10. Statistical Analysis

The results were analyzed by using GraphPad Prism.9 and SPSS 19.0 software. Measurements are presented as the mean ± standard deviation. Differences between groups were analyzed by one-way ANOVA, and two-way comparisons were performed by *t*-test; statistical significance was set as $\alpha = 0.05$.

3. Results

3.1. Reproductive System of Male Offspring

As illustrated in Figure 3a, the duration of foreskin separation in male mice from the F1 and F2 generations was extended as the exposure doses increased, with the most pronounced impact seen in the 500 mg/kg/d group ($p < 0.05$). Body weight at the time of foreskin separation did not change much between dose groups (Figure 3b). Anal–genital distances of male offspring were measured at postnatal days 14, 19, and 24, and showed a gradual decrease with increasing doses in male offspring ($p < 0.05$, Figure 3c,d).

The weights of reproductive organs were included in the evaluation of reproductive system injuries, with testicular and epididymal weights measured and organ coefficients calculated for both F1- and F2-generation male mice. It was observed that testis weight and organ coefficient decreased with increasing dose in male offspring ($p < 0.05$, Figure 3e,f).

Moreover, although the weight of the epididymis decreased in F1 male mice, the organ coefficient did not exhibit any notable differences. In F2 male mice, both epididymis weight and organ coefficient tended to decrease, but again, no significant difference was noted (Figure 3g,h). These findings clearly indicate that paternal exposure to DEHP adversely impacts the development and maturation of the reproductive organ of male offspring.

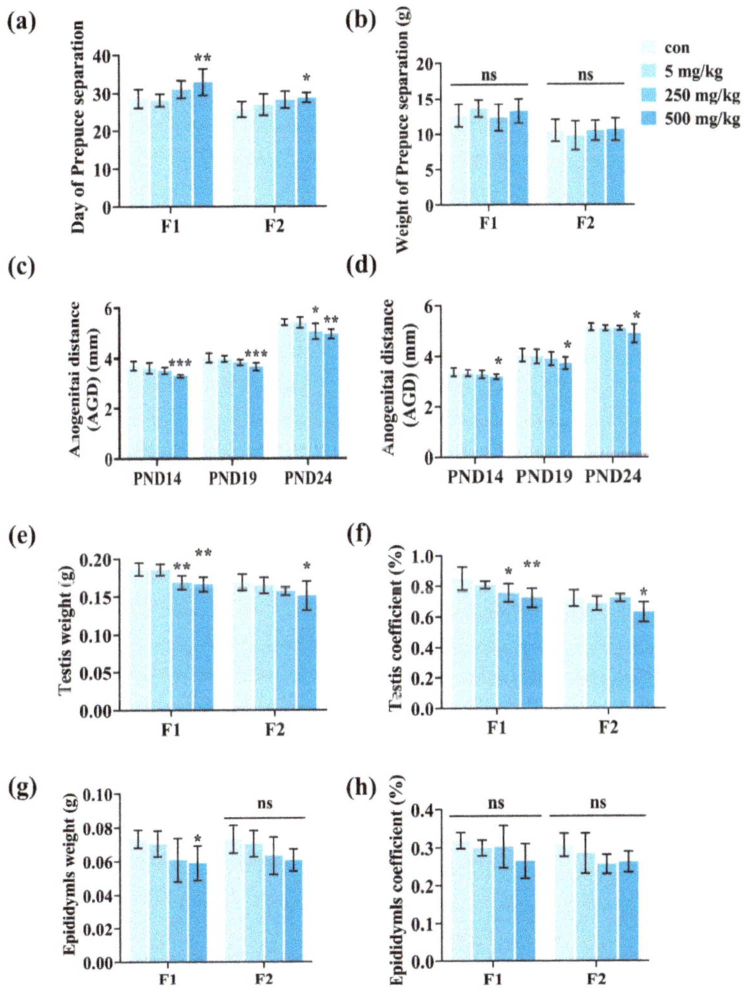

Figure 3. Reproductive system evaluation of male mice in F1 and F2 generations after paternal DEHP exposure. (**a**) F1 and F2 male foreskin separation time. (**b**) Weight of F1 and F2 male foreskin at separation. (**c**) Anogenital distances (mm) of F1 males PND14, 19, and 24. (**d**) Anogenital distances (mm) of F2 males PND14, 19, and 24. (**e**) Testis weight of F1 and F2 males. (**f**) Testicular coefficients for F1 and F2 males. (**g**) Epididymal weights of F1 and F2 males. (**h**) Epididymal coefficients for F1 and F2 males ((**a–d**), n = 9, (**e–h**), n = 6, *** $p < 0.001$, ** $p < 0.01$, * $p < 0.05$, and ns indicates no difference).

3.2. Male Offspring Sperm Parameters

To examine how paternal exposure to DEHP affects the sperm quality in male offspring, we assessed four sperm parameters: sperm density, curvilinear velocity (VCL), straight-line velocity (VSL), and percentage of forward movement (PR%). In Figure 4, the findings revealed a significant reduction in sperm density, VCL, VSL, and PR% with increasing doses in the F1 generation ($p < 0.05$). Even in the F2 generation, the sperm density along with VCL and VSL also diminished with escalating doses, with the most significant impacts noted in the 500 mg/kg/d group ($p < 0.05$). Conversely, there was no significant difference in PR% when compared to the control. This suggests that exposure of fathers to DEHP has a negative impact on the sperm quality of their male offspring.

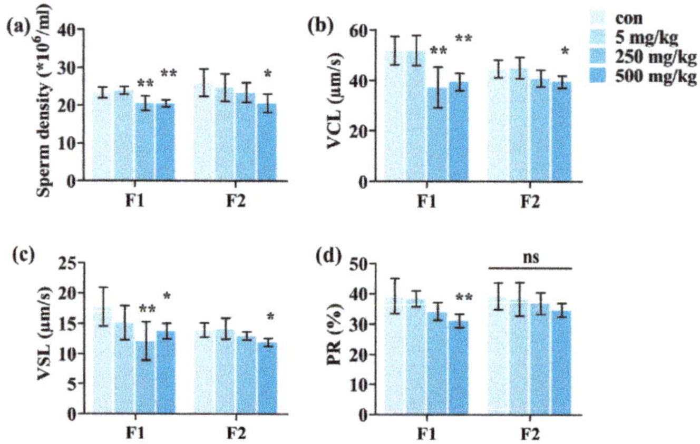

Figure 4. Evaluation of sperm quality in F1- and F2-generation male mice after paternal exposure to DEHP. (**a**) F1 and F2 male sperm density. (**b**) F1 and F2 male sperm curvilinear velocity (VCL). (**c**) F1 and F2 male sperm straight-line velocity (VSL). (**d**) F1 and F2 male percentage of spermatozoa with forward motile spermatozoa (PR%) (n = 6, ** $p < 0.01$, * $p < 0.05$, and ns indicates no difference).

3.3. Histology of Male Offspring Testes

We examined the morphology of testicular tissues in male offspring. The testicular tissues of the male offspring in the DEHP-contaminated group exhibited disorganized spermatogenic tubules, vacuolization, detachment of the spermatogenic epithelium, breakage of the basement membrane, and other pathological damages. In contrast, the control group displayed intact spermatogenic epithelium and spermatogenic tubules arranged in an orderly manner (Figure 5a). Additionally, the lumen area within testicular tissues in the F1 generation demonstrated a notable increase as the dosage of the DEHP rose, while the increase in the lumen area for the F2 generation was not statistically significant (Figure 5b). The testicular tissue seminiferous tubular area, epithelial height, and diameter tended to decrease in the F1 and F2 generations, with a significant decrease in the high-dose group ($p < 0.05$, Figure 5c–e). Taken together, the results suggest that paternal exposure to DEHP significantly impairs the structure of the male testis in the offspring.

3.4. Male Offspring Reproductive Hormone Levels

Exposure to DEHP influences testosterone production. To explore the impact of paternal DEHP exposure on reproductive hormone levels in male offspring, we examined several important hormones. The findings indicated that testosterone levels exhibited a tendency to decrease in both generations of mice, with a notable reduction observed in the 500 mg/kg/d group ($p < 0.05$, Figure 6a). Androgen binding protein levels dropped in the F1 generation ($p < 0.05$, Figure 6b) and showed little variation in the F2 generation. In the F1 generation, levels of luteinizing hormone and follicle-stimulating hormone rose in 250 and 500 mg/kg/d groups ($p < 0.05$, Figure 6c,d), while remaining stable in the F2 generation.

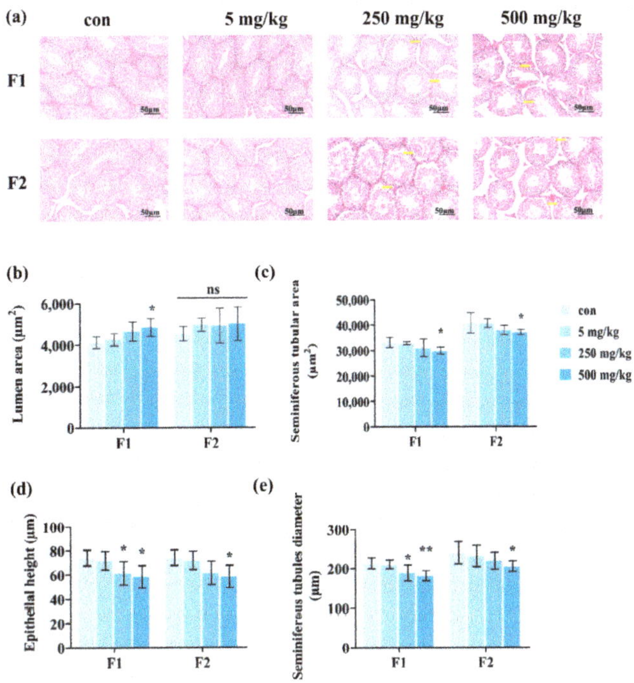

Figure 5. Testicular histology in F1- and F2-generation male mice after paternal exposure to DEHP. (**a**) Representative images of F1 and F2 male testis histology with a scale bar of 50 μM; yellow arrows indicate detachment of the spermatogenic epithelium. (**b**) Testicular lumen area in F1 and F2 males. (**c**) Testicular seminiferous tubular area in F1 and F2 males. (**d**) Epithelial height of spermatogenic tubules in F1 and F2 male testes. (**e**) Diameter of testicular seminiferous tubules in F1 and F2 males (n = 6, ** $p < 0.01$, * $p < 0.05$, and ns indicates no difference).

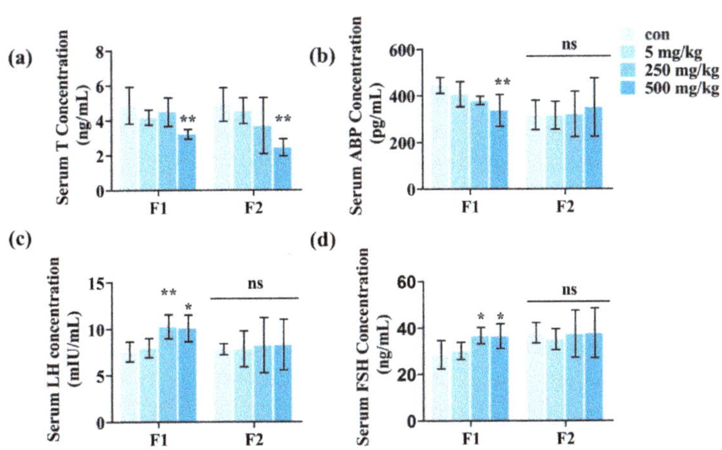

Figure 6. Changes in reproductive hormones in male offspring after paternal DEHP exposure. (**a**) Testosterone (T) levels in serum of F1 and F2 males. (**b**) Androgen-binding protein (ABP) levels in serum of F1 and F2 males. (**c**) Luteinizing hormone (LH) levels in serum of F1 and F2 males. (**d**) Follicle-stimulating hormone (FSH) levels in serum of F1 and F2 males (n = 5, ** $p < 0.01$, * $p < 0.05$, and ns indicates no difference).

3.5. Apoptosis in Male Offspring Testis Cells

TUNEL staining (Figure 7a) revealed that male offspring showed an increased count of TUNEL-positive cells in the 250 and 500 mg/kg/d groups. This observation indicates that exposure of the parental to DEHP leads to apoptosis in the testicular cells of their offspring. MEHP is a metabolite of DEHP in vivo, which has a toxic effect on testes, and because of the continuous decrease in the testosterone level we chose TM3 cells for further experimental studies. Flow results showed that after 24 h of MEHP treatment of TM3 cells, the rate of apoptosis increased significantly with increasing dose ($p < 0.05$, Figure 7b), indicating that MEHP induced apoptosis in TM3 cells.

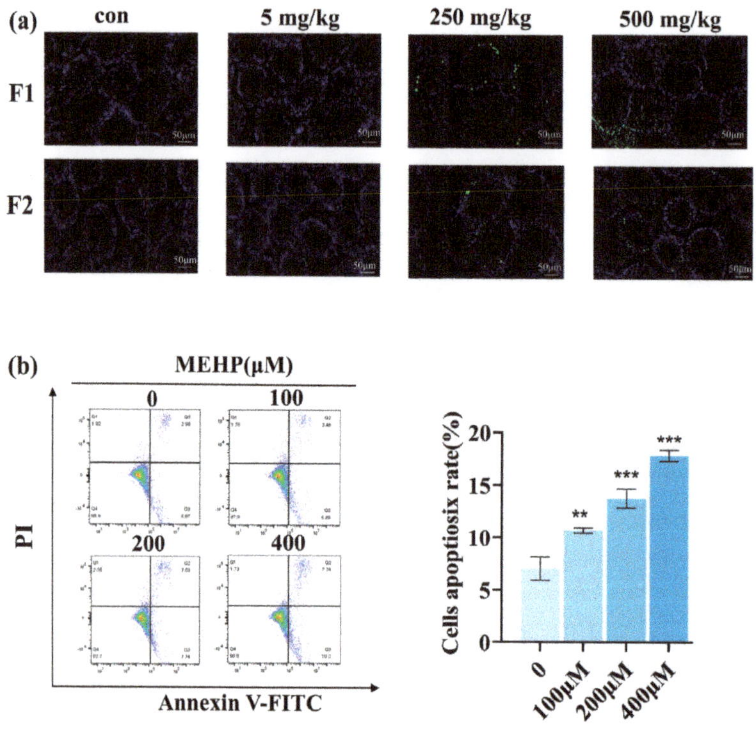

Figure 7. Testicular cell apoptosis in male offspring following paternal DEHP exposure. (a) TUNEL staining of F1 and F2 male testis tissues with a scale bar of 50 μM. TUNEL green fluorescent cells are apoptotic cells. (b) The apoptosis of TM3 cells treated with MEHP for 24 h was detected by flow cytometry. On the left is the representative flow scatter plot, and on the right is the percentage of apoptosis of TM3 cells (n = 3, *** $p < 0.001$, ** $p < 0.01$).

3.6. H3K27me3 Mediates DEHP Paternal Exposure-Induced Apoptosis in Male Offspring Testis Cells

To further elucidate the occurrence of apoptosis at the molecular level in testicular cells following staining, Western blot analysis was conducted on animal and cell staining models. The results of the analysis show that the expression of Bax was elevated, while Bcl-2 expression was reduced after MEHP treatment of TM3 cells for 24 h (Figure 8a). Similarly, the protein Bax, which is linked to apoptosis, showed increased expression, and Bcl-2 exhibited decreased levels in the testicular tissues of male offspring following their fathers' exposure to DEHP (Figure 8b,c). Furthermore, it has been established that the histone H3K27me3, an epigenetic modification, can inhibit Bcl-2 expression in response to environmental stressors, thereby promoting apoptosis. The findings of our study demonstrated an increase in

H3K27me3 expression after 24 h of MEHP treatment in TM3 cells (Figure 8a), alongside heightened levels of H3K27me3 in the testicular tissues of male offspring (Figure 8b,c). To further elucidate the regulation of Bcl-2 by H3K27me3, we administered GSK126, an H3K27me3 inhibitor, to the TM3-treated group, effectively inhibiting the expression of H3K27me3 (Figure 8d). Subsequently, we observed a reduction in apoptosis, along with decreased expression of Bax and H3K27me3, and an increase in Bcl-2 expression (Figure 8d). The findings indicate that histone H3K27me3 is necessary for apoptosis in male offspring testis cells after paternal exposure to DEHP.

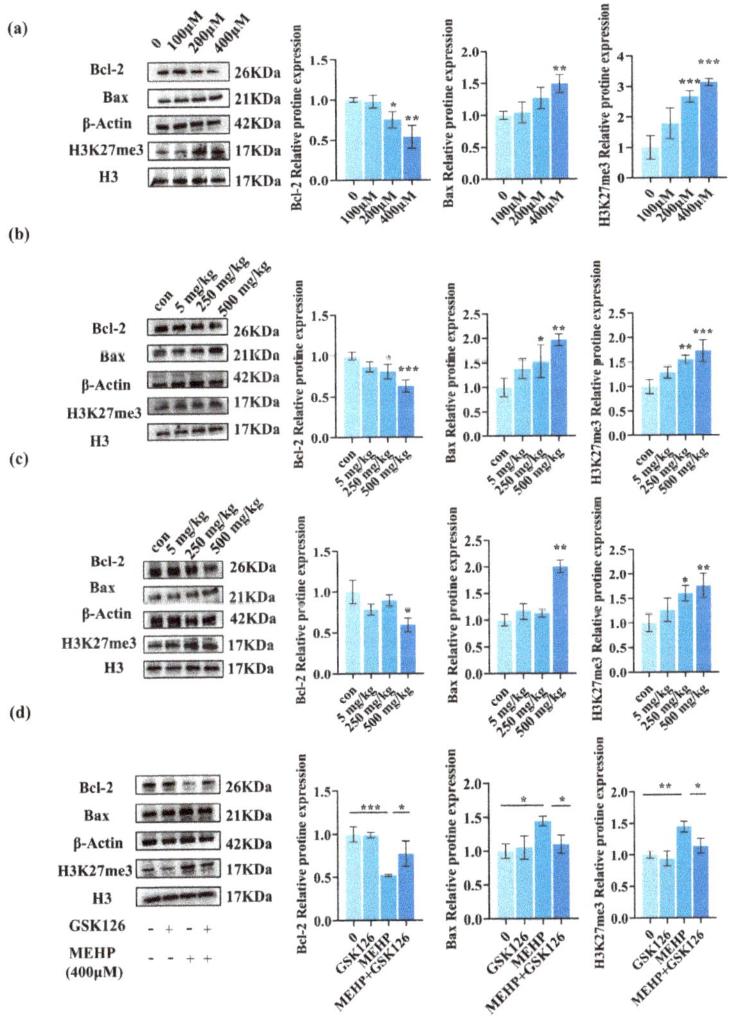

Figure 8. H3K27me3 mediates apoptosis in male offspring testis cells due to DEHP paternal exposure. (**a**) Immunoblot images and quantification of Bax, Bcl-2, and H3K27me3 levels in TM3 cells 24 h after MEHP treatment. (**b**) Immunoblot images and quantification of Bax, Bcl-2, and H3K27me3 levels in testicular tissue from F1 males. (**c**) Immunoblot images and quantification of Bax, Bcl-2, and H3K27me3 levels in testicular tissue from F2 males. (**d**) The "+" indicates treatment with MEHP/GSK126; "-" indicates no treatment. Immunoblot images and quantification of Bax, Bcl-2, and H3K27me3 after simultaneous treatment of TM3 cells with GSK126 inhibitor and MEHP for 24 h compared to MEHP-treated group (n = 3, *** $p < 0.001$, ** $p < 0.01$, * $p < 0.05$).

4. Discussion

DEHP is a well-known environmental endocrine disruptor that exerts detrimental effects on male reproductive health [25]. Numerous animal studies and analyses of population data have demonstrated that DEHP exposure leads to reproductive impairments [26,27]. Furthermore, exposure during pregnancy adversely impacts the growth, development, and fertility of offspring [28]. Studies involving Caenorhabditis elegans have shown that exposure to DEHP results in decreased offspring numbers and reproductive senescence across generations [29]. Nonetheless, the impacts and processes related to paternal exposure on male offspring have not been thoroughly examined. Thus, elucidating the effects of paternal DEHP exposure on male offspring and underlying mechanisms is essential. The concentration at which no adverse effects were observed for DEHP exposure in the EU risk assessment was 4.8 mg/kg/d. Additionally, SD rats exposed to 5 mg/kg/d DEHP did not result in adverse effects on testicular or developmental toxicity across three consecutive generations of male rats [30]. Conversely, subjecting pubertal male mice to a dosage of 250 mg/kg caused damage to testicular cells and disrupted normal testicular functions [31]. Additionally, decreased testosterone levels and hindered spermatogenesis has been found in the F1 male offspring of pregnancy exposure to a mixture of phthalates at 500 mg/kg [32]. In light of these results, we developed an experimental study that included a control group (corn oil) and exposure groups with DEHP doses of 5, 250, and 500 mg/kg/d.

The growth and development of offspring may indicate reproductive developmental toxicity resulting from paternal exposure. Anogenital distance (AGD) has been utilized as a marker for exposure to environmental endocrine disruptors, reflecting early androgenic effects and predicting reproductive health in adulthood [33]. Jorge's study revealed that low-dose benzo(a)pyrene exposure in the rat father led to a significant decrease in AGD and reduced fertility in the F2 generation of male rats [34]. Furthermore, exposure to DEHP in mothers prior to conception has been linked to a delay in foreskin separation, a reduction in anogenital distance (AGD), and disrupted activation and functioning of the gonadotropic axis in male offspring [23]. Similarly, our study demonstrated that DEHP exposure resulted in delayed foreskin separation and decreased AGD in male mice across both F1 and F2 generations. Prepuce separation is a marker of the onset of male puberty, and the delay suggests that paternal exposure to DEHP causes delayed puberty in male offspring, which may be induced by antiandrogenic activity, as evidenced by the decline in AGD we detected [35]. Reproductive organ weight and sperm quality are critical indicators for assessing reproductive toxic effects in males, and direct exposure of male rats to DEHP has been shown to decrease sperm viability [8]. In this research, exposure of male mice to DEHP led to a decrease in both testicular and epididymal weights, along with decreased sperm quality in the F1 generation, and the weight loss of testis and epididymis and the decrease in sperm quality were still observed in the 500 mg/kg/d group of the F2 generation. This may be due to the fact that the H3K27me3 protein escapes epigenetic reprogramming events during transgenerational inheritance in the high-dose group, conferring conditions for the transmission of high-dose transgenerational reproductive damage [36]. Thus, partial reproductive impairment was still observed in the high-dose group. The difference in effects between the F2 and F1 generations may be due to the different intergenerational and transgenerational effects resulting from different exposure doses in the F0 generation [37]. Collectively, these data show that paternal exposure to DEHP contributes to reproductive damage in male offspring.

Normal endocrine function is crucial for male reproductive health. Our study showed that FSH and LH levels were elevated in the F1 generation, while testosterone levels were decreased in both the F1 and F2 generations. The results of the present study suggest that DEHP directly damages TM3 cells, resulting in decreased testosterone levels. The decrease in testosterone level activates the negative feedback regulation mechanism of the hypothalamic–pituitary–gonadal axis, which results in the upward elevation of FSH and LH levels secreted by the pituitary gland [38,39]. Testosterone promotes the formation of the male reproductive phenotype and facilitates spermatogenesis [32]. Given that TM3 cells are responsible for testosterone production, we opted to utilize the TM3 cell line in our in vitro studies. Numerous research efforts have shown that DEHP triggers apoptosis in testicular cells [40]. Our research revealed that paternal exposure to DEHP led to pathological harm in the offspring, which encompassed testicular tissue atrophy and TUNEL positivity observed in testicular cells, indicative of apoptosis. The result of changed expression levels of apoptosis-related proteins Bcl-2 and Bax within the testicular tissues of both F1 and F2 generations offer molecular support for the assertion that paternal DEHP exposure initiates testicular apoptosis in the progeny.

Exposure of parents to environmental endocrine disruptors leads to modifications in the epigenetic traits of all somatic cells derived from them by changing the epigenetic information in the germ cells, which subsequently affects the phenotype of their offspring [41]. H3K27me3 is a well-established epigenetic modification primarily associated with gene repression. Different cell types inhibit the expression of Bcl-2 anti-apoptotic molecules through high levels of H3K27me3 in the promoter region, which enhances the expression of the downstream pro-apoptotic molecule Bax, and finally induces cell apoptosis [42]. To explore the potential function of H3K27me3 in a transgenerational model of parental exposure to DEHP, we examined H3K27me3 expression levels in testicular tissues of the F1 and F2 generations, and showed that expression was elevated in both generations. Furthermore, we observed increased H3K27me3 expression and apoptosis in MEHP-treated TM3 cells after 24 h. The H3K27me3 protein level in the MEHP group was not completely restored after using the inhibitor GSK126, indicating that the GSK126 inhibitor could not completely inhibit the expression of the H3K27me3 protein. In addition to H3K27me3, Bcl-2 may also be affected by epigenetic modifications such as small noncoding RNAs and DNA methylation [43,44] Thus, Bcl-2 protein levels were not completely reversed in the MEHP-stained group after addition of the inhibitor.

As research on the reproductive toxicity of DEHP progresses, the exposure doses selected in animal studies are increasingly reflective of actual human exposure levels in daily life. Nonetheless, it is important to evaluate the effects of long-term exposure of DEHP, particularly on transgenerational aftermath, due to its significant persistence and bioaccumulation in the environment. In this study we initially explored the role that histone methylation plays in a transgenerational model of paternal exposure to DEHP, without exploring more fully whether DNA methylation and small noncoding RNAs play a role in this, and how histone methylation is maintained. In the animal experiments, no intervention group was established concurrently, and the intervention experiments were ultimately conducted using an in vitro cellular model; we did not go further to investigate the regulation of Bcl-2 by H3K27me3 in our in vitro cellular experiments, and we will consider this work to enrich our study in the future. Our present study found that reproductive toxicity associated with paternal exposure to DEHP persisted into the F2 generation but the effect was not significant relative to the F1 generation; however, we did not conduct experiments with the F3 and F4 generations. Consequently, we cannot determine whether the reproductive system toxicity resulting from DEHP paternal exposure in male offspring recovers in subsequent generations and the mechanisms involved.

5. Conclusions

Our research indicated that exposure of fathers to DEHP leads to impaired growth and development, as well as reproductive dysfunction in male offspring. Furthermore, the modification of H3K27me3 is implicated as one of the epigenetic mechanisms contributing to offspring testicular cell apoptosis induced by paternal DEHP exposure. These findings indicate that reproductive system damage resulting from paternal DEHP exposure can be transmitted across generations, extending to the F2 generation, and has long-term implications for reproductive health and fertility in animals. This research deepens our comprehension of the negative impacts of DEHP exposure from fathers on their male offspring. Additionally, it may provide a foundation for future studies on reproductive toxicity and the underlying mechanisms affecting male offspring due to paternal DEHP exposure.

Author Contributions: Conceptualization, methodology and writing—original draft preparation L.Z., R.Y. and G.X.; software and validation, L.W.; formal analysis, W.C. and Y.T.; methodology and data curation, W.L. and G.Z. (Guowei Zhang); investigation, review and editing, G.Z. (Guanghui Zhang); writing—review and editing, project administration and supervision J.L. and Z.Z. All authors have read and agreed to the published version of the manuscript.

Funding: This research was funded by the Key Joint Project of the National Natural Science Foundation of China (U23A20494), the National Key Research and Development Program of China (No 2022YFC2702902), and the Natural Science Foundation of Chongqing (CSTB2024NSCQLZX0142).

Institutional Review Board Statement: All animal studies were authorized by the Laboratory Animal Welfare and Ethical Committee of the Army Medical University (AMUWEC20226243) on 3 November 2022.

Informed Consent Statement: Not applicable.

Data Availability Statement: The data used to support the findings of this study are available from the corresponding author upon reasonable request.

Conflicts of Interest: The authors declare no conflicts of interest.

References

1. Barakat, R.; Lin, P.C.; Park, C.J.; Zeineldin, M.; Zhou, S.; Rattan, S.; Brehm, E.; Flaws, J.A.; Ko, C.J. Germline-dependent transmission of male reproductive traits induced by an endocrine disruptor, di-2-ethylhexyl phthalate, in future generations. *Sci. Rep.* **2020**, *10*, 5705. [CrossRef] [PubMed]
2. Ferrero, G.; Festa, R.; Follia, L.; Lettieri, G.; Tarallo, S.; Notari, T.; Giarra, A.; Marinaro, C.; Pardini, B.; Marano, A.; et al. Small noncoding RNAs and sperm nuclear basic proteins reflect the environmental impact on germ cells. *Mol. Med.* **2024**, *30*, 12. [CrossRef]
3. Marinaro, C.; Lettieri, G.; Chianese, T.; Bianchi, A.R.; Zarrelli, A.; Palatucci, D.; Scudiero, R.; Rosati, L.; De Maio, A.; Piscopo, M. Exploring the molecular and toxicological mechanism associated with interactions between heavy metals and the reproductive system of Mytilus galloprovincialis. *Comp. Biochem. Physiol. C Toxicol. Pharmacol.* **2024**, *275*, 109778. [CrossRef]
4. Thacharodi, A.; Hassan, S.; Acharya, G.; Vithlani, A.; Hoang Le, Q.; Pugazhendhi, A. Endocrine disrupting chemicals and their effects on the reproductive health in men. *Environ. Res.* **2023**, *236*, 116825. [CrossRef]
5. Vested, A.; Giwercman, A.; Bonde, J.P.; Toft, G. Persistent organic pollutants and male reproductive health. *Asian J. Androl.* **2014**, *16*, 71–80. [CrossRef] [PubMed]
6. Mohajer, N.; Culty, M. IMPACT OF REAL-LIFE ENVIRONMENTAL EXPOSURES ON REPRODUCTION: Impact of human-relevant doses of endocrine-disrupting chemical and drug mixtures on testis development and function. *Reproduction* **2025**, *169*, e240155. [CrossRef] [PubMed]
7. Zhang, Y.; Lyu, L.; Tao, Y.; Ju, H.; Chen, J. Health risks of phthalates: A review of immunotoxicity. *Environ. Pollut.* **2022**, *313*, 120173. [CrossRef] [PubMed]
8. XueXia, L.; YaNan, L.; Zi, T.; YuSheng, Z.; ZeLin, W.; Peng, Z.; MeiNa, X.; FuJun, L. Di-2-ethylhexyl phthalate (DEHP) exposure induces sperm quality and functional defects in mice. *Chemosphere* **2023**, *312*, 137216. [CrossRef] [PubMed]

9. Liu, C.; Qian, P.; Yang, L.; Zhang, L.; Chen, C.; He, M.; Lu, Y.; Feng, W.; Li, M.; Zhang, Y.; et al. Pubertal exposure to di-(2-ethylhexyl)-phthalate inhibits G9a-mediated histone methylation during spermatogenesis in mice. *Arch. Toxicol.* **2016**, *90*, 955–969. [CrossRef] [PubMed]
10. Tando, Y.; Hiura, H.; Takehara, A.; Ito-Matsuoka, Y.; Arima, T.; Matsui, Y. Epi-mutations for spermatogenic defects by maternal exposure to di(2-ethylhexyl) phthalate. *Elife* **2021**, *10*, e70322. [CrossRef] [PubMed]
11. Cintado, E.; Tezanos, P.; De Las Casas, M.; Muela, P.; McGreevy, K.R.; Fontán-Lozano, Á.; Sacristán-Horcajada, E.; Pignatelli, J.; de Ceballos, M.L.; Del Hierro, M.J.; et al. Grandfathers-to-Grandsons Transgenerational Transmission of Exercise Positive Effects on Cognitive Performance. *J. Neurosci.* **2024**, *44*, e2061232024. [CrossRef]
12. Watkins, A.J.; Dias, I.; Tsuro, H.; Allen, D.; Emes, R.D.; Moreton, J.; Wilson, R.; Ingram, R.J.M.; Sinclair, K.D. Paternal diet programs offspring health through sperm- and seminal plasma-specific pathways in mice. *Proc. Natl. Acad. Sci. USA* **2018**, *115*, 10064–10069. [CrossRef] [PubMed]
13. Molangiri, A.; Varma, S.; Boga, N.S.; Das, P.; Duttaroy, A.K.; Basak, S. Gestational exposure to BPA alters the expression of glucose and lipid metabolic mediators in the placenta: Role in programming offspring for obesity. *Toxicology* **2024**, *509*, 153957. [CrossRef] [PubMed]
14. Singh, S.; Li, S.S. Epigenetic effects of environmental chemicals bisphenol A and phthalates. *Int. J. Mol. Sci.* **2012**, *13*, 10143–10153. [CrossRef]
15. Hsu, P.C.; Jhong, J.Y.; Huang, L.P.; Lee, K.H.; Chen, H.P.; Guo, Y.L. Transgenerational Effects of Di(2-Ethylhexyl) Phthalate on Anogenital Distance, Sperm Functions and DNA Methylation in Rat Offspring. *Int. J. Mol. Sci.* **2021**, *22*, 4131. [CrossRef] [PubMed]
16. Liu, J.; Wang, W.; Zhu, J.; Li, Y.; Luo, L.; Huang, Y.; Zhang, W. Di(2-ethylhexyl) phthalate (DEHP) influences follicular development in mice between the weaning period and maturity by interfering with ovarian development factors and microRNAs. *Environ. Toxicol.* **2018**, *33*, 535–544. [CrossRef] [PubMed]
17. Zhang, T.; Zhou, Y.; Li, L.; Zhao, Y.; De Felici, M., Reiter, R.J.; Shen, W. Melatonin protects prepuberal testis from deleterious effects of bisphenol A or diethylhexyl phthalate by preserving H3K9 methylation. *J. Pineal Res.* **2018**, *65*, e12497. [CrossRef] [PubMed]
18. Kaneshiro, K.R.; Rechtsteiner, A.; Strome, S. Sperm-inherited H3K27me3 impacts offspring transcription and development in C. elegans. *Nat. Commun.* **2019**, *10*, 1271. [CrossRef] [PubMed]
19. Yang, J.; Tang, R.; Chen, S.; Chen, Y., Yuan, K.; Huang, R.; Wang, L. Exposure to high-sugar diet induces transgenerational changes in sweet sensitivity and feeding behavior via H3K27me3 reprogramming. *Elife* **2023**, *12*, e85365. [CrossRef]
20. Raas, M.W.D.; Zijlmans, D.W.; Vermeulen, M.; Marks, H. There is another: H3K27me3-mediated genomic imprinting. *Trends Genet.* **2022**, *38*, 82–96. [CrossRef] [PubMed]
21. Tran, M.; Kuo, F.C.; Low, J.T.; Chuang, Y.M.; Sultana, S.; Huang, W.L.; Lin, Z.Y.; Lin, G.L.; Wu, C.F.; Li, S.S.; et al. Prenatal DEHP exposure predicts neurological disorders via transgenerational epigenetics. *Sci. Rep.* **2023**, *13*, 7399. [CrossRef] [PubMed]
22. Oluwayiose, O.A.; Marcho, C.; Wu, H.; Houle, E.; Krawetz, S.A.; Suvorov, A.; Mager, J.; Pilsner, R.J. Paternal preconception phthalate exposure alters sperm methylome and embryonic programming. *Environ. Int.* **2021**, *155*, 106693. [CrossRef] [PubMed]
23. Adam, N.; Desroziers, E.; Hanine, R.; Bascarane, K.; Naulé, L.; Mhaouty-Kodja, S. Developmental exposure to environmentally relevant doses of phthalates alters the neural control of male and female reproduction in mice. *Environ. Res.* **2024**, *258*, 119476. [CrossRef]
24. Shen, J.; Perveen, A.; Kaka, N.; Li, Z.; Dai, P.; Li, C. Maternal Exposure to T-2 Toxin Induces Changes in Antioxidant System and Testosterone Synthesis in the Testes of Mice Offspring. *Animals* **2019**, *10*, 74. [CrossRef] [PubMed]
25. Mondal, S.; Bandyopadhyay, A. Antioxidants in mitigating phthalate-induced male reproductive toxicity: A comprehensive review. *Chemosphere* **2024**, *364*, 143297. [CrossRef] [PubMed]
26. Mínguez-Alarcón, L.; Burns, J.; Williams, P.L.; Korrick, S.A.; Lee, M.M.; Bather, J.R.; Kovalev, S.V.; Sokolov, S.A.; Lebedev, A.T.; Smigulina, L.; et al. Urinary phthalate metabolite concentrations during four windows spanning puberty (prepuberty through sexual maturity) and association with semen quality among young Russian men. *Int. J. Hyg. Environ. Health* **2022**, *243*, 113977. [CrossRef]
27. Oluwayiose, O.A.; Houle, E.; Whitcomb, B.W.; Suvorov, A.; Rahil, T.; Sites, C.K.; Krawetz, S.A.; Visconti, P.E.; Pilsner, J.R. Urinary phthalate metabolites and small non-coding RNAs from seminal plasma extracellular vesicles among men undergoing infertility treatment. *Environ. Pollut.* **2023**, *329*, 121529. [CrossRef]
28. Yin, J.; Liu, S.; Li, Y.; Hu, L.; Liao, C.; Jiang, G. Exposure to MEHP during Pregnancy and Lactation Impairs Offspring Growth and Development by Disrupting Thyroid Hormone Homeostasis. *Environ. Sci. Technol.* **2024**, *58*, 3726–3736. [CrossRef] [PubMed]
29. Zhang, Y.; Li, J.; Shi, W.; Lu, L.; Zhou, Q.; Zhang, H.; Liu, R.; Pu, Y.; Yin, L. Di(2-ethylhexyl) phthalate induces reproductive toxicity and transgenerational reproductive aging in Caenorhabditis elegans. *Environ. Pollut.* **2023**, *336*, 122259. [CrossRef] [PubMed]

30. Tassinari, R.; Tait, S.; Busani, L.; Martinelli, A.; Narciso, L.; Valeri, M.; Gastaldelli, A.; Deodati, A.; La Rocca, C.; Maranghi, F. Metabolic, reproductive and thyroid effects of bis(2-ethylhexyl) phthalate (DEHP) orally administered to male and female juvenile rats at dose levels derived from children biomonitoring study. *Toxicology* **2021**, *449*, 152653. [CrossRef]
31. Wang, J.; Wei, Y.; Wu, Y.; Zhao, T.; Kang, L.; Han, L.; Chen, J.; Long, C.; Wei, G.; Shen, L.; et al. Di-(2-ethylhexyl) phthalate induces prepubertal testicular injury through MAM-related mitochondrial calcium overload in Leydig and Sertoli cell apoptosis. *Toxicology* **2024**, *509*, 153956. [CrossRef]
32. Barakat, R.; Seymore, T.; Lin, P.P.; Park, C.J.; Ko, C.J. Prenatal exposure to an environmentally relevant phthalate mixture disrupts testicular steroidogenesis in adult male mice. *Environ. Res.* **2019**, *172*, 194–201. [CrossRef] [PubMed]
33. Li, K.; Zhang, Y.; Li, L.; Cui, K.; Li, Y.; Li, C.; Dai, Y.; Xiao, W.; Wang, Q. Identification of sensitive endpoints for the assessment of phthalates-induced reproductive and developmental toxicity: A literature mining study. *Food Chem. Toxicol.* **2024**, *188*, 114686. [CrossRef] [PubMed]
34. Jorge, B.C.; Stein, J.; Reis, A.C.C.; Bueno, J.N.; Paschoalini, B.R.; Moreira, S.D.S.; Manoel, B.M.; Arena, A.C. Paternal low-dose benzo(a)pyrene exposure in rats impairs sexual development and fertility of the paternal lineage in F2 generation: A transgenerational study. *Toxicology* **2023**, *494*, 153585. [CrossRef]
35. Fischer, M.B.; Mola, G.; Priskorn, L.; Scheel, L.; Hegaard, H.K.; Sundberg, K.; Frederiksen, H.; Andersson, A.M.; Juul, A.; Hagen, C.P. Longitudinal Evaluation of Fetal and Infant AGD in Healthy Children: Association With Penile Size, Testosterone, and DHT. *J. Clin. Endocrinol. Metab.* **2024**, *109*, 3087–3095. [CrossRef] [PubMed]
36. Xavier, M.J.; Roman, S.D.; Aitken, R.J.; Nixon, B. Transgenerational inheritance: How impacts to the epigenetic and genetic information of parents affect offspring health. *Hum. Reprod. Update* **2019**, *25*, 518–540. [CrossRef] [PubMed]
37. Van Cauwenbergh, O.; Di Serafino, A.; Tytgat, J.; Soubry, A. Transgenerational epigenetic effects from male exposure to endocrine-disrupting compounds: A systematic review on research in mammals. *Clin. Epigenetics* **2020**, *12*, 65. [CrossRef]
38. Plunk, E.C.; Richards, S.M. Endocrine-Disrupting Air Pollutants and Their Effects on the Hypothalamus-Pituitary-Gonadal Axis. *Int. J. Mol. Sci.* **2020**, *21*, 9191. [CrossRef] [PubMed]
39. Zhu, X.; Hu, M.; Ji, H.; Huang, T.; Ge, R.S.; Wang, Y. Exposure to di-n-octyl phthalate during puberty induces hypergonadotropic hypogonadism caused by Leydig cell hyperplasia but reduced steroidogenic function in male rats. *Ecotoxicol. Environ. Saf.* **2021**, *208*, 111432. [CrossRef] [PubMed]
40. Chen, J.; Zhao, T.; Zheng, X.; Kang, L.; Wang, J.; Wei, Y.; Wu, Y.; Shen, L.; Long, C.; Wei, G.; et al. Protective effects of melatonin on DEHP-induced apoptosis and oxidative stress in prepubertal testes via the PI3K/AKT pathway. *Environ. Toxicol.* **2024**, *39*, 952–964. [CrossRef]
41. McSwiggin, H.; Magalhães, R.; Nilsson, E.E.; Yan, W.; Skinner, M.K. Epigenetic transgenerational inheritance of toxicant exposure-specific non-coding RNA in sperm. *Environ. Epigenet* **2024**, *10*, dvae014. [CrossRef] [PubMed]
42. Gao, J.; Gu, J.; Pan, X.; Gan, X.; Ju, Z.; Zhang, S.; Xia, Y.; Lu, L.; Wang, X. Blockade of miR-142-3p promotes anti-apoptotic and suppressive function by inducing KDM6A-mediated H3K27me3 demethylation in induced regulatory T cells. *Cell Death Dis.* **2019**, *10*, 332. [CrossRef] [PubMed]
43. Tian, F.; Zhan, Y.; Zhu, W.; Li, J.; Tang, M.; Chen, X.; Jiang, J. MicroRNA-497 inhibits multiple myeloma growth and increases susceptibility to bortezomib by targeting Bcl-2. *Int. J. Mol. Med.* **2019**, *43*, 1058–1066. [CrossRef] [PubMed]
44. Zeng, H.; Li, T.; He, X.; Cai, S.; Luo, H.; Chen, P.; Chen, Y. Oxidative stress mediates the apoptosis and epigenetic modification of the Bcl-2 promoter via DNMT1 in a cigarette smoke-induced emphysema model. *Respir. Res.* **2020**, *21*, 229. [CrossRef] [PubMed]

toxics

MDPI

Article

The Relationship Between PM2.5 and Eight Common Lung Diseases: A Two-Sample Mendelian Randomization Analysis

Yuhang Jiang [1,†], Jingwen Si [2,†], Yuhang Wang [3], Han Zhang [1], Fang Zhou [1,3], Xike Lu [3], Xin Li [1,3], Daqiang Sun [1,3,*] and Zheng Wang [3,*]

1 Department of Clinical Medicine, Medical School, Tianjin University, Tianjin 300072, China
2 Department of Pathology, Tianjin Central Hospital of Obstetrics and Gynecology, Tianjin 300100, China
3 Department of Thoracic, Tianjin Chest Hospital Affiliated to Tianjin University, Tianjin 300051, China
* Correspondence: sdqmdsr@163.com (D.S.); emre_schlager@163.com (Z.W.)
† These authors contributed equally to this work.

Abstract: Air pollutants have both acute and chronic impacts on human health, affecting multiple systems and organs. While PM2.5 exposure is commonly assumed to be strongly associated with all respiratory diseases, this relationship has not been systematically analyzed. This study employed a two-sample Mendelian randomization approach to investigate the effects of PM2.5 on eight common lung diseases, using data from GWAS. Additionally, multivariable Mendelian randomization was applied to assess the direct effects of various air pollutants and the mediating roles of common factors such as BMI and smoking. At a significance threshold of 5×10^{-8}, PM2.5 showed a significant causal relationship with both asthma and COPD. When the screening threshold was relaxed to 5×10^{-6}, this exposure continued to demonstrate significant associations not only with asthma and COPD, but also with other respiratory diseases, including pneumonia, emphysema/chronic bronchitis, and lung cancer. In the multivariable Mendelian randomization analysis, which controlled for smoking and bacterial infections, the association with pneumonia became non-significant, while the relationships with the other four diseases persisted. This study provides a systematic exploration of the relationship between PM2.5 and eight pulmonary diseases from a new perspective, deepening our understanding of the impact of air pollution on health and laying the foundation for future efforts to mitigate these effects.

Keywords: air pollution; PM2.5; COPD; asthma; chronic bronchitis; lung cancer; MR

1. Introduction

Human activities continuously release various pollutants into the atmosphere, and their accumulation not only threatens the environment, but also has numerous negative impacts on human health. Air pollution is the leading environmental cause of death worldwide, with household air pollution causing from approximately 3.5 to 4 million deaths annually. Women and children living in extreme poverty are the most affected by household air pollution. Ref. [1] These significant changes in atmospheric composition are primarily driven by the widespread combustion of fossil fuels in industries such as power generation and transportation. Given the wide-ranging sources and complex composition of air pollutants, their chemical properties, reactivity, emission methods, and persistence in the environment vary. As a result, the ultimate effects on human health and ecosystems depend on the specific type of pollutant.

Particulate matter (PM) is a broad term for air pollutants composed of a complex and varied mixture of particles suspended in the air. These particles differ in size and composition, originating from both natural processes and human activities [2]. The primary sources of particulate pollution include factories, power plants, and natural dust storms. It can also appear at high concentrations in kitchens. A systematic review by Lin and colleagues [3] provides strong evidence that using gas for cooking and heating can lead to pollutant levels—such as nitrogen dioxide, carbon monoxide, and PM2.5—that exceed the World Health Organization's indoor air quality guidelines. Particle pollutants vary in size. PM2.5 refers to particles with an aerodynamic diameter of less than 2.5 μm, while PM10 refers to particles with a diameter between 2.5 and 10 μm. Based on these measurements, particles are categorized into ultrafine, fine, and coarse particles. The size of the particles determines where they deposit in the respiratory tract and is closely related to their ability to penetrate the system [4]. PM10 particles primarily deposit in the upper respiratory tract, whereas ultrafine particles can reach the alveoli and even enter the circulatory system.

To date, no single component can fully explain the health effects caused by particulate matter. Factors such as particle size, surface properties, quantity, and chemical composition all play important roles. Particulate matter (PM) is highly complex, as it can adsorb and carry various pollutants. Thus, the composition of PM may differ significantly depending on the environment. There is strong evidence suggesting that ultrafine and fine particles are more hazardous than larger particles (coarse particles) in terms of mortality and cardiovascular and respiratory impacts. Because of their tiny size, they can penetrate deeply into the respiratory system undetected, reaching the alveoli and potentially entering the bloodstream [5]. Consequently, fine particles can cause chronic, long-term effects on the respiratory and immune systems, increasing the risk of disease. Notably, research shows that individuals with asthma, pneumonia, diabetes, respiratory diseases, and cardiovascular conditions are more vulnerable to the harmful effects of particulate matter. Both PM2.5 and PM10 are strongly linked to various respiratory diseases [6]. For example, in the United States, for every 10 $\mu g/m^3$ increase in PM2.5, the incidence rate ratio (IRR) for lung cancer is 1.19 (95% CI: 1.09, 1.30) [7]. In conclusion, PM2.5, due to its small size, poses more significant health risks. These fine particles suspended in the air are also a major contributor to the formation of "smog" in many cities [8,9].

In recent years, rapid industrial development and overpopulation have made China one of the Asian countries facing serious air pollution challenges [10,11].There is evidence suggesting that air pollution may contribute to the onset of asthma, which is also highlighted in ref. [12]. However, not all studies support a definitive causal link between air pollution and asthma. A recent meta-analysis [13] of cross-sectional studies comparing communities with varying levels of pollution found that long-term exposure to pollution did not affect asthma prevalence. Some studies also suggest that environmental air pollution increases the risk of respiratory-related mortality, though the evidence for its impact on lung function and chronic obstructive pulmonary disease (COPD) remains inconclusive [14]. Numerous epidemiological studies, such as ref. [15], have been conducted globally on the health effects of particulate matter. For instance, both short- and long-term exposure to PM2.5 have been positively associated with acute nasopharyngitis [16], a significant correlation has been found between PM2.5 exposure and COPD, and lung cancer mortality has been linked to fine particulate matter exposure [8]. However, most of these epidemiological studies rely on PM2.5 monitors, which lack sufficient spatial resolution. This makes it difficult to accurately measure the actual daily inhalation of PM2.5. Furthermore, the limited placement of monitors within specific study areas or urban regions does not accurately represent the true PM2.5 exposure experienced by the broader population. A recent epidemiological study conducted by the Department of Environmental Health at the Harvard T.H. Chan School of Public Health (Boston, MA) [17] highlighted that the spatial variability in PM2.5 concentrations results in exposure measurement errors. Additionally, in regions with severe PM2.5 pollution, other pollutants are often also present in significant quantities, leading to confounding factors that further diminish the accuracy of study conclusions.

Mendelian randomization (MR) is a statistical method that utilizes genetic variations as instrumental variables to assess the causal relationship between exposure and outcomes [18]. This approach is considered to be a natural simulation of a randomized controlled trial, free from confounding factors and reverse causality biases. Unlike traditional randomized controlled trials—the gold standard for causal inference—MR assigns individuals based on their genotype, thereby avoiding reverse causality and confounding influences such as ethical, socioeconomic, and measurement biases. Our goal is to employ a two-sample MR analysis to investigate the causal relationship between PM2.5 exposure and eight common lung diseases. Multivariable Mendelian randomization (MVMR), a recent extension of MR, uses genetic variations linked to multiple potentially related exposures to estimate the effect of each exposure on a single outcome, resulting in more accurate insights. MVMR also allows for mediation analysis within the MR framework, making it possible to estimate mediation effects [19]. Mediation analysis can identify the factors that mediate the relationship between exposure and an outcome, enabling targeted interventions to reduce the impact of this exposure. This method retains the advantages of using genetic instruments for causal inference, such as eliminating bias from confounding variables while allowing for the estimation of mediation effects. We hypothesize that PM2.5 may either increase or decrease susceptibility to lung diseases. Our study aims to bridge the current knowledge gap regarding the effects of PM2.5 on common lung diseases, guide prevention and treatment strategies for vulnerable populations, and further validate previous findings, offering more comprehensive preventive measures from a new perspective.

2. Materials and Methods

2.1. Data Source

The study design and data source for this methodological research were based on a genome-wide association study (GWAS) summary obtained from the OpenGWAS data infrastructure. The data cover PM2.5 air pollution and its association with common lung diseases such as chronic obstructive pulmonary disease (COPD), asthma, pneumonia, bronchitis, emphysema/chronic bronchitis, pulmonary fibrosis, bronchiectasis, and lung cancer. A genome-wide association study (GWAS) is a method used to detect gene variations associated with complex human diseases or traits, and its objective is to reveal the impact of genetic variations on the risk of complex diseases, thereby providing new clues and strategies for prevention, diagnosis, and treatment [20]. OpenGWAS is an open genomic-wide association study (GWAS) data infrastructure designed to provide access to a vast collection of publicly available GWAS datasets. The exposure factor under investigation was PM2.5 air pollution, with a sample size of 423,796 individuals, all of European ancestry. A total of 9,851,867 single-nucleotide polymorphisms (SNPs) were analyzed. The summary statistics for the GWAS were sourced from the MRC-IEU. The original lung cancer data were obtained from the UK Biobank, the pulmonary fibrosis data were sourced from Neale Lab, while the remaining datasets were derived from the MRC-IEU. The UK Biobank aggregates genetic data related to PM2.5 exposure from 423,796 European participants. This study was based on the ESCAPE project (European Study of Cohorts for Air Pollution Effects), which utilized a land-use regression (LUR) model to estimate the PM2.5 pollution levels at participants' residential addresses [21]. The average PM2.5 concentration in the GWAS data was 9.99 ($\pm$1.06) $\mu g/m^3$. This dataset is publicly available from MRC IEU OpenGWAS and MR-Base, with the GWAS-ID being ukb-b-10817. The GWAS pipeline output iwa derived from phesant variables from the UK Biobank.

2.2. Screening and Extraction Methods

We extracted a GWAS summary dataset for exposure (Table 1). Following previous studies, we selected single-nucleotide polymorphisms (SNPs) within the gene locus that had a significance level ($p < 5 \times 10^{-8}$) as instrumental variables. If no valid instrumental variables were identified, the p-value threshold was relaxed to 5×10^{-6}. A key principle of MR is that there should be no linkage disequilibrium (LD) among the selected instrumental variables, as a strong LD can lead to biased results. In this study, we applied clumping ($R^2 < 0.001$, clumping distance = 10,000 kb) to evaluate the LD between SNPs.

Table 1. Outcome and exposure GWAS samples used in this study.

GWAS ID	Trait	Consortium	Sample Size	Year	Category
ukb-b-10817	Particulate matter air pollution (PM2.5); 2010	MRC-IEU	423,796	2018	Continuous
ukb-b-20208	Diagnoses—main ICD10: J45.9 Asthma, unspecified	MRC-IEU	463,010	2018	Binary
ukb-b-16751	Diagnoses—secondary ICD10: J44.9 Chronic obstructive pulmonary disease, unspecified	MRC-IEU	463,010	2018	Binary
ieu-b-4976	Pneumonia	MRC-IEU	486,484	2018	Disease
ukb-b-3467	Non-cancer illness code, self-reported: bronchitis	MRC-IEU	462,933	2018	Binary
ukb-b-7280	Non-cancer illness code, self-reported: emphysema/chronic bronchitis	MRC-IEU	462,933	2018	Binary
ukb-a-358	Underlying (primary) cause of death: ICD10: J84.1 Other interstitial pulmonary diseases with fibrosis	Neale Lab	7637	2017	NA
ukb-b-18163	Non-cancer illness code, self-reported: bronchiectasis	MRC-IEU	462,933	2018	Binary
ieu-b-4954	Lung cancer	UK Biobank	374,687	2021	Disease
ukb-b-19953	Body mass index (BMI)	MRC-IEU	461,460	2018	Continuous
ukb-b-20261	Ever smoked	MRC-IEU	461,066	2018	Binary
ebi-a-GCST90038709	Bacterial infection	NA	484,598	2021	PMID: 33959723

2.3. Statistical Methods

The Mendelian randomization (MR) model, which uses genetic variants as instrumental variables (IVs), relies on three core assumptions. ① IV Assumption I (Relevance Assumption): The genetic variant (G) is associated with the exposure (X). ② IV Assumption II (Independence Assumption): The genetic variant (G) is independent of any confounding factors (U). ③ IV Assumption III (Exclusivity Assumption): The genetic variant (G) affects the outcome (Y) only through the exposure (X) and not via any other pathways. Assumptions II and III are collectively referred to as being independent of pleiotropy. Due to the inherent biological characteristics of genetic variants, MR models can be prone to estimation failures, often caused by the inadequate representativeness of genetic variants for the exposure or by pleiotropy. This inadequate representativeness of the genetic variants typically reduces the statistical power of the MR model, while pleiotropy can lead to biased effect estimates.

The relevance of Assumption I was evaluated using the F-statistic [22]. An F-statistic greater than 10 indicates that IV Assumption I is satisfied, meaning that there is no weak instrument bias.

2.4. Two-Sample MR Method

We initially performed the Mendelian randomization (MR) analysis using the "TwosampleMR" R package [23,24] with inverse variance weighting [25] (IVW) [26] as the primary method to assess the causal relationship between PM2.5 air pollution and common lung diseases. The IVW method regressed the SNP–outcome associations on the SNP–exposure associations, weighting the results by the inverse of the squared standard errors of the SNP–outcome associations, providing an overall weighted estimate of the causal effect. To ensure the robustness of our findings, we also applied several other MR methods for sensitivity analysis, as follows: MR-Egger regression [27], weighted median [28], and maximum likelihood [29]. Additionally, we employed multivariable Mendelian randomization (MVMR) to account for potential confounders. The MVMR analysis was carried out using the mr_mvivw, mr_mvegger, and mr_mvlasso functions from the "mendelianrandomization" R package.

2.5. Sensitivity Analysis Methods

To ensure the accuracy of the results, the MR-Egger regression model was employed to test IV Assumption III (the exclusivity assumption). The intercept of the MR-Egger regression provides an estimate of the average pleiotropic effect of all SNPs under the InSIDE assumption. If the intercept differs from zero, this indicates the presence of horizontal pleiotropy [30]. Horizontal pleiotropy was tested using the mr_pleiotropy_test function from the R package "TwoSampleMR." In cases where the MR-Egger detected pleiotropy, the MR PRESSO method was used to identify and remove potential outliers. Additionally, a leave-one-out analysis was conducted to determine whether any single SNP was driving the causal effect. The Cochran Q statistic was used to test for heterogeneity among the SNPs. If the p-value of the Q statistic is greater than 0.05, this suggests that no heterogeneity exists, and the study results do not need to account for heterogeneity effects. However, if the p-value was less than 0.05, a random effects model was applied, with the IVW method serving as the primary reference for the results. Pleiotropy testing was performed using the MR-Egger method, and heterogeneity was assessed through both the IVW and MR-Egger methods. The MR-Egger method was used to estimate the impact of pleiotropy, producing more robust pleiotropy-corrected causal estimates under the assumptions of no measurement error and an instrument strength independent of direct effects [31]. The instrument strength was also evaluated using the following formula to calculate the F-statistic:

$$F = \frac{R^2(N-1-k)}{(1-R^2)k} \quad (1)$$

where R^2 represents the variance in the exposure explained by the selected SNPs, N is the sample size, and k is the number of instrumental variables. If $F < 10$, it suggests a higher likelihood of a weak instrument bias, indicating a weaker association between the instrumental variable and the exposure.

2.6. Analysis Software

All two-sample analyses were conducted using the TwoSampleMR package (v0.5.8) in R software (version 4.2.3, R Foundation). For multivariable analyses, the mendelianrandomization package (v1.0.0) was used in R software (version 4.4.1, R Foundation).

3. Results and Analysis

3.1. Selection of Instrumental Variables

After removing palindromic SNPs, performing clumping, and harmonizing the data, the number of SNPs associated with the outcomes ranged from one to seven. The R^2 and F statistic values for the exposures are summarized in Table S1. To increase the number of SNPs and improve the stability and accuracy of the analysis, we lowered the extraction threshold to 5×10^{-6}, resulting in the extraction of 58 SNPs in total. The R^2 values and F-statistics for the exposure variables are summarized in Table S1. All F-statistics were greater than 10, indicating no evidence of weak instrument bias and confirming the validity of the SNPs. Each SNP under the 5×10^{-6} threshold was further screened using LDtrait (https://ldlink.nih.gov/?tab=ldtrait) (accessed on September 10, 2024) to ensure that there were no confounding factors.

3.2. Sensitivity Analysis

To assess the robustness of the results, a sensitivity analysis was performed, as detailed in Supplementary Table S2. By examining Cochran's Q statistic and its p-value, heterogeneity was identified in the two-sample Mendelian randomization involving chronic obstructive pulmonary disease (COPD) and emphysema/chronic bronchitis. As a result, we applied the random-effects IVW model for analysis. No outliers were detected in either the MR-Egger or IVW tests during the sensitivity analysis.

The MR-Egger intercept revealed a p-value of 0.037 in the two-sample Mendelian randomization analysis with COPD, which is less than 0.05, indicating potential horizontal pleiotropy. However, for all other analyses, the intercept p-values were above 0.05, suggesting no evidence of horizontal pleiotropy. We used MR-PRESSO to exclude outlier SNPs, and after their removal, the corrected p-value continued to show a significant association between PM2.5 and COPD, with the association becoming stronger. While the MR-PRESSO Global test detected outlier SNPs in some analyses, the MR-PRESSO Distortion test indicated no significant difference between the results before and after correcting for outliers.

3.3. Results

The IVW method was employed as the primary analytical approach to evaluate the relationship between PM2.5 and common lung diseases. To minimize potential confounding factors, we carefully selected SNPs based on stringent criteria and conducted two-sample MR analyses using different instrumental variable extraction thresholds (5×10^{-8}). At the 5×10^{-8} threshold, seven SNPs were identified for the exposure (particulate matter air pollution (PM2.5) | | id: ukb-b-10817) in a genome-wide association study. We performed the two-sample MR analysis with these extracted instrumental variables. However, due to the limited number of SNPs, we adjusted the extraction threshold to 5×10^{-6} to gather more instrumental variables, aiming to provide a more comprehensive analysis by lowering the threshold.

At a significance threshold of 5×10^{-8}, there was a strong indication of a causal relationship between PM2.5 exposure and both asthma and chronic obstructive pulmonary disease (COPD). Specifically, a weighted median analysis of the PM2.5 dataset and the asthma dataset from MRC-IEU demonstrated a significant association (OR = 1.013224, 95% CI: 1.0030398–1.023512, p = 0.01080753). Likewise, a significant link was observed between the PM2.5 dataset and a COPD database comprising 463,010 samples (OR = 1.027142, 95% CI: 1.0035843–1.051254, p = 0.0236828). The MR Egger analysis further supported this association with a p-value of 0.02063981. While no significant associations were found between PM2.5 exposure and emphysema/chronic bronchitis in the IVW and MR-Egger tests, both the weighted median and weighted mode tests suggested a potential association, though with a weaker statistical power. As a result, a definitive causal link could not be conclusively established in this case.

However, after performing the MR-PRESSO analysis, the p-values for the two-sample Mendelian randomization tests for asthma and chronic obstructive pulmonary disease (COPD) were 0.06338194 and 0.09279563, respectively, indicating no significant association. Interestingly, following the MR-PRESSO analysis, a clear association was found between PM2.5 exposure and pulmonary interstitial fibrosis, without excluding any SNPs, with a p-value of 0.03590268. In the two-sample analysis for COPD, Cochran's Q-test detected heterogeneity, leading to the use of a random-effects IVW-MR model to improve the accuracy of the data analysis. To enhance the accuracy of our analysis, we adjusted the SNP selection criteria by lowering the threshold to 5×10^{-6}. As a result, we successfully identified 58 SNPs associated with respiratory diseases. These SNPs continued to demonstrate significant associations with asthma (OR = 1.005819, 95% CI: 1.0012449–1.010414, p = 0.01259716) and chronic obstructive pulmonary disease (COPD, OR = 1.0118626, 95% CI: 1.0049928–1.018779, p = 0.0006916272), and also revealed strong links to other respiratory conditions, including pneumonia (OR = 1.337119, 95% CI: 1.0361446–1.72552, p = 0.02555535), emphysema/chronic bronchitis (OR = 1.012886, 95% CI: 1.004885–1.02095, p = 0.0015536956), and lung cancer (OR = 1.006532, 95% CI: 1.0016285–1.011459, p = 0.008972278) (Figures 1 and 2, Table S1). The scatter plot can help to check whether the selected instrumental variable has a sufficiently strong association. If the distribution of points in the scatter plot shows a clear linear trend, it indicates a strong linear relationship between asthma and PM2.5 exposure (Figure 1). Notably, these associations remained statistically significant even after the MR-PRESSO test, further confirming the robustness and reliability of the findings. We conducted a leave-one-out analysis of the IVW results (Figure 3). By removing each SNP individually, we obtained p-values of < 0.05, which were consistent with the IVW method's causal effect estimates, indicating that no single SNP significantly influenced the results. Additionally, the funnel plots for PM2.5 and the eight diseases (Figure 4) were symmetrical, suggesting that pleiotropy did not impact our analysis. The F-statistics, ranging from 20.88 to 69.92 (Table S1), ruled out bias from weak instruments. Given the absence of horizontal pleiotropy, we selected IVW as the primary method for evaluating causal relationships. We conclude that PM2.5 is a risk factor for asthma, COPD, pneumonia, emphysema/chronic bronchitis, and lung cancer. To further explore potential interactions between these SNPs and environmental factors, and to eliminate the influence of other exposures, we performed multivariable Mendelian randomization analyses for smoking and bacterial infections, validated using a LASSO regression model. The results indicated that the association between PM2.5 and pneumonia became non-significant after adjusting for confounding factors, suggesting that PM2.5 may not be a direct risk factor for pneumonia (Table S3). However, the associations with asthma, COPD, emphysema/chronic bronchitis, and lung cancer remained significant. We then investigated potential mediators in the relationship between PM2.5 and these four diseases. Using BMI and smoking as mediators, we found evidence of reverse causality between PM2.5 exposure and these two common factors, indicating that neither BMI nor smoking serves as a mediator in the association between PM2.5 and these common lung diseases.

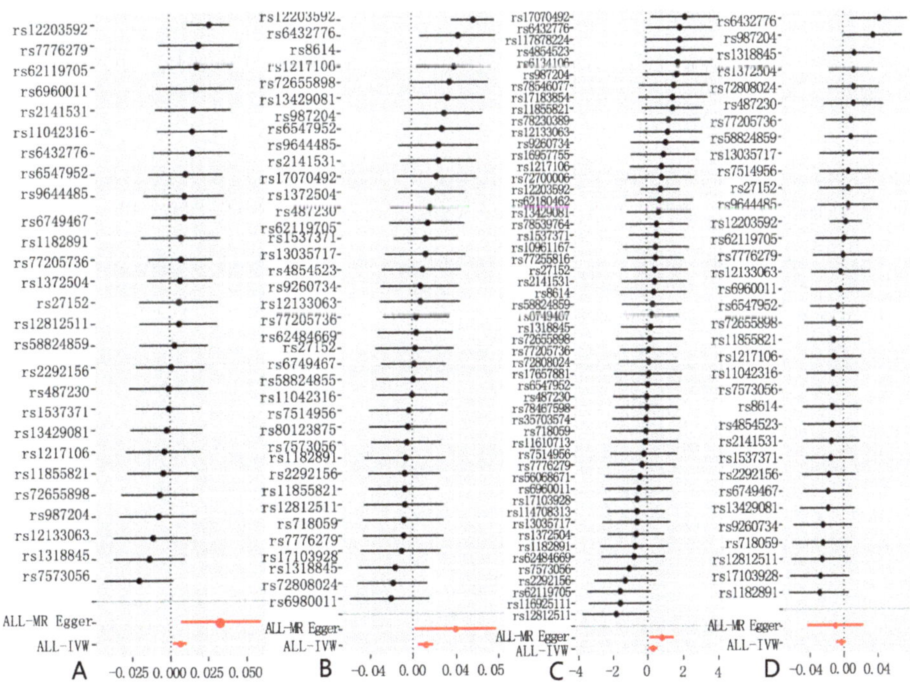

Figure 1. *Cont.*

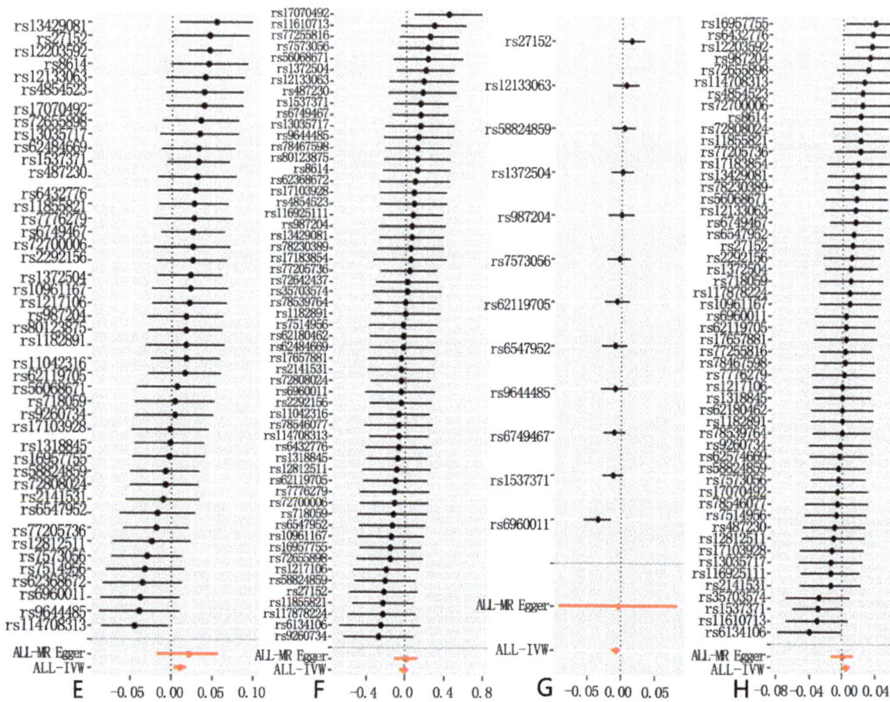

Figure 1. Forest plot of causal associations between PM2.5 and eight common lung diseases in the analysis (5×10^{-6}). (**A**): PM2.5 and asthma, unspecified; (**B**): PM2.5 and chronic obstructive pulmonary disease; (**C**): PM2.5 and pneumonia; (**D**): PM2.5 and bronchitis; (**E**): PM2.5 and emphysema/chronic bronchitis; (**F**): PM2.5 and interstitial pulmonary diseases with fibrosis; (**G**): PM2.5 and bronchiectasis; and (**H**): PM2.5 and lung cancer. NSNP, number of SNPs; OR, odds ratio; IVW, inverse variance weighted; CI, confidence interval.

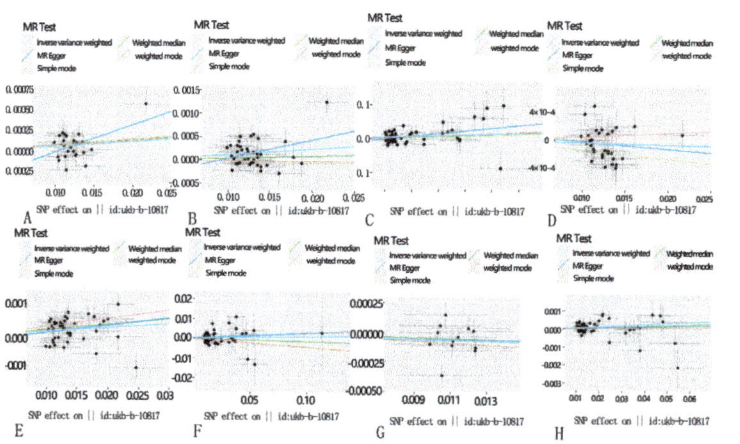

Figure 2. Scatter plot showing the causal estimate for different MRs of PM2.5 on eight common lung diseases. (**A**): PM2.5 and asthma, unspecified; (**B**): PM2.5 and chronic obstructive pulmonary disease; (**C**): PM2.5 and pneumonia; (**D**): PM2.5 and bronchitis; (**E**): PM2.5 and emphysema/chronic bronchitis; (**F**): PM2.5 and interstitial pulmonary diseases with fibrosis; (**G**): PM2.5 and bronchiectasis; and (**H**): PM2.5 and lung cancer.

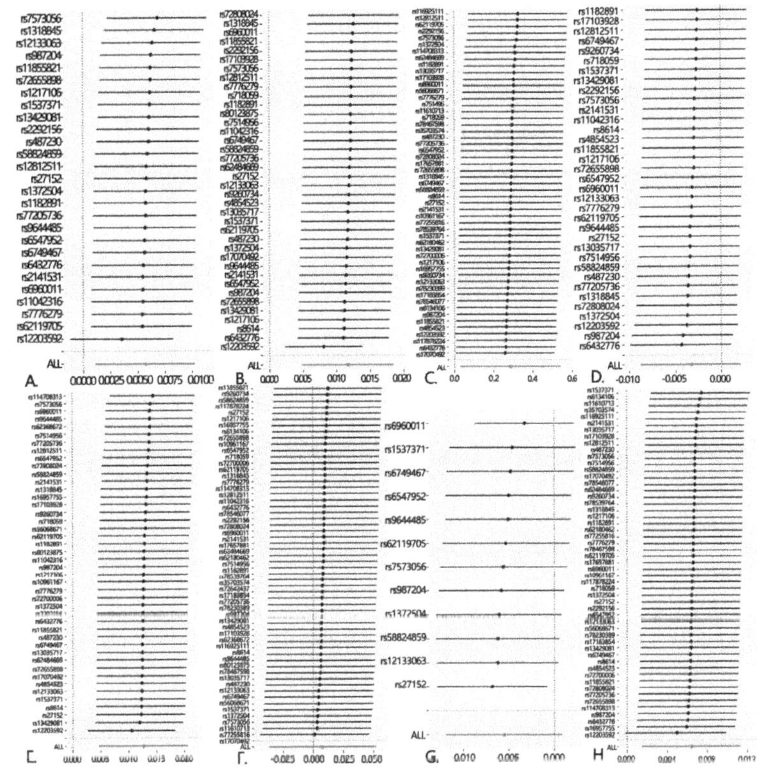

Figure 3. Forest plot of the "leave-one-out" sensitivity analysis method to show the influence of individual SNPs on the results. The red point indicates the IVW estimates using all SNPs. (**A**): PM2.5 and aAsthma, unspecified; (**B**): PM2.5 and cChronic obstructive pulmonary disease; (**C**): PM2.5 and pPneumonia; (**D**): PM2.5 and bronchitis; (**E**): PM2.5 and emphysema/chronic bronchitis; (**F**): PM2.5 and interstitial pulmonary diseases with fibrosis; (**G**): PM2.5 and bronchiectasis; and (**H**): PM2.5 and lLung cancer.

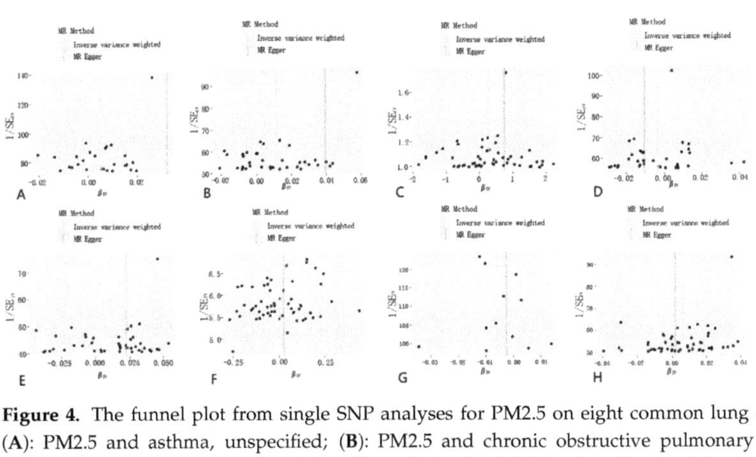

Figure 4. The funnel plot from single SNP analyses for PM2.5 on eight common lung diseases. (**A**): PM2.5 and asthma, unspecified; (**B**): PM2.5 and chronic obstructive pulmonary disease; (**C**): PM2.5 and pneumonia; (**D**): PM2.5 and bronchitis; (**E**): PM2.5 and emphysema/chronic bronchitis; (**F**): PM2.5 and interstitial pulmonary diseases with fibrosis; (**G**): PM2.5 and bronchiectasis; and (**H**): PM2.5 and lung cancer.

4. Discussion

In the current study, we conducted a Mendelian randomization (MR) analysis to assess the causal relationships between PM2.5 exposure and common lung diseases. Utilizing large-scale summary statistics for PM2.5 and various common pulmonary diseases, our primary MR analysis revealed a significant positive association between PM2.5 exposure and asthma, chronic obstructive pulmonary disease (COPD), pneumonia, emphysema/chronic bronchitis, and lung cancer, consistent with previous studies. We also found no significant association between PM2.5 and bronchitis, interstitial lung disease, or bronchiectasis, an area that currently lacks relevant clinical trials.

Based on the two-sample Mendelian randomization results, PM2.5 exposure showed a clear association with pneumonia, aligning with current mainstream perspectives. DARROW et al. [32] analyzed emergency department visits for bronchiolitis, pneumonia, and upper respiratory infections in children aged 0–4 years from Atlanta and Georgia between 1993 and 2010. They studied the effects of short-term exposure to atmospheric PM2.5 on the emergency department visit rates for pediatric respiratory infections and found that PM2.5 significantly exacerbated upper and lower respiratory tract infections. However, after performing multivariable Mendelian randomization and a LASSO regression analysis adjusting for smoking and bacterial infections, they found no significant association between PM2.5 exposure and pneumonia. This may be related to the complex composition of PM2.5, which contains various bacterial components, and after controlling for relevant confounders, no significant association with pneumonia was observed. It is likely that the induction of pneumonia by PM2.5 mainly relies on its bacterial components, but further research is needed to clarify the exact mechanism. Therefore, this study also emphasizes the validity and necessity of multivariable MR in MR analyses, particularly when a large number of genetic variables are used as instrumental variables. Multivariable Mendelian randomization should be employed to improve the accuracy of experimental results.

Researchers have long been concerned with the effects of PM2.5 on the respiratory system. As early as 2014, TSAI et al. [33] utilized hospitalization data for respiratory diseases from 2006 to 2010 in Kaohsiung, Taiwan, along with atmospheric PM2.5 monitoring data, to explore the relationship between PM2.5 exposure and hospital admissions for respiratory diseases. They found a significant correlation between increased respiratory disease admissions and high PM2.5 concentrations during the colder seasons. The associations between PM2.5 and the eight diseases studied in this article have also been reported in previous research. However, most studies have focused on the relationships between PM2.5 and chronic obstructive pulmonary disease (COPD), asthma, pulmonary inflammation, and lung cancer. The connection between PM2.5 and diseases like pulmonary fibrosis has not received sufficient attention. Observational studies have shown that, in prospective cohorts of both children and adults with asthma, short-term exposure to environmental PM2.5 is associated with asthma symptoms [34]. In a key analysis of COPD prevalence, PM2.5 showed a significant association (OR = 1.52 [95% CI: 1.42, 1.62] per 5 $\mu g/m^3$) [14]. Long-term exposure to PM2.5 has also been significantly linked to an increased risk of lower respiratory tract infections, including a higher pneumonia mortality [35] and chronic bronchitis symptoms. Goobie's study highlighted that particulate matter smaller than 2.5 μm (PM2.5) is associated with adverse outcomes in idiopathic pulmonary fibrosis, although the exact relationship remains unclear [36]. Lung cancer has been a major focus of research. A meta-analysis of 14 outdoor air pollution studies, mostly conducted in North America and Europe, found that, for every 10 $\mu g/m^3$ increase in PM2.5, the risk of developing or dying from lung cancer rises by 9% (95% CI, 4%–14%) [37].GUO et al. [38] used a spatio-temporal cohort model to assess the relative risk of lung cancer associated with PM2.5 exposure. The results indicated that an increased incidence of lung cancer was significantly correlated with PM2.5 levels. However, there is still a limited understanding of the biological and molecular mechanisms underlying these diseases. There are several hypotheses regarding the impact of PM2.5 on respiratory health, including the oxidative damage theory involving reactive oxygen species (ROS) and the inflammation-related factor activation theory, each supported by their own theoretical framework. Studies have shown that PM2.5 exposure elevates the levels of reactive oxygen species (ROS) [39], which may lead to the development of these diseases by promoting oxidative stress, allergic inflammation, or increasing the efficiency of gene translation in the glycolysis pathway [34,40]. In 2013, Honda et al. [41] collected PM2.5 extracts from industrial and urban areas in Japan. Their study found that organic extracts of PM2.5 could stimulate airway epithelial cells to produce IL-6, thereby triggering an inflammatory response. PM2.5 significantly impacts the occurrence and development of obstructive respiratory diseases, infectious diseases, allergic diseases, and tumors, markedly increasing the incidence and mortality of respiratory diseases. The underlying mechanisms may involve oxidative stress, inflammatory responses, and genotoxicity. However, the effects of PM2.5 on the respiratory system and its mechanisms of action require further investigation.

Our study has several key advantages. To our knowledge, while most existing research on the relationship between air pollution and lung diseases relies on cohort studies, this is the first to systematically use two-sample Mendelian randomization (MR) to explore the causal links between PM2.5 exposure and multiple lung diseases. Previous epidemiological studies have suggested associations between PM2.5 and various common lung diseases, a widely accepted view. However, no prior research has investigated these associations using Mendelian randomization, which helps to address confounding factors and reverse causality. The composition of PM2.5 is often highly complex and frequently coexists with other air pollutants, such as ozone, nitrogen oxides, and sulfur oxides, as shown in ref. [37]. This close interaction with other pollutants can complicate and obscure the understanding of these relationships. PM2.5's spatial distribution varies, and it often coexists with other pollutants, which can raise doubts about the reliability of past findings.

MR analysis, by using genetic variants as proxies for exposure based on Mendel's law of independent assortment, strengthens the reliability of results. Since genetic variants exist before the onset of disease, this approach eliminates the influence of reverse causality and provides a long-term perspective on exposure—reflecting an individual's lifetime biological traits, unlike traditional studies that often focus on short-term exposure. Moreover, by using data from large-scale GWAS meta-analyses, we increased the statistical power of our MR analysis, something clinical trials often cannot achieve. Our findings offer new theoretical and experimental insights into the prevention of air-pollution-related health risks, supporting previous research from a fresh perspective. Additionally, this study provides a foundation for identifying mediating factors, which could further inform strategies for mitigating the impact of air pollution on lung diseases.

Our study has several limitations. First, the GWAS datasets used in the MR analysis were derived from European populations, which may not be representative of other ethnic groups. To enhance the generalizability of our findings, future research should include populations from other regions and countries. Second, we used the LDtrait tool to ensure that the instrumental variables (IVs) met the assumptions of the MR analysis, specifically that the IVs are not directly associated with the lung diseases studied. However, some unpublished SNPs may still be associated with the diseases analyzed, which could affect our results. Our findings were based on a significance threshold of 5×10^{-6}. While there were not enough SNPs reaching the genome-wide significance threshold of 5×10^{-8}, we still conducted two-sample MR analyses, and the association between increased PM2.5 levels and asthma and COPD remained consistent with our conclusions. Third, our estimates may be subject to the inherent limitations of MR analysis, such as selection bias. For example, GWAS studies often do not account for the effects of other air pollutants, which may influence the selection of the genetic instruments used in our MR analysis. Since the GWAS data do not provide specific information on the sample's gender and age composition, the potential impacts of factors such as gender and age have not been further explored in this study. This aspect will be addressed in future work. Fourth, the impact of genetic variants on exposure factors is typically small, meaning that MR analysis may only capture part of the exposure's effect, making it difficult to fully reflect its influence on disease outcomes. Therefore, further research with larger and more diverse studies is necessary to gather more comprehensive evidence and explore the full range of PM2.5's effects and mechanisms. It is clear that air pollutants like PM2.5 not only cause short-term, visible harm to the human body, but also have long-term impacts on the respiratory and immune systems. Furthermore, PM2.5 may exert chronic, persistent effects on ecosystems such as water environments, plants, and animals, which, in turn, may cause unforeseen harm to human health. Although these indirect effects may not be immediately apparent, they represent important areas for future research and warrant careful attention. It is believed that, in the near future, with increased participation from various research disciplines and a growing body of studies on PM2.5, our understanding of PM2.5 will be further enhanced. Research on its relationship with respiratory diseases will continue to make new breakthroughs, leading to more practical and effective strategies for preventing and mitigating its harmful effects.

5. Conclusions

In summary, our study shows that increased PM2.5 concentrations are significantly associated with a higher risk of asthma, chronic obstructive pulmonary disease (COPD), emphysema/chronic bronchitis, and lung cancer. However, no significant associations were found between elevated PM2.5 levels and pneumonia, bronchitis, interstitial lung disease, or bronchiectasis. Further clinical and foundational research is needed to confirm and strengthen the validity of these findings.

Supplementary Materials: The following supporting information can be downloaded at: https://www.mdpi.com/article/10.3390/toxics12120851/s1, Table S1: Causal Estimates of PM2.5 on Common Pulmonary Diseases from Two-Sample Mendelian Randomization. Table S2: Sensitivity analyses of Mendelian randomization for PM2.5 and eight common lung diseases. Table S3: Results of Multivariable Mendelian Randomization.

Author Contributions: J.S., conceptualization and project administration; Y.J., data curation and formal analysis; D.S., X.L. (Xin Li), funding acquisition; F.Z., investigation; X.L. (Xike Lu), methodology; D.S. and Z.W., supervision; Z.W. and H.Z., validation; Y.W., visualization; Y.J., writing—original draft; Z.W., writing—review and editing. All authors have read and agreed to the published version of the manuscript.

Funding: All authors report that this study was funded by the Tianjin Medical Key Specialty Construction Project (grant number TJYXZDXK-018A), the Tianjin Metrology Science and Technology Project (grant number 2024TJMT001), and the Tianjin Health Research Project (grant number TJWJ2024QN063).

Institutional Review Board Statement: This study was based on a published database and did not require ethical approval.

Informed Consent Statement: Not applicable.

Data Availability Statement: Publicly available datasets were analyzed in this study. These data can be found in the UK Biobank and Neale Lab.

Acknowledgments: We want to acknowledge the participants and investigators of the MRC-IEU study. We would also like to thank the UK Biobank and Open GWAS Database.

Conflicts of Interest: The authors declare no conflicts of interest.

References

1. Gordon, S.B.; Bruce, N.G.; Grigg, J.; Hibberd, P.L.; Kurmi, O.P.; Lam, K.H.; Mortimer, K.; Asante, K.P.; Balakrishnan, K.; Balmes, J.; et al. Respiratory risks from household air pollution in low and middle income countries. *Lancet Respir. Med.* **2014**, 2, 823–860. [CrossRef] [PubMed]
2. Pöschl, U. Atmospheric Aerosols: Composition, Transformation, Climate and Health Effects. *Angew. Chem. Int. Ed.* **2005**, *44*, 7520–7540. [CrossRef] [PubMed]
3. Lin, W.; Brunekreef, B.; Gehring, U. Meta-analysis of the effects of indoor nitrogen dioxide and gas cooking on asthma and wheeze in children. *Int. J. Epidemiol.* **2013**, *42*, 1724–1737. [CrossRef]

4. Wilson, W.E.; Suh, H.H. Fine Particles and Coarse Particles: Concentration Relationships Relevant to Epidemiologic Studies. *J. Air Waste Manag. Assoc.* **1997**, *47*, 1238–1249. [CrossRef]
5. Kelishadi, R.; Poursafa, P. Air pollution and non-respiratory health hazards for children. *Arch. Med. Sci.* **2010**, *4*, 483–495. [CrossRef] [PubMed]
6. Kappos, A.D.; Bruckmann, P.; Eikmann, T.; Englert, N.; Heinrich, U.; Höppe, P.; Koch, E.; Krause, G.H.M.; Kreyling, W.G.; Rauchfuss, K.; et al. Health effects of particles in ambient air. *Int. J. Hydrogen Environ. Health* **2004**, *207*, 399–407. [CrossRef]
7. Coleman, N.C.; Burnett, R.T.; Ezzati, M.; Marshall, J.D.; Robinson, A.L.; Pope, C.A. Fine Particulate Matter Exposure and Cancer Incidence: Analysis of SEER Cancer Registry Data from 1992–2016. *Environ. Health Perspect.* **2020**, *128*, 107004. [CrossRef]
8. Kan, H.; Chen, R.; Tong, S. Ambient air pollution, climate change, and population health in China. *Environ. Int.* **2012**, *42*, 10–19. [CrossRef]
9. Burroughs Peña, M.S.; Rollins, A. Environmental Exposures and Cardiovascular Disease. *Cardiol. Clin.* **2017**, *35*, 71–86. [CrossRef]
10. Guo, Y.; Zeng, H.; Zheng, R.; Li, S.; Pereira, G.; Liu, Q.; Chen, W.; Huxley, R. The burden of lung cancer mortality attributable to fine particles in China. *Sci. Total Environ.* **2017**, *579*, 1460–1466. [CrossRef]
11. Hou, Q.; An, X.Q.; Wang, Y.; Guo, J.P. An evaluation of resident exposure to respirable particulate matter and health economic loss in Beijing during Beijing 2008 Olympic Games. *Sci. Total Environ.* **2010**, *408*, 4026–4032. [CrossRef] [PubMed]
12. Dong, G.-H.; Chen, T.; Liu, M.-M.; Wang, D.; Ma, Y.-N.; Ren, W.-H.; Lee, Y.L.; Zhao, Y.-D.; He, Q.-C. Gender Differences and Effect of Air Pollution on Asthma in Children with and without Allergic Predisposition: Northeast Chinese Children Health Study. *PLoS ONE* **2011**, *6*, e22470. [CrossRef] [PubMed]
13. Anderson, H.R.; Favarato, G.; Atkinson, R.W. Long-term exposure to outdoor air pollution and the prevalence of asthma: Meta-analysis of multi-community prevalence studies. *Air Qual. Atmos. Health* **2013**, *6*, 57–68. [CrossRef]
14. Doiron, D.; De Hoogh, K.; Probst-Hensch, N.; Fortier, I.; Cai, Y.; De Matteis, S.; Hansell, A.L. Air pollution, lung function and COPD: Results from the population-based UK Biobank study. *Eur. Respir. J.* **2019**, *54*, 1802140. [CrossRef]
15. Cheung, K.; Daher, N.; Kam, W.; Shafer, M.M.; Ning, Z.; Schauer, J.J.; Sioutas, C. Spatial and temporal variation of chemical composition and mass closure of ambient coarse particulate matter (PM10–2.5) in the Los Angeles area. *Atmos. Environ.* **2011**, *45*, 2651–2662. [CrossRef]
16. Zhang, L.; Yang, Y.; Li, Y.; Qian, Z.M.; Xiao, W.; Wang, X.; Rolling, C.A.; Liu, E.; Xiao, J.; Zeng, W.; et al. Short-term and long-term effects of PM2.5 on acute nasopharyngitis in 10 communities of Guangdong, China. *Sci. Total Environ.* **2019**, *688*, 136–142. [CrossRef]
17. Kloog, I.; Ridgway, B.; Koutrakis, P.; Coull, B.A.; Schwartz, J.D. Long- and Short-Term Exposure to PM2.5 and Mortality: Using Novel Exposure Models. *Epidemiology* **2013**, *24*, 555–561. [CrossRef]
18. Davey Smith, G.; Hemani, G. Mendelian randomization: Genetic anchors for causal inference in epidemiological studies. *Hum. Mol. Genet.* **2014**, *23*, R89–R98. [CrossRef]
19. Sanderson, E. Multivariable Mendelian Randomization and Mediation. *Cold Spring Harb. Perspect. Med.* **2021**, *11*, a038984. [CrossRef]
20. Visscher, P.M.; Brown, M.A.; McCarthy, M.I.; Yang, J. Five Years of GWAS Discovery. *Am. J. Hum. Genet.* **2012**, *90*, 7–24. [CrossRef]
21. Eeftens, M.; Beelen, R.; De Hoogh, K.; Bellander, T.; Cesaroni, G.; Cirach, M.; Declercq, C.; Dėdelė, A.; Dons, E.; De Nazelle, A.; et al. Development of Land Use Regression Models for PM2.5, PM2.5 Absorbance, PM $_{10}$ and PM $_{coarse}$ in 20 European Study Areas; Results of the ESCAPE Project. *Environ. Sci. Technol.* **2012**, *46*, 11195–11205. [CrossRef] [PubMed]
22. Burgess, S.; Thompson, S.G. CRP CHD Genetics Collaboration Avoiding bias from weak instruments in Mendelian randomization studies. *Int. J. Epidemiol.* **2011**, *40*, 755–764. [CrossRef] [PubMed]
23. Huang, Y.; Ognjenovic, J.; Karandur, D.; Miller, K.; Merk, A.; Subramaniam, S.; Kuriyan, J. A molecular mechanism for the generation of ligand-dependent differential outputs by the epidermal growth factor receptor. *eLife* **2021**, *10*, e73218. [CrossRef]
24. Hemani, G.; Tilling, K.; Davey Smith, G. Orienting the causal relationship between imprecisely measured traits using GWAS summary data. *PLoS Genet.* **2017**, *13*, e1007081. [CrossRef]
25. Burgess, S.; Butterworth, A.; Thompson, S.G. Mendelian Randomization Analysis With Multiple Genetic Variants Using Summarized Data. *Genet. Epidemiol.* **2013**, *37*, 658–665. [CrossRef] [PubMed]
26. Fu, S.; Zhang, L.; Ma, F.; Xue, S.; Sun, T.; Xu, Z. Effects of Selenium on Chronic Kidney Disease: A Mendelian Randomization Study. *Nutrients* **2022**, *14*, 4458. [CrossRef]
27. Bowden, J.; Davey Smith, G.; Burgess, S. Mendelian randomization with invalid instruments: Effect estimation and bias detection through Egger regression. *Int. J. Epidemiol.* **2015**, *44*, 512–525. [CrossRef]
28. Bowden, J.; Davey Smith, G.; Haycock, P.C.; Burgess, S. Consistent Estimation in Mendelian Randomization with Some Invalid Instruments Using a Weighted Median Estimator. *Genet. Epidemiol.* **2016**, *40*, 304–314. [CrossRef] [PubMed]
29. Pierce, B.L.; Burgess, S. Efficient Design for Mendelian Randomization Studies: Subsample and 2-Sample Instrumental Variable Estimators. *Am. J. Epidemiol.* **2013**, *178*, 1177–1184. [CrossRef]
30. The LifeLines Cohort Study; The InterAct Consortium; kConFab/AOCS Investigators; Endometrial Cancer Association Consortium; Ovarian Cancer Association Consortium; PRACTICAL consortium; Day, F.R.; Thompson, D.J.; Helgason, H.; Chasman, D.I.; et al. Genomic analyses identify hundreds of variants associated with age at menarche and support a role for puberty timing in cancer risk. *Nat. Genet.* **2017**, *49*, 834–841. [CrossRef]

31. Burgess, S.; Thompson, S.G. Interpreting findings from Mendelian randomization using the MR-Egger method. *Eur. J. Epidemiol.* **2017**, *32*, 377–389. [CrossRef] [PubMed]
32. Darrow, L.A.; Klein, M.; Flanders, W.D.; Mulholland, J.A.; Tolbert, P.E.; Strickland, M.J. Air Pollution and Acute Respiratory Infections Among Children 0–4 Years of Age: An 18-Year Time-Series Study. *Am. J. Epidemiol.* **2014**, *180*, 968–977. [CrossRef] [PubMed]
33. Tsai, S.-S.; Chiu, H.-F.; Liou, S.-H.; Yang, C.-Y. Short-Term Effects of Fine Particulate Air Pollution on Hospital Admissions for Respiratory Diseases: A Case-Crossover Study in a Tropical City. *J. Toxicol. Environ. Health Part A* **2014**, *77*, 1091–1101. [CrossRef] [PubMed]
34. Mann, J.K.; Balmes, J.R.; Bruckner, T.A.; Mortimer, K.M.; Margolis, H.G.; Pratt, B.; Hammond, S.K.; Lurmann, F.W.; Tager, I.B. Short-Term Effects of Air Pollution on Wheeze in Asthmatic Children in Fresno, California. *Environ. Health Perspect.* **2010**, *118*, 1497–1502. [CrossRef] [PubMed]
35. Pun, V.C.; Kazemiparkouhi, F.; Manjourides, J.; Suh, H.H. Long-Term PM2.5 Exposures and Respiratory, Cancer and Cardiovascular Mortality in American Older Adults. *Am. J. Epidemiol.* **2017**, *186*, 961–969. [CrossRef]
36. Goobie, G.C.; Carlsten, C.; Johannson, K.A.; Khalil, N.; Marcoux, V.; Assayag, D.; Manganas, H.; Fisher, J.H.; Kolb, M.R.J.; Lindell, K.O.; et al. Association of Particulate Matter Exposure With Lung Function and Mortality Among Patients With Fibrotic Interstitial Lung Disease. *JAMA Intern. Med.* **2022**, *182*, 1248. [CrossRef]
37. Turner, M.C.; Andersen, Z.J.; Baccarelli, A.; Diver, W.R.; Gapstur, S.M.; Pope, C.A.; Prada, D.; Samet, J.; Thurston, G.; Cohen, A. Outdoor air pollution and cancer: An overview of the current evidence and public health recommendations. *CA A Cancer J. Clin.* **2020**, *70*, 460–479. [CrossRef]
38. Guo, Y.; Zeng, H.; Zheng, R.; Li, S.; Barnett, A.G.; Zhang, S.; Zou, X.; Huxley, R.; Chen, W.; Williams, G. The association between lung cancer incidence and ambient air pollution in China: A spatiotemporal analysis. *Environ. Res.* **2016**, *144*, 60–65. [CrossRef]
39. Choe, S.-A.; Kauderer, S.; Eliot, M.N.; Glazer, K.B.; Kingsley, S.L.; Carlson, L.; Awad, Y.A.; Schwartz, J.D.; Savitz, D.A.; Wellenius, G.A. Air pollution, land use, and complications of pregnancy. *Sci. Total Environ.* **2018**, *645*, 1057–1064. [CrossRef]
40. Chen, Q.; Wang, Y.; Yang, L.; Sun, L.; Wen, Y.; Huang, Y.; Gao, K.; Yang, W.; Bai, F.; Ling, L.; et al. PM2.5 promotes NSCLC carcinogenesis through translationally and transcriptionally activating DLAT-mediated glycolysis reprograming. *J. Exp. Clin. Cancer Res.* **2022**, *41*, 229. [CrossRef]
41. Honda, A.; Fukushima, W.; Oishi, M.; Tsuji, K.; Sawahara, T.; Hayashi, T.; Kudo, H.; Kashima, Y.; Takahashi, K.; Sasaki, H.; et al. Effects of Components of PM2.5 Collected in Japan on the Respiratory and Immune Systems. *Int. J. Toxicol.* **2017**, *36*, 153–164. [CrossRef] [PubMed]

toxics

MDPI

Article

Consumption of Native Fish Associated with a Potential Carcinogenic Risk for Indigenous Communities in the Peruvian Amazon

Magaly Alejandra Brousett-Minaya [1,*], Fred William Chu-Koo [1], Juvenal Napuchi-Linares [1], Cynthia Elizabeth Zambrano Panduro [1], Juan Amilcar Reyes-Larico [2], Adriana Edith Larrea-Valdivia [2] and Ivan Edward Biamont-Rojas [3,4]

1 Faculty of Sciences, National Autonomous University of Alto Amazonas (UNAAA), Prolongación Libertad 1220-1228, Yurimaguas 16501, Loreto, Peru; fchu@unaaa.edu.pe (F.W.C.-K.); jnapuchi@unaaa.edu.pe (J.N.-L.); 1261903137@unaaa.edu.pe (C.E.Z.P.)
2 Faculty of Natural Sciences, National University of San Agustin—Arequipa (UNSA), Santa Catalina No. 117, Arequipa 04000, Arequipa, Peru; jreyesl@unsa.edu.pe (J.A.R.-L.)
3 Institute of Science and Technology, State University of São Paulo (UNESP), Av. Três de Março 511, Alto da Boa Vista, Sorocaba 18087-180, SP, Brazil; biamont.ivan@gmail.com
4 Oceanographic Institute, University of São Paulo (USP), Praça do Oceanográfico, 191, São Paulo 05508-120, SP, Brazil
* Correspondence: mbrousett@unaaa.edu.pe

Abstract: Aquatic environments, such as fluvial environments, play an important role in the transport of material from throughout the basin, and this material partially sediments along the way. The objective of this study was to analyze, from an ecotoxicological point of view, the concentrations of arsenic and heavy metals in sediment and the muscle of native fish, to correlate their interaction and to evaluate the potential risk to public health using carcinogenic risk indices in four rivers of the Peruvian Amazon. There were 27 sampling sites where sediment and fish (except for five points) samples were collected. A sampling pool was created with fish muscles from all species collected at each sampling site. Concentrations of As, Cd, Cr, Cu, Ni, Pb, Zn, and Hg were analyzed in both sediment and fish muscle, in duplicate. The results indicate the presence of concentrations higher than those recommended by international guidelines for sediment and food. Mercury (Hg) concentrations in the Tigre, Morona, and Pastaza rivers are up to six times higher than the recommended value for daily consumption. The carcinogenic risk due to the regular consumption of native species in the indigenous communities living on the banks of the four studied rivers is high.

Keywords: human health risk assessment; fluvial sediment; fish muscle; carcinogenic index; heavy metals

1. Introduction

The minerals found in the basins are transported to water bodies due to natural and artificial actions. Some of these elements are essential for the dynamics in aquatic environments, and for life itself [1,2]. A significant part of the rivers in the Amazon basin originates in the Peruvian and Ecuadorian Andes, draining their waters through steep and rocky volcanic terrain, carrying metals or soluble chemical compounds in their path [3]. Minerals, because of their polar properties, are adsorbed to particles (e.g., organic matter, dead cells, etc.), making them heavier and causing them to sediment [4–6]. This results in a natural sink for all of the material derived from natural or anthropic sources in the basin [7]. The sedimented material can easily be resuspended due to physical phenomena (e.g., wind, precipitation, current alteration, etc.), which increases their negative impact on the aquatic environment [2].

When metals and metalloids, as part of the minerals, are found in high concentrations in different environmental compartments, such as sediment, they become an environmental threat [8,9] to the aquatic system and to public health. The Amazon Basin is susceptible to these fluctuations, especially for human communities settled in riverside zones that culturally have a major food dependency on aquatic ecosystems for fishing and drinking water [10].

Artisanal mining is one of the main activities in the upper basin area (Peru and Ecuador). In this type of mining, chemicals such as mercury and cyanide 8 are frequently employed without supervision. Additionally, mining activity in the Ecuadorian Amazon tripled in size from 2015 to 2021 (7495 ha) across various provinces (Chinchipe, Napo, Morona Santiago, and Sucumbíos) [11–14]. The major concern is that not just mining activities but also petroleum extraction in the area jeopardizes indigenous communities in the Pastaza, Corrientes, Tigre, and Marañón rivers [15,16]. Both activities endanger the ichthyological diversity in the Amazonian rivers, considered the world's highest diversity (2406 species) [17].

The persistence of minerals in aquatic bodies leads to their accumulation in living organisms. Some of these elements are difficult to metabolize and, therefore, remain in the organism, a phenomenon known as bioaccumulation. Another issue to consider is the process of accumulation within the food web itself, which can be related to each species' feeding habits (detritivores, carnivores, benthonic, etc.) [18,19]. When some species feed on contaminated organisms, there is an increasing concentration of a particular metal or metalloid in the predator, a process known as biomagnification. These hydrobiological resources, many of which are essential in the diet of Amazonian people, are increasingly exposed to higher concentrations of elements in fluvial and lacustrine environments.

People of the Peruvian Amazon fish a wide variety of species (approximately 60 species), and fish consumption in this area is almost three times the national average, reaching 50 kg/person/year [10]. Indigenous people (105,900 inhabitants) [20] live in this area. Ethnic groups such as the Kichwa, Achuar, Wampis, Shapra, and Kandozi are mainly settled along the sides of the Pastaza, Morona, Tigre, and Corrientes rivers, with a traditional dependence on fish.

In this context, the presence of metals or metalloids in fluvial sediments, due to physical disturbances, can resuspend and increase bioaccumulation and biomagnification processes that affect fish, turning them into potential carriers of toxic substances in the food web. As far as is known, this is the first study in the Peruvian Amazon that relates the presence of metals and metalloids in fish muscles to their concentrations in fluvial sediments in areas affected by mining and petroleum activities. This study makes a significant contribution to environmental toxicology and geochemistry in Amazonian fluvial environments. Finally, the results explore the probable carcinogenic and non-carcinogenic risk occurrences due to fish consumption in human communities settled along four rivers in the Peruvian Amazon.

Therefore, the objective was to analyze the arsenic and heavy metal concentrations in both the sediment and native fish muscles from the ecotoxicological perspective, to correlate their interaction and assess their potential risk to public health, employing carcinogenic risk indices in four rivers of the Peruvian Amazon (Tigre, Morona, Corrientes, and Pastaza).

2. Material and Methods

During February and March 2023, sediment and fish samples were collected from four rivers in two provinces: Loreto (Corrientes and Tigre rivers) and Datém del Marañón (Pastaza and Morona rivers), both in the department of Loreto, Peru. The collections coincided with the time of high water, so all of the rivers were navigable, with considerable daily fluvial transit among rural areas where small indigenous communities are settled. These native communities are established along the riversides, with fish being their main food source.

Sediments were collected from 27 sites along the Tigre (T1–T7), Corrientes (C1–C6), Pastaza (P1–P6), and Morona (M1–M7) rivers (Figure 1 and Table 1). Petroleum storage reservoirs were observed at some sampling sites, which belong to PetroPeru. Fish samples were collected at the same sites as the sediments, from a total of 22 sites in fishing zones, except at C2, C5, T2, T3, and T5. Sediment and fish sampling sites are represented by orange dots, while sediment-only sampling sites are represented by green dots (Figure 1).

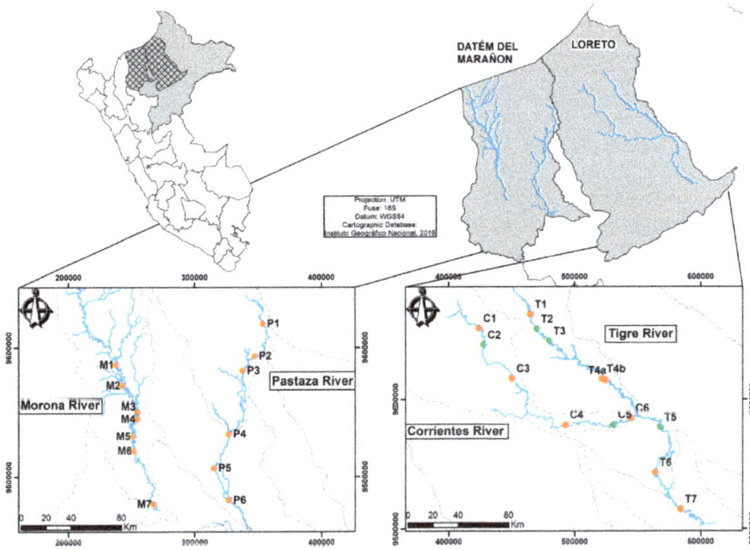

Figure 1. The Morona, Pastaza, Corrientes, and Tigre rivers are located in the northeast of Peru, in the department of Loreto. These rivers have their headwaters in Ecuadorian territory; from there, they flow into the Peruvian Amazon, joining the Marañón River, which, in confluence with the Ucayali River, forms the Amazon River. Sediment and fish sampling sites are in orange; sediment only sampling sites are in green.

Table 1. Sampling sites, geographical information, and daily fish intake for the Corrientes, Tigre, Morona, and Pastaza rivers. Data on daily fish consumption were obtained through interviews with residents.

Site	Small Town or Village	No. of Fish Specimens per Pool	River	District/Province	Human Daily Fish Intake (g/Person/Day)
C1	Nueva Valencia	18	Corrientes	Trompeteros/Loreto	103.00
C3	Pucacuro	19	Corrientes	Trompeteros/Loreto	103.23
C4	Trompeteros	17	Corrientes	Trompeteros/Loreto	82.94
C6	Providencia	31	Corrientes	Trompeteros/Loreto	60.00
T1	Paiche Playa	16	Tigre	Tigre/Loreto	146.14
T4a	Intuto	19	Tigre	Tigre/Loreto	122.45
T4b	28 de Julio	28	Tigre	Tigre/Loreto	175.68
T6	Piura	11	Tigre	Tigre/Loreto	134.46
T7	Nueva York	30	Tigre	Tigre/Loreto	56.62
M1	Inka Roca-Tigreyacu	10	Morona	Morona/Datém del Marañón	302.36
M2	Caballito-Tipishcacocha	19	Morona	Morona/Datém del Marañón	383.00
M3	Shoroya nuevo	10	Morona	Morona/Datém del Marañón	382.11
M4	Pinshacocha	17	Morona	Morona/Datém del Marañón	63.01

Table 1. *Cont.*

Site	Small Town or Village	No. of Fish Specimens per Pool	River	District/Province	Human Daily Fish Intake (g/Person/Day)
M5	San Martin	41	Morona	Morona/Datém del Marañón	62.53
M6	Puerto Alegría	13	Morona	Morona/Datém del Marañón	63.15
M7	Puerto América	15	Morona	Morona/Datém del Marañón	64.24
P1	Nuevo Soplín	13	Pastaza	Morona/Datém del Marañón	60.00
P2	Loboyacu	18	Pastaza	Morona/Datém del Marañón	302.37
P3	Sungache	18	Pastaza	Morona/Datém del Marañón	100.00
P4	San Fernando	10	Pastaza	Morona/Datém del Marañón	101.20
P5	Musakarusha	12	Pastaza	Morona/Datém del Marañón	82.41
P6	Nueva Alianza	8	Pastaza	Morona/Datém del Marañón	84.43

2.1. Fish Sampling

Fish were collected from different fishing areas located in the four rivers. These fish included carnivorous, omnivorous, and detritivore species (Table 2). The collection followed the protocols established by the Peruvian Ministry of Environment [21]. This method involved setting up fishing nets that remained in place for 24 h. These nets were periodically checked to ensure that predator fish did not damage the captured samples, and to prevent major vertebrates (reptiles, aquatic mammals, etc.) from being accidentally trapped. A total of 404 individuals were collected from the four rivers. Approximately 500 to 800 g of fish muscle was collected at the different sampling sites, according to the number of individuals captured (Table 1).

Table 2. Basic biological information of fish collected from the four Amazonian rivers in this study.

Scientific Name	Name	River				Total	Feeding Regime	Habitat
		Corrientes	Tigre	Morona	Pastaza			
Acestrorhynchus falcirostris	Big-eyed cachorro	1	2		1	4	Piscivorous	Benthopelagic
Adontosternarchus balaenops	Ghost knifefish		4			4	Carnivorous	Benthopelagic
Ageneiosus inermis	Manduba	1		2	1	4	Piscivorous	Pelagic
Amblydoras affinis	Rego rego			7		7	Omnivore	Demersal
Ancistrus dolichopterus	Bushymouth catfish			1		1	Omnivore	Demersal
Ancistrus temminckii	Carachama			4		4	Omnivore	Demersal
Anodus elongatus	Yulilla	1	3			4	Omnivore	Pelagic
Astronatus ocellatus	Oscar				2	2	Omnivore	Benthopelagic
Biotodoma cupido	Greenstreaked eartheater			1	2	3	Omnivore	Benthopelagic
Brachyplatytoma vaillantii	Laulao catfish				1	1	Piscivorous	Demersal
Brycon amazonicus	Sábalo		1	3		4	Omnivore	Benthopelagic
Bunocephalus coraoideus	Banjo catfish			1		1	Omnivore	Demersal
Calophysus macropterus	Zamurito				1	1	Carnivorous	Demersal
Chaetobranchus flavescens	Bujurqui vaso		15	1	5	21	Omnivore	Benthopelagic
Cheirodon interruptus	Uruguay tetra		2			2	Omnivore	Benthopelagic
Chilodus punctatus	Spotted headstander		5			5	Omnivore	Pelagic
Cichla monoculus	Peacock bass	1			2	3	Carnivorous	Benthopelagic
Cichla ocellaris	Peacock cichlid		1			1	Carnivorous	Benthopelagic
Corydoras arcuatus	Skunk corydoras			1		1	Detritivore	Demersal
Curimatella meyeri	Yahuarachi				1	1	Detritivore	Benthopelagic
Cynodon gibbus	Chambira				1	1	Carnivorous	Pelagic
Hemiodus microlepis	Yulilla				1	1	Omnivore	Benthopelagic
Hemisorubim platyrhynchos	Porthole shovelnose catfish	1				1	Carnivorous	Demersal
Heros efasciatus	Bujurqui acha vieja				1	1	Omnivore	Benthopelagic

Table 2. *Cont.*

Scientific Name	Name	River				Total	Feeding Regime	Habitat
		Corrientes	Tigre	Morona	Pastaza			
Heros severus	Banded cichlid			1		1	Omnivore	Benthopelagic
Hoplerythrinus unitaeniatus	Aimara		2	1	9	12	Carnivorous	Pelagic
Hoplias malabaricus	Trahira	3	5	7	7	22	Carnivorous	Benthopelagic
Hoplosternum littorale	Atipa				4	4	Detritivore	Demersal
Hyphessobrycon copelandi	Wira mojara			5		5	Omnivore	Benthopelagic
Hypophthalmus edentatus	Highwaterman catfish	16	1			17	Herbivore	Pelagic
Hypselecara temporalis	Emerald cichlid				5	5	Omnivore	Benthopelagic
Lamontichthys stibaros	Shitari	1				1	Detritivore	Demersal
Leporinus friderici	Threespot leporinus			6		6	Omnivore	Benthopelagic
Megaleporinus trifasciatus	Lisa	1	1			2	Omnivore	Benthopelagic
Myleus rubripinnis	Redhook myleus	10	7	1	6	24	Omnivore	Benthopelagic
Pimelodus blochii	Bloch's catfish	1	2	1		4	Omnivore	Benthopelagic
Pinirampus pirinampu	Flatwhiskered catfish	1				1	Carnivorous	Demersal
Potamorhina altamazonica	Yahuarachi	6	22	5	4	37	Detritivore	Benthopelagic
Potamotrygon magdalenae	Magdalena river stingray		2			2	Detritivore	Benthopelagic
Prochilodus nigricans	Black prochilodus	1	11	21	12	45	Detritivore	Benthopelagic
Psalidodon fasciatus	Banded astyanax			1		1	Omnivore	Benthopelagic
Psectrogaster amazonica	Chio Chio	11	26	4		41	Detritivore	Benthopelagic
Pseudorinelepis genibarbis	Carachama negra		1			1	Detritivore	Benthopelagic
Pterodoras granulosus	Granulated catfish		2	2		4	Omnivore	Demersal
Pterygoplichthys pardalis	Amazon sailfin catfish			16		16	Detritivore	Demersal
Pygocentrus nattereri	Red piranha			4	1	5	Carnivorous	Pelagic
Rhaphiodon vulpinus	Biara			1		1	Carnivorous	Pelagic
Rhytiodus microlepis	Lisa			1		1	Herbivorous	Benthopelagic
Roeboides myersii	Dentón	2	1	4	1	8	Carnivorous	Benthopelagic
Satanoperca jurupari	Demon eartheater				5	5	Carnivorous	Benthopelagic
Schizodon fasciatus	Characin			5	4	9	Omnivore	Benthopelagic
Semaprochilodus insignis	Kissing prochilodus	1	2		2	5	Detritivore	Benthopelagic
Serrasalmus rhombeus	Red-eye piranha	1		10	3	14	Carnivorous	Benthopelagic
Squaliforma emarginata	Carachama blanca			2		2	Detritivore	Demersal
Trachelyopterus galeatus	Novia cunchi	2		2	4	8	Omnivore	Demersal
Triportheus angulatus	Sardina	3	3	4	7	17	Omnivore	Benthopelagic

Fish muscle extraction was performed according to the Peruvian Technical Standard 700.002 (NTP, 2021). A sampling pool was created with fish muscles from all species collected at each sampling site. Sample pooling is a method where units that were supposed to be measured individually are processed together, making separate analyses impossible, because human residents of the indigenous communities did not consume only one species of fish per day but a variety of species existing in their catches. Sampling pool analyses were carried out, since the indigenous people do not have a preference for a particular fish species, nor do they select them in their daily diet for reasons of the place they occupy in the water column or because of the fish's diet. The sample pools were stored at −20 °C until their evaluation in the laboratory.

2.2. Sediment Sampling

A total of 50 samples were collected from the Tigre (12 samples), Corrientes (12 samples), Pastaza (12 samples), and Morona (14 samples) (Figure 1). Samples were extracted from the upper layer (0–10 cm), extracted using a Van Veen sediment sampler (1000 cm^3). The sediment was stored in plastic flasks (300 cm^3) in the dark and kept at 4 °C until analysis in the laboratory.

2.3. Daily Fish Intake

To calculate the daily fish intake in riverside indigenous communities, census data from the National Institute of Statistics and Informatics [22] were used, indicating a total of 29,084 people living in the areas of interest. With this total number, and using finite population sampling ($p = 0.05$) [23], a representative sample of 1356 people from different indigenous communities was calculated and interviewed.

2.4. Metal Concentration Analysis

Fish muscle: The biological sample analysis was performed at the National University of San Agustín, following the method mentioned by Qin et al. (2015) [24], with partial modifications. This process took 0.5 g of the homogenized samples (epaxial muscle without skin), which were then subjected to microwave digestion in Teflon vessels (Milestone, Sorisole, Italy, Ethos Easy model). In the vessels, 10 mL of a HNO_3:H_2O_2 mixture (at an 8:2 ratio) received the homogenized sample, which was heated to 280 °C in a thirty-minute ramp. The resulting sample was filtered through a PVDF membrane filter (Whatman, Maidstone, UK, 0.45 μm), and then it was diluted with Milli-Q water up to 50 mL and stored at 4 °C. Metals, except mercury, were analyzed via inductively coupled plasma mass spectrometry (ICP-MS) (PerkinElmer, Waltham, MA, USA, NexION 2000C model). Mercury was analyzed directly in an automatized mercury analyzer (Milestone, DMA-80 evo model).

Sediment: Eleven elements were studied (As, Cd, Cr, Cu, Ni, Pb, Al, Ba, Fe, Zn, and Hg). Metals, except Hg, were analyzed using inductively coupled plasma optical spectrometry (ICP-OES). This procedure requires a previous digestion of the sample, following the method of SW 846 US EPA 3050 [25]. It consisted of acid digestion, with the addition of HNO_3, H_2O_2, and HCl in 4.5 h at 90 °C. In the case of mercury (Hg), it was analyzed via cold vapor atomic absorption spectroscopy (CVAAS), following the USEPA 7471B method [26], where the sample must be digested by a sequence of reactions employing H_2SO_4, HNO_3, and $KMnO_4$ in 2 h. Metal and metalloid data are expressed as milligrams per kilogram of dry weight (mg/kg dw).

2.5. QA/QC

Quality control was performed through the evaluation of the precision and accuracy of the methodology, as follows: Analytical-grade reagents (obtained from PerkinElmer) were used in all of the analyses. All glassware items and equipment used to store and process the samples for metal assessment were left in 10% nitric acid for at least 24 h, followed by rinsing with ultrapure water.

Fish muscle: Blank and control samples were analyzed in a 10-sample batch, assuring the standards. The results were between 80% and 120%, which is the recommended range [25]. During calibration, we obtained an $R^2 > 0.999$, which indicates a strong correlation of the signal. The quantification limits for the metals analyzed were as follows: Cr (0.216 mg/kg), Ni (0.016 mg/kg), Cu (0.066 mg/kg), Zn (0.712 mg/kg), As (0.007 mg/kg), Cd (0.001 mg/kg), Hg (0.01 mg/kg), and Pb (0.016 mg/kg).

Sediments: Recovery control varied between 93.9% and 116%, which is in the recommended range [25]. The linearity and strong correlation of the signal were assured, with an $R^2 > 0.999$. The quantification limits for the elements were as follows: Cr (1.0 mg/kg), Ni (1.0 mg/kg), Cu (0.8 mg/kg), Zn (0.6 mg/kg), As (3.6 mg/kg), Cd (0.3 mg/kg), Hg (0.01 mg/kg), and Pb (3.0 mg/kg), Fe (2.5 mg/kg), Al (3.0 mg/kg), and Ba (0.3 mg/kg).

2.6. Risk Assessment

2.6.1. Estimated Daily Intake (EDI)

The daily intake was calculated for each element (Cr, Ni, Cu, Zn, As, Cd, Pb, and Hg) using the following equation:

$$EDI = \frac{FIR \times Ci}{BW}$$

where FIR is the fish intake ratio (g/person/day, wet weight), Ci is the mean concentration of the element in fish muscle (mg/kg), and BW is the mean corporal weight of an adult (70 kg in this study) [27]. For adults living in rural areas, such as the ones in this study (Datém del Marañón and Loreto), the FIR was calculated for each particularly small town or village in the study, employing the data collected from the interviews, to present a more reliable measurement. This was merely to highlight that, since these small towns or villages are located far from major urban centers (1–2 days of navigating), fish intake represents a major percentage of the diet compared to other kinds of meat.

2.6.2. Non-Carcinogenic Risk

The target hazard quotient (THQ) was employed to measure the non-carcinogenic risk. The THQ is the ratio of EDI to the oral reference dose (RfD, mg/kg·day); this RfD was established by the US Environmental Protection Agency (U.S. EPA 2023). This quotient was calculated as follows:

$$THQ = \frac{EDI}{RfD}$$

On this basis, there are three scenarios according to Hossain et al. (2018) [28] and Huang et al. (2019) [29]:

THQ < 1, the population will not experience any adverse health hazards.
THQ = 1, the receptors of concern may experience non-carcinogenic health effects.
THQ > 1, there is an increasing probability of adverse health hazard occurrences.

2.6.3. Carcinogenic Risk (CRI)

This index is used to assess potential carcinogenic risks of fish consumption [30]. This calculation was performed only for Cr, As, and Cd, using the following equation:

$$CRI = \frac{FIR \times E_F \times E_D}{BW \times T_A} \times SF_i \times C_i$$

where E_F is the exposure frequency (365 day per year), ED is the exposure duration (70 years), TA is the average time (365 × ED d), and SFi is the oral slope factor (mg/kg·day) for a single element. The oral intake of carcinogenic slope factors for Cr, As, and Cd was 0.50, 0.38, and 1.50, respectively [29].

This brings three classifications based on the outcomes, according to [30]:
$CRI < 10^{-6}$, the compound is safe for humans.
$10^{-6} < CRI < 10^{-4}$, there are potential carcinogenic risks to the exposed population.
$CRI > 10^{-4}$, the exposed people would encounter excess carcinogenic risk.

2.7. Statistical Analysis

Descriptive statistics was used to analyze the fish muscle and sediment concentrations. A principal component analysis (PCA) was performed to identify the relations among sample sites and the assessed elements, for both fish muscle and sediments. PCA reduces all datasets to a lower number of variables (usually the first two components) for plotting purposes. The graphical biplot correlation in the PCA was based on [31]; this analysis was performed using the free statistical software Paleontological Statistics (PAST) Version 4.03. Data analyzed in PCA were previously log-transformed; subsequently, the PCA was performed. A Spearman correlation was performed ($p < 0.05$) between fish muscle and sediments [32].

3. Results

3.1. Metal(loid)s in Fish Muscles

Regarding the element outcomes in fish (Table 3), the mean concentrations of Ni, Cu, Zn, As, Cd, and Pb demonstrated the presence of these metals at all sampling sites, with Ni, Cd, Pb, and Hg showing higher variation in at least one of the four rivers assessed. On the other hand, zinc is the metal that presented the highest mean concentrations in all four rivers, reaching a maximum of 9.88 mg/kg in the Tigre River (Table 3). Although the mean Zn concentrations were higher, they did not surpass the limits established by the FAO and ANVISA. However, the mean chromium concentrations registered in all rivers were higher than the WHO/FAO, EU, and ANVISA guidelines [27,33–36] (Table 4).

Table 3. Metal(loid)s' descriptive statistics in fish muscle (mg/kg wet weight); mean, standard deviation, range, and coefficient of variation (expressed in %) for the four rivers assessed.

Element	Tigre (n = 104)			Morona (n = 125)			Corrientes (n = 85)			Pastaza (n = 79)		
	Mean ± SD	Range	CV	Mean ± SD	Range	CV	Mean ± SD	Range	CV	Mean ± SD	Range	CV
Cr	0.73 ± 0.34	0.32–1.29	51.95	0.46 ± 0.24	0.23–0.93	53.2	0.53 ± 0.10	0.43–0.67	19.01	0.40 ± 0.16	0.29–0.72	40.88
Ni	0.22 ± 0.19	0.04–0.64	94.74	0.10 ± 0.03	0.04–0.13	32.07	0.19 ± 0.09	0.08–0.32	45.8	0.06 ± 0.05	0.02–0.13	92.2
Cu	0.54 ± 0.19	0.22–0.89	33.36	0.46 ± 0.13	0.22–0.67	28.89	0.47 ± 0.11	0.32–0.68	24.31	0.41 ± 0.13	0.28–0.59	32.74
Zn	6.30 ± 1.76	3.91–9.88	25.19	5.34 ± 0.96	4.37–7.42	15.79	6.58 ± 0.85	5.60–7.64	12.98	5.49 ± 1.32	4.17–7.72	24.03
As	0.02 ± 0.02	ND–0.07	109.67	0.02 ± 0.02	ND–0.07	104.79	0.02 ± 0.01	ND–0.03	60.61	0.01 ± 0.002	ND–0.01	21.02
Cd	0.006 ± 0.002	0.002–0.01	40.53	0.006 ± 0.01	0.001–0.02	94.68	0.005 ± 0.002	0.003–0.01	31.11	0.01 ± 0.004	0.004–0.01	32.6
Pb	0.05 ± 0.02	0.03–0.07	31.91	0.04 ± 0.02	0.01–0.07	54.98	0.06 ± 0.04	0.02–0.12	70.6	0.06 ± 0.03	0.03–0.13	53.29
Hg	0.31 ± 0.10	0.20–0.43	33.43	0.18 ± 0.10	0.10–0.39	54.9	0.11 ± 0.01	0.10–0.13	11.24	0.28 ± 0.14	0.12–0.52	50.02

ND = not detected; n: the number of samples of fish muscle.

Table 4. Limit concentrations of metals in fish muscle according to international guidelines (mg/kg).

Guideline/Reference	Cr	Ni	Cu	Pb	Zn	Hg	As	Cd
FAO [27]				0.2	50	0.5		0.05
FAO/WHO [33]	0.05	8.97	30	0.05				0.015
China QS [34]	2.0			0.5		0.5	0.1	
European Union [35]	0.5			0.3		0.5		0.05
ANVISA [36]	0.1	5.0	30		50	0.5	0.5	

Even though the mean Hg concentrations did not surpass the guideline values in the Tigre and Pastaza rivers (0.31 and 0.28 mg/kg, respectively), the maximum values showed concentrations that are close to or even higher than the probable harmful concentration according to international guidelines. The percentage of the near and upper samples of Hg in the Tigre River was 40%, and in the Pastaza it was 16.7%.

The PCA for fish muscle (Figure 2) shows that there are no clear differences among the assessed rivers; however, the relationship of the sample sites to certain metals can be observed. There is a group composed of sample sites from the Pastaza (P1, P4, P5, and P6) and Tigre (T4a) rivers demonstrating a positive relation to mercury (Hg). Additionally, sample sites in the Corrientes, Tigre, and Morona rivers (C4, T6, and M5, respectively) show a positive relation to cadmium (Cd), while P2, P3, M1, and M2 (Pastaza and Morona rivers) are related to lead (Pb). Sample sites in the Morona (M3 and M7) exhibit a positive relation to arsenic (As), whereas sites in the Corrientes (C1, C3, and C6) and Tigre (T4b) show a relation to copper (Cu) and iron (Fe).

The correlation analysis among fish muscle samples indicates positive relationships between Cu and Zn, Ni and Zn, and Cr and Ni. On the other hand, there is an inverse relationship of Hg with Pb and Fe. A weak relationship between As and Cd can also be observed.

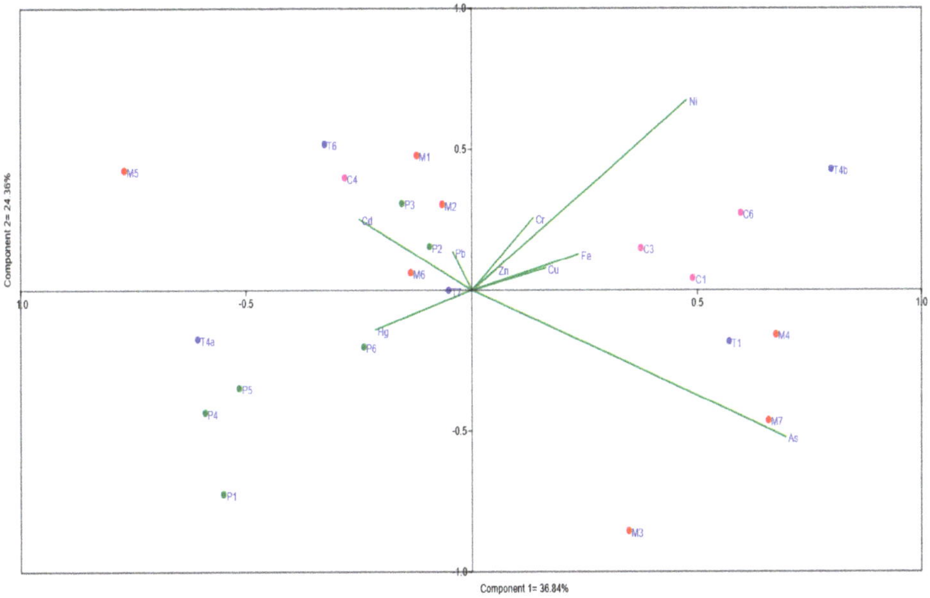

Figure 2. Principal component analysis of fish muscle.

3.2. Sediments

Among all elements assessed in the four basins (Table 5), the highest mean concentrations of Cr, Ni, and Cu (17.85, 47.10, and 9.31 mg/kg, respectively) were observed in the Morona River. Additionally, the Morona River showed the highest mean concentration of Zn (52.19 mg/kg), with a maximum value reaching 99.80 mg/kg. In contrast, the Tigre River presented the lowest mean concentrations of Cr, Ni, Cu, and Zn (7.53, 7.00, 4.24, and 16.89 mg/kg, respectively).

Table 5. Descriptive statistical data of the metal(loid)s found in sediments. Standard deviation and range (min–max) values in mg/kg, and coefficient of variation (CV) expressed in %.

Element	Tigre (n = 12)			Morona (n = 14)			Corrientes (n = 12)			Pastaza (n = 12)			Guidelines		
	Mean ± SD	Range	CV	Mean ± SD	Range	CV	Mean ± SD	Range	CV	Mean ± SD	Range	CV	NOAAA	ISQG	SQG-EPA
Cr	7.53 ± 1.77	1.90–16.00	63.34	12.74 ± 1.51	8.30–21.80	35.43	11.58 ± 2.23	3.20–35.30	79.65	17.85 ± 3.06	12.50–24.00	22.77	13	37.2	43.4
Ni	7 ± 1.28	3.60–10.40	32.63	10.83 ± 2.39	7.20–18.0	31.28	10.57 ± 5.77	3.10–21.10	54.59	47.10 ± 8.67	27.5–95.10	39.62	9.9	18	22.7
Cu	4.24 ± 0.49	2.20–8.40	58.67	7.48 ± 1.25	1.90–21.00	96.95	4.58 ± 1.98	2.10–8.70	65.05	9.31 ± 1.95	5.80–18.00	42.42	25	35.7	31.6
Zn	16.89 ± 2.52	5.40–38.40	62.26	52.19 ± 13.58	29.70–99.80	45.18	20.78 ± 2.32	8.90–37.60	44.86	31.94 ± 3.19	25.0–39.50	13.13	38	123	121
Al	2523.78 ± 378.2	626.6–7447.0	79.45	9489.71 ± 1239.4	4467.0–21,160.0	62.98	2988.03 ± 206.5	941.4–7365	63.71	5714.92 ± 379.2	3404.0–8674.0	25.76	2600		
Fe	5671.50 ± 424.1	1911.0–12,585.0	62.94	14,114.14 ± 2921.6	8664.0–23,352.0	34.65	7160.2 ± 322.2	2366–14,375	56.69	15,543.0 ± 1077.5	12,993.0–19,773.0	12.99	18,000		20,000
Ba	26.80 ± 2.1	8.60–71.8	71.48	89.93 ± 11.55	52.7–158.1	38.86	35.9 ± 2.88	16.9–51.7	35.88	34.97 ± 7.1	19.40–47.70	22.58	0.70		
As	<3.6	0	0.00	<3.6	0	0	<3.6	0	0	<3.6	0	0	1.1	5.9	<3
Cd	<0.3	0	0.00	<0.3	0	0	<0.3	0	0	<0.3	0	0	0.3	0.6	0.99
Pb	<3.0	0	0.00	<3.0	0	0	<3.0	0	0	<3.0	0	0	17	35	35.8
Hg	0.02 ± 0.01	0.01–0.06	70.46	0.04 ± 0.02	0.01–0.07	55.22	0.02 ± 0.01	0.01–0.03	50.65	0.02 ±0.01	0.01–0.04	83.85	0.05	0.17	0.18

n: the number of samples of sediment. NOAA: National Oceanic and Atmospheric Administration (USA). ISQG: Interim Sediment Quality Guidelines (Canada). SQG-EPA: Small Quantity Generator U.S. Environmental Protection Agency (USA).

Regarding the PCA (Figure 3), differences among the four assessed rivers were observed, with Morona River showing the clearest distinction, where the sample sites were related to Al, Ba, and Zn. The Pastaza River exhibited correlations with Ni and Cr. The Tigre and Corrientes rivers showed some similarities in certain sample sites; generally, these rivers were inversely related to Fe and Cr.

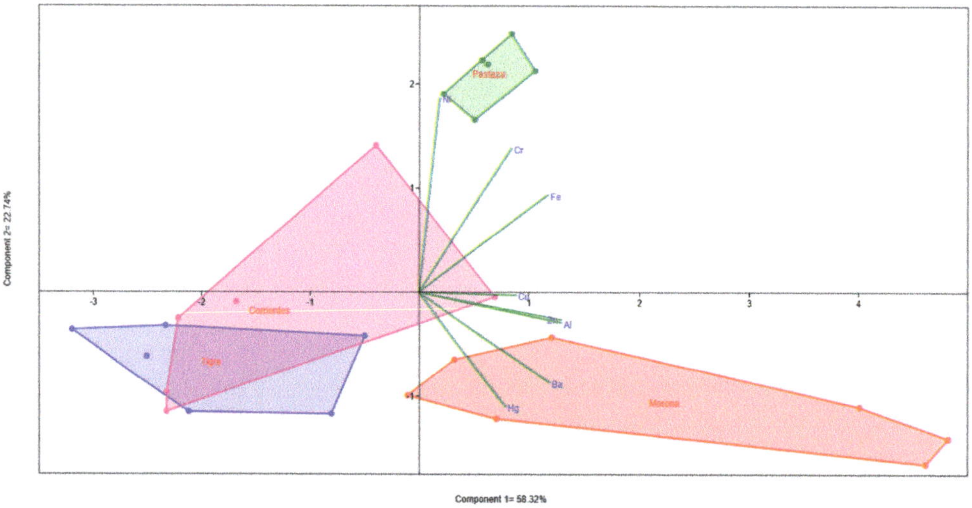

Figure 3. Principal component analysis for sediment.

According to the Spearman correlation analyses performed, the metalloid contents obtained from the analyzes of fish and sediments showed significantly high ratios of Ni (Corrientes River) and Zn (Morona and Pastaza rivers), moderate ratios of Cr and Ni (Río Pastaza), and a low ratio of Cr (Río Morona) (Figure 4).

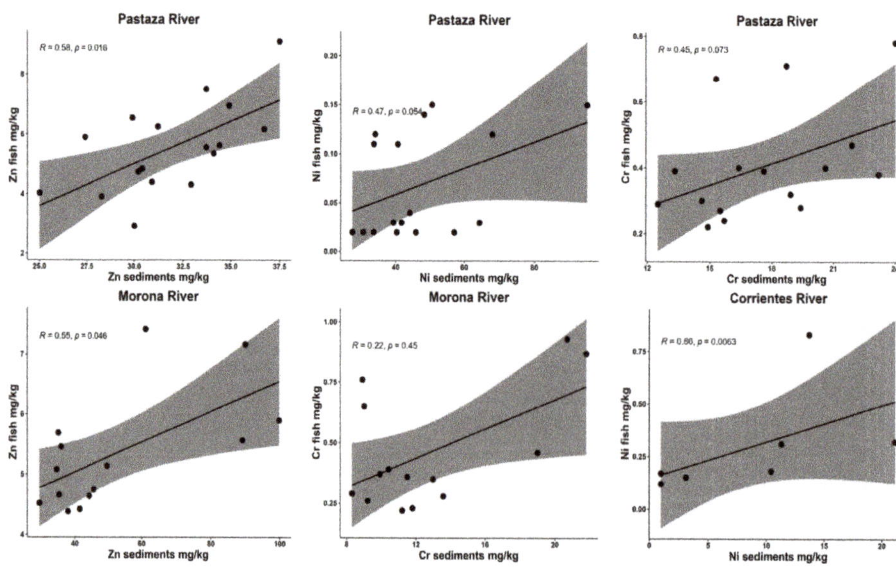

Figure 4. Spearman correlation analyses for sediments and fish tissues.

3.3. Carcinogenic and Non-Carcinogenic Analysis

The oral reference doses (RfD) for Ni, Cu, Zn, Cr, As, Cd, and Hg were 20, 40, 300, 3, 0.3, 1 and 0.3 µg/kg·d, respectively [37]. Following the European Food Safety Authority's guidelines, the RfD for Pb was set to 1.5 µg/kg·d [38].

Table 6 shows the results for RfD, EDI, THQ, and CRI for the analyzed elements in different fish muscles collected from the four river basins. Concerning THQ, Hg is the only metal that exceeds the USEPA-recommended levels in the Tigre, Morona, and Pastaza rivers (1.92, 1.83, and 1.50, respectively). When examining the CRI, Cr is the only metal that poses a potential carcinogenic risk in all four basins, with maximum values even higher in the Tigre and Morona rivers.

Table 6. Carcinogenic and non-carcinogenic risk analysis of elements in fish consumed in Loreto, and carcinogenic risk index for Cr (10^{-4}), As, and Cd (10^{-6}). RfDs (µg/kg·day), CRI range (min–max).

Elements	RfDs	Tigre			Morona			Corrientes			Pastaza		
		EDI	THQ	CRI	EDI	THQ	CRI	EDI	THQ	CRI	EDI	THQ	CRI
Cr	1	1.33	0.44	6.6 (1.3–13.1)	1.58	0.53	7.8 (1.01–21.5)	0.68	0.23	3.3 (1.8–4.8)	0.72	0.24	3.5 (1.3–9)
Ni	20	0.40	0.02		0.26	0.01		0.22	0.01		0.14	0.01	
Cu	40	0.97	0.02		1.38	0.03		0.57	0.01		0.67	0.02	
Zn	300	11.31	0.04		14.66	0.05		8.11	0.03		9.08	0.03	
As	* 0.3	0.05	0.16	71.6 (8.6–183.8)	0.05	0.17	78.4 (2.99–312.9)	0.02	0.08	35.5 (5.47–64.4)	0.02	0.07	30.3 (14.9–85.2)
Cd	1	0.01	0.01	4.6 (0.7–7.6)	0.01	0.01	4.8 (0.8–14.6)	0.01	0.01	2.2 (1.7–2.7)	0.02	0.02	8.2 (1.4–24.1)
Pb	1.5	0.09	0.06		0.10	0.07		0.09	0.06		0.11	0.07	
Hg	** 0.3	0.57	1.92		0.55	1.83		0.14	0.45		0.45	1.50	

* Inorganic arsenic; ** elemental mercury, and mercury compounds.

4. Discussion

The findings of this study highlight a concerning scenario regarding potential carcinogenic risks associated with mercury (Hg) and chromium (Cr) for indigenous communities in the Peruvian Amazon. The high concentrations of metals and metalloids found in the Tigre, Pastaza, and Morona rivers imply risks to public health and the well-being of communities residing in these areas. It is crucial to recognize that remote communities, situated far from urban centers, rely heavily on local resources for their livelihoods.

However, the disruption caused by human activities directly impacts aquatic environments, leading to scenarios of bioaccumulation and biomagnification.

4.1. Fish Muscle Analysis

It is evident that the more remotely a community is located, the higher its fish consumption, as shown in Table 1 and Figure 1. This trend can be observed at sites like T1 and C1 in Loreto, or M2 and P2 in Datém del Marañón. The prevalence of fish in the diets of these communities is notable not only on the Peruvian side, but also in Ecuador, where it reaches up to 623 g/day in the Pastaza River [39]. Regarding the metal and metalloid concentrations in fish muscle, chromium (Cr) exceeds the established reference concentrations set out by the WHO, FAO, EU, and ANVISA in all four rivers (Table 4). Although chromium naturally originates from rocks in the basin, its presence is also linked to human activities such as petroleum extraction [40]. Additionally, the concentration of Cr can vary depending on its geological source [41], and its use in the paint industry (Cr_2O_3) provides chemical resistance to abrasion [42]. This type of paint is commonly used on boats in these areas.

When comparing data from the Tigre River with other global rivers (Table 7), it is evident that the maximum Cr values are higher than those observed in the Sinos and Northeast China rivers [29,43], and similar to those found in the Paraopeba [44] and Piracicaba [45] rivers in Brazil, where significant anthropogenic pollution has been reported.

In contrast, the outcomes for the Tigre and Pastaza rivers are considerably lower than those observed in the Houjin River [46].

Table 7. Comparison of metal(loid) concentrations (mg/kg ww) in fish among different riverine environments.

River	Country	Cr	Ni	Cu	Zn	As	Cd	Pb	Hg	References
Tigre	Peru	0.32–1.29	0.04–0.49	0.28–0.75	4.14–8.28	0.003–0.06	0.002–0.01	0.03–0.07	0.20–0.41	This study
Pastaza	Peru	0.29–0.72	0.02–0.13	0.28–0.59	4.17–7.72	ND–0.01	0.004–0.01	0.03–0.13	0.12–0.52	This study
Abaeté and Paraopeba	Brazil	0.42–1.7		5.62–32.2	8.88–21.1		0.02–0.33	0.17–2.11		[44]
Piracicaba	Brazil	0.05- 1.11	0.05–2.83	0.03–4.18		0.73–0.93	0.02–0.92	0.66–3.25		[45]
Sinos	Brazil	0.09–0.38	-	1.43–5.4	22.9–34.6	1.47–8.79	0.07–0.8	1.2–2.5	-	[43]
Northeast of China	China	ND–0.49	ND–0.78	0.067–0.97	2.49–51.38	ND–0.39	ND–0.009	ND–0.70	ND–0.82	[29]
Yangtze	China	0.10–0.24	-	0.77–1.22	2.8–7.55	-	0.046–0.12	0.21–0.81	-	[47]
Houjin	Taiwan	ND–83.44	ND–34.59	ND–380	ND–107	ND–3.11	ND–14.5	ND–13.5	ND–0.38	[46]
Gomti	Bangladesh	0.004	-	-	-	0.002	BDL	BDL	0.006	[28]
Alto Solimões	Brazil								0.081–0.33	[48]
Rio Amazonas–Manaos	Brazil								0.0–2.18	[49]
Bajo Napo–Loreto	Perú								0.04–1.94	[50]

ND: not detected; BDL: below detectable level.

A similar pattern was observed with Cu, the levels of which were comparable to the Yangtze River [47] but much lower than the Paraopeba River. Regarding Zn, the Tigre and Pastaza rivers showed lower concentrations compared to the Paraopeba, Sinos [43], and Northeast China rivers [29], possibly due to agricultural activities. Mercury in the Tigre and Pastaza Rivers presents maximum concentrations that exceed the values reported in the Northeast China [29] and Gomti [28] Rivers. In the case of Peru, fish in other Amazonian rivers have registered higher values than the FEPA and WHO guidelines [50].

4.2. Sediment Analysis

The outcomes indicate that the Cr, Ni, and Zn concentrations surpass the NOAA, ISQG, and EPA international guidelines (Table 5). According to the statistical analysis, significant correlations between sediment and fish muscle were identified for Ni, Zn, and Cr (Figure 4). This phenomenon could be related to bioaccumulation occurrences, particularly noticeable in the case of Cr.

4.3. Human Health Risks

The findings of this study highlight a concerning scenario regarding possible carcinogenic risks related to mercury (Hg) and chromium (Cr) for indigenous communities in the Peruvian Amazon. The recommended daily intake limits for metals [33,51] are 0.2 mg/day for Cr, 1.5 mg/day for Cu, 0.002 mg/day for As, 0.007 mg/day for Cd, and 0.0001 mg/day for Hg per person. It is evident from the findings that the EDI calculated for metals (except Hg) in this study did not exceed the recommended values. However, the Hg concentrations in the Tigre River (0.00057 mg/kg·person), Morona River (0.00055 mg/kg·person), and Pastaza River (0.00045 mg/kg·person) are 5 to 6 times higher than the recommended values.

Regarding the risks to human health, it is noteworthy that, among the areas assessed in this study, three basins are more likely to pose negative health effects due to high THQ values for Hg and Cr. Sampling sites such as T4, M1, M3, and P3 have THQ values above 1 for Hg, while T1, T6, M2, P2, and P4 reach values of almost 3, indicating an increased probability of adverse health effects. Of particular concern is sampling site M3, which reports a THQ of 6.43, indicating a substantial potential health impact. Similar studies have also shown high THQ values in Amazonian fish species, ranging from 1.04 to 4.18 [52,53], categorizing them as unsuitable for human consumption.

Regarding the mean THQ value for Cr, it did not exceed the reference value in any of the four basins. However, it is important to note that M1 and M2 registered 1.18 and 1.44, respectively. This is a health alert for the Morona River Basin, as well as for the Shapra and Wampis indigenous communities, which should be continuously monitored by the appropriate authorities. Additionally, the CRI values for Cr were higher than the reference values in all four basins, indicating that fish consumption may expose people to excess carcinogenic risk. The Morona River Basin shows the highest CRI values, with sites like M1, M2, and M4 having CRI values of 0.0018, 0.0022, and 0.001, respectively.

In the case of Hg, THQ's potential risks to the environment are probably the result of human activities developed in the watershed, which includes Ecuadorian territory. In Peru, there are no official reports of legal gold exploitation in the three basins; however, a metallogenic gold map was recently published in Peru [54]. This map clearly establishes that certain Amazonian rivers (Santiago River, the Marañón, the middle part of the Morona River, and the lower part of the Pastaza River are favorable for placer, alluvial, and moraine-type gold deposits. Therefore, the possible presence of informal or illegal dredgers furtively exploiting gold with unsafe techniques and acting as potential sources of Hg in these rivers cannot be ruled out. On the other hand, studies indicate the presence of mining activities, mainly illegal gold mining, including the upper basin of the Morona and Pastaza rivers [11,12,55].

5. Conclusions

The sediment and fish muscle assessment in the four rivers revealed the actual concentrations of metals in the environment. In the case of sediments, Cr, Ni, and Zn exceeded the concentrations of international standards (NOAAA and ISQG). Similarly, high concentrations of Cr and Hg were found in fish muscle in the Tigre, Morona, and Pastaza rivers.

On the other hand, the non-carcinogenic risk analysis indicates that Hg is considered to be a health threat, especially in the Tigre, Morona, and Pastaza rivers, which means that there is an increasing likelihood of adverse health events related to this metal. Meanwhile, the carcinogenic risk assessment shows that Cr is a potential driver in all four rivers, so exposed people would face an excess carcinogenic risk due to this metal. Thus, the evidence found regarding the high concentrations of metals (Hg, Cr) could become chronic accumulation in human organisms, resulting in a public health problem.

The results presented in this study provide information that will serve as a basis for decision-making in future management plans that would help maintain or restore the riparian environment in the Department of Loreto.

Author Contributions: M.A.B.-M. performed conceptualization, formal analysis, investigation, methodology, project administration, supervision, writing—original draft, writing—review and editing, and fund acquisition; F.W.C.-K., formal analysis, investigation, data curation, writing—original draft, writing—review and editing; C.E.Z.P., investigation; J.N.-L., conceptualization, investigation, methodology; A.E.L.-V., investigation, methodology; J.A.R.-L., investigation, methodology; I.E.B.-R., conceptualization, methodology, investigation, formal analysis, writing—original draft, writing—review and editing. All authors have read and agreed to the published version of the manuscript.

Funding: This study was funded by the National Autonomous University of Alto Amazonas through the Research Institute (Resolución Presidencial No. 292-2022-UNAAA/P).

Institutional Review Board Statement: Not applicable.

Informed Consent Statement: Not applicable.

Data Availability Statement: Data available on request due to ethical restrictions.

Acknowledgments: The authors would like to thank to Hans Marbel Pashanase Melo and Carlos Javier Valenzuela Huillca, who helped in the field and laboratory phases; We also wish to thank that Programa de Estudantes-Convênio de Pós-Graduação (PEC-PG), CAPES/CNPq—Brasil (process 190216/2017-4), for having provided a scholarship to Ivan Edward Biamont-Rojas.

Conflicts of Interest: The authors declare no conflicts of interest.

References

1. Zoroddu, M.A.; Aaseth, J.; Crisponi, G.; Medici, S.; Peana, M.; Nurchi, V.M. The Essential Metals for Humans: A Brief Overview. *J. Inorg. Biochem.* **2019**, *195*, 120–129. [CrossRef] [PubMed]
2. Biamont-Rojas, I.E.; Cardoso-Silva, S.; Alves de Lima Ferreira, P.; Alfaro-Tapia, R.; Figueira, R.; Pompêo, M. Chronostratigraphy Elucidates Environmental Changes in Lacustrine Sedimentation Rates and Metal Accumulation. *Environ. Sci. Pollut. Res.* **2023**, *30*, 72430–72445. [CrossRef]
3. McClain, M.E.; Naiman, R.J. Andean Influences on the Biogeochemistry and Ecology of the Amazon River. *Bioscience* **2008**, *58*, 325–338. [CrossRef]
4. Biamont-Rojas, I.E.; Cardoso-Silva, S.; Pompêo, M. Heterogeneidade Espacial e Ecotoxicidade de Metais No Sedimento Em Três Reservatorios Paulistas Aplicando Um Enfoque Geoestatístico. In *Aspectos da Ecotoxicidade em Ambientes Aquáticos*; Pompêo, M., Moschini-Carlos, V., López-Doval, J.C., Eds.; Instituto de Biociências, Universidade de São Paulo: São Paulo, Brazil, 2022; pp. 43–57.
5. Martins, T.; Ferreira, K.; Rani-Borges, B.; Biamont-Rojas, I.; Cardoso-Silva, S.; Moschini-Carlos, V.; Pompêo, M. Land Use, Spatial Heterogeneity of Organic Matter, Granulometric Fractions and Metal Complexation in Reservoir Sediments. *Acta Limnol. Bras.* **2021**, *33*, e23. [CrossRef]
6. Biamont-Rojas, I.E.; Mamani Villalba, B.A. Mercurio Derivado de La Actividad Minera Artesanal Evidencia Un Alto Potencial Tóxico En Una Subcuenca Del Lago Titicaca, Perú. In *Minería, Mercurio y Salud. Aportes de la Comunidad Académica*; Cabrera Jaramillo, A., Arango Ruiz, Á., Eds.; Editorial Lasallista: Caldas, Colombia, 2022; pp. 43–75.
7. Khan, R.; Saxena, A.; Shukla, S. Evaluation of Heavy Metal Pollution for River Gomti, in Parts of Ganga Alluvial Plain, India. *SN Appl. Sci.* **2020**, *2*, 1451. [CrossRef]
8. Brousett-Minaya, M.A.; Rondan-Sanabria, G.G.; Chirinos-Marroquín, M.; Biamont-Rojas, I. Impacto de La Minería En Aguas Superficiales de La Región Puno—Perú. *Fides Ratio—Rev. Difusión Cult. Científica Univ. Salle Boliv.* **2021**, *21*, 187–208.
9. Biamont-Rojas, I.E.; Cardoso-Silva, S.; Figueira, R.C.L.; Kim, B.S.M.; Alfaro-Tapia, R.; Pompêo, M. Spatial Distribution of Arsenic and Metals Suggest a High Ecotoxicological Potential in Puno Bay, Lake Titicaca, Peru. *Sci. Total Environ.* **2023**, *871*, 162051. [CrossRef]
10. Heilpern, S.A.; Sethi, S.A.; Barthem, R.B.; Batista, V.D.S.; Doria, C.R.C.; Duponchelle, F.; Vasquez, A.G.; Goulding, M.; Isaac, V.; Naeem, S.; et al. Biodiversity Underpins Fisheries Resilience to Exploitation in the Amazon River Basin. *Proc. R. Soc. B Biol. Sci.* **2022**, *289*, 20220726. [CrossRef]
11. Passarelli, I.; Villacis Verdesoto, M.V.; Jiménez-Oyola, S.; Flores Huilcapi, A.G.; Mora-Silva, D.; Anfuso, G.; Esparza Parra, J.F.; Jimenez-Gutierrez, M.; Carrera Almendáriz, L.S.; Avalos Peñafiel, V.G.; et al. Analysis of Mercury in Aquifers in Gold Mining Areas in the Ecuadorian Amazon and Its Associated Risk for Human Health. *Toxics* **2024**, *12*, 162. [CrossRef]
12. Mestanza-Ramón, C.; Cuenca-Cumbicus, J.; D'Orio, G.; Flores-Toala, J.; Segovia-Cáceres, S.; Bonilla-Bonilla, A.; Straface, S. Gold Mining in the Amazon Region of Ecuador: History and a Review of Its Socio-Environmental Impacts. *Land* **2022**, *11*, 221. [CrossRef]
13. Sánchez-Vázquez, L.; Espinosa-Quezada, M.G.; Eguiguren-Riofrío, M.B. "Golden Reality" or the "Reality of Gold": Artisanal Mining and Socio-Environmental Conflict in Chinapintza, Ecuador. *Extr. Ind. Soc.* **2016**, *3*, 124–128. [CrossRef]
14. Villacís, S.; Ochoa, J.; Borja, M.O.; Josse, C.; Finer, M.; Mamani, N. MAAP #151: Minería Ilegal En La Amazonía Ecuatoriana. Available online: https://www.maaproject.org/2022/mineria-ecuador/ (accessed on 10 July 2024).
15. Ulfe, M.E.; Vergara, R. Measuring Incommensurability: Compensations in Judicial Processes of Oil Spills in Northern Peruvian Amazon. *Tapuya Lat. Am. Sci. Technol. Soc.* **2022**, *5*, 2144004. [CrossRef]
16. MINSA. Ministerio de Salud; Instituto Nacional de Salud. *Niveles y Factores de Riesgo de Exposición a Metales Pesados e Hidrocarburos En Los Habitantes de Las Comunidades de Las Cuencas de Los Ríos Pastaza, Tigre, Corrientes y Marañón Del Departamento de Loreto*; Ministerio de Salud: Lima, Peru, 2017.
17. Jézéquel, C.; Tedesco, P.A.; Bigorne, R.; Maldonado-Ocampo, J.A.; Ortega, H.; Hidalgo, M.; Martens, K.; Torrente-Vilara, G.; Zuanon, J.; Acosta, A.; et al. A Database of Freshwater Fish Species of the Amazon Basin. *Sci. Data* **2020**, *7*, 96. [CrossRef] [PubMed]
18. Al-Homaidan, A.A.; Al-Otaibi, T.G.; El-Sheikh, M.A.; Al-Ghanayem, A.A.; Ameen, F. Accumulation of Heavy Metals in a Macrophyte Phragmites Australis: Implications to Phytoremediation in the Arabian Peninsula Wadis. *Environ. Monit. Assess.* **2020**, *192*, 202. [CrossRef] [PubMed]
19. Basallote, M.D.; Zarco, V.; Macías, F.; Cánovas, C.R.; Hidalgo, P.J. Metal Bioaccumulation in Spontaneously Grown Aquatic Macrophytes in Fe-Rich Substrates of a Passive Treatment Plant for Acid Mine Drainage. *J. Environ. Manag.* **2023**, *345*, 118495. [CrossRef] [PubMed]
20. INEI. Censos Nacionales 2017. Resultados Definitivos de los Censos Nacionales 2017—Puno. Available online: https://www.inei.gob.pe/media/MenuRecursivo/publicaciones_digitales/Est/Lib1563/ (accessed on 30 July 2022).
21. MINAM; Ministerio del Ambiente. *Métodos de Colecta, Identificación y Análisis de Comunidades Biológicas: Plancton, Perifiton, Bentos (Macroinvertebrados) y Necton (Peces) En Aguas Continentales Del Perú*; Zona Comunicaciones S.A.C.: Lima, Peru, 2014.
22. INEI. *Perú: Proyecciones de Población, Según Departamento, Provincia y Distrito, 2021-2022*; McGraw-Hill Interamericana: Lima, Peru, 2020.

23. López-Alvarenga, J.C.; Reding-Berrnal, A. Cálculo Del Tamaño de La Muestra: Enfoque Práctico de Sus Elementos Necesarios. In *Introducción a la Metodología de la Investigación en Ciencias de la Salud*; McGraw-Hill Interamericana: Ciudad de México, Mexico, 2011; pp. 67–76.
24. Qin, D.; Jiang, H.; Bai, S.; Tang, S.; Mou, Z. Determination of 28 Trace Elements in Three Farmed Cyprinid Fish Species from Northeast China. *Food Control* **2015**, *50*, 1–8. [CrossRef]
25. U.S. EPA. *Method 3050B: Acid Digestion of Sediments, Sludges, and Soils, Revision 2*; U.S. EPA: Washington, DC, USA, 1996.
26. U.S. EPA. *Method: 7471B Mercury in Solid or Semisolid Waste (Manual Cold-Vapor Technique)*; U.S. EPA: Washington, DC, USA, 2007.
27. FAO. *Heavy Metals Regulations Legal Notice No 66/2003*; FAO: Rome, Italy, 2003.
28. Hossain, M.B.; Ahmed, A.S.S.; Sarker, M.S.I. Human Health Risks of Hg, As, Mn, and Cr through Consumption of Fish, Ticto Barb (Puntius Ticto) from a Tropical River, Bangladesh. *Environ. Sci. Pollut. Res.* **2018**, *25*, 31727–31736. [CrossRef] [PubMed]
29. Huang, X.; Qin, D.; Gao, L.; Hao, Q.; Chen, Z.; Wang, P.; Tang, S.; Wu, S.; Jiang, H.; Qiu, W. Distribution, Contents and Health Risk Assessment of Heavy Metal(Loid)s in Fish from Different Water Bodies in Northeast China. *RSC Adv.* **2019**, *9*, 33130–33139. [CrossRef]
30. U.S. EPA. *Guidance for Assessing Chemical Contaminant Data for Use in Fish Advisories*, 3rd ed.; United States Environmental Protection Agency: Washington, DC, USA, 2000; Volume 2.
31. Legendre, P.; Legendre, L. *Numerical Ecology*, 2nd ed.; Elsevier: Amsterdam, The Netherlands, 1998. [CrossRef]
32. R Core Team. *R: A Language and Environment for Statistical Computing*; R Foundation for Statistical Computing: Vienna, Austria, 2023; Available online: https://www.R-project.org/ (accessed on 9 July 2024).
33. WHO. *Evaluation of Certain Food Additives and Contaminants: Thirty-Third Report of the Joint FAO/WHO Expert Committee on Food Additives*; WHO: Geneva, Switzerland, 1989.
34. *GB2762-2017*; National Food Safety Standard: Limits of Contaminants in Food. Office of Agricultural Affairs: Beijing, China, 2017.
35. EU. *Commission Regulation EC No. 629/2008. Setting Maximum Levels for Certain Contaminants in Foodstuffs*; EU: Brussels, Belgium, 2008.
36. ANVISA. *Agência Nacional de Vigilância Sanitária. Decreto No. 55.871. Modifica o Decreto No 50.040, de 24 de Janeiro de 1961, Referente a Normas Reguladoras do Emprêgo de Aditivos para Alimentos, Alterado Pelo Decreto No 691, de 13 de Março de 1962*, Presidência da República: Brasília, Brazil, 1965.
37. U.S. EPA. *Regional Screening Level (RSL)—Generic Tables*; U.S. EPA: Washington, DC, USA, 2024.
38. EFSA. Scientific Opinion on Lead in Food. *EFSA J.* **2010**, *8*, 1570. [CrossRef]
39. Vasco, C.; Sirén, A. Determinants of Wild Fish Consumption in Indigenous Communities in the Ecuadorian Amazon. *Soc. Nat. Resour.* **2019**, *32*, 21–33. [CrossRef]
40. Islam, M.A.; Angove, M.J.; Morton, D.W. Recent Innovative Research on Chromium (VI) Adsorption Mechanism. *Environ. Nanotechnol. Monit. Manag.* **2019**, *12*, 100267. [CrossRef]
41. Ullah, S.; Liu, Q.; Wang, S.; Jan, A.U.; Sharif, H.M.A.; Ditta, A.; Wang, G.; Cheng, H. Sources, Impacts, Factors Affecting Cr Uptake in Plants, and Mechanisms behind Phytoremediation of Cr-Contaminated Soils. *Sci. Total Environ.* **2023**, *899*, 165726. [CrossRef] [PubMed]
42. Bolelli, G.; Steduto, D.; Kiilakoski, J.; Varis, T.; Lusvarghi, L.; Vuoristo, P. Tribological Properties of Plasma Sprayed Cr_2O_3, Cr_2O_3–TiO_2, Cr_2O_3–Al_2O_3 and Cr_2O_3–ZrO_2 Coatings. *Wear* **2021**, *480–481*, 203931. [CrossRef]
43. Weber, P.; Behr, E.R.; Knorr, C.D.L.; Vendruscolo, D.S.; Flores, E.M.M.; Dressler, V.L.; Baldisserotto, B. Metals in the Water, Sediment, and Tissues of Two Fish Species from Different Trophic Levels in a Subtropical Brazilian River. *Microchem. J.* **2013**, *106*, 61–66. [CrossRef]
44. Savassi, L.A.; Paschoalini, A.L.; Arantes, F.P.; Rizzo, E.; Bazzoli, N. Heavy Metal Contamination in a Highly Consumed Brazilian Fish: Immunohistochemical and Histopathological Assessments. *Environ. Monit. Assess.* **2020**, *192*, 542. [CrossRef] [PubMed]
45. Meche, A.; Martins, M.C.; Lofrano, B.E.S.N.; Hardaway, C.J.; Merchant, M.; Verdade, L. Determination of Heavy Metals by Inductively Coupled Plasma-Optical Emission Spectrometry in Fish from the Piracicaba River in Southern Brazil. *Microchem. J.* **2010**, *94*, 171–174. [CrossRef]
46. Vu, C.T.; Lin, C.; Yeh, G.; Villanueva, M.C. Bioaccumulation and Potential Sources of Heavy Metal Contamination in Fish Species in Taiwan: Assessment and Possible Human Health Implications. *Environ. Sci. Pollut. Res.* **2017**, *24*, 19422–19434. [CrossRef] [PubMed]
47. Yi, Y.J.; Zhang, S.H. The Relationships between Fish Heavy Metal Concentrations and Fish Size in the Upper and Middle Reach of Yangtze River. *Procedia Environ. Sci.* **2012**, *13*, 1699–1707. [CrossRef]
48. Ferreira da Silva, S.; de Oliveira Lima, M. Mercury in Fish Marketed in the Amazon Triple Frontier and Health Risk Assessment. *Chemosphere* **2020**, *248*, 125989. [CrossRef]
49. Basta, P.C.; de Vasconcellos, A.C.S.; Hallwass, G.; Yokota, D.; Pinto, D.d.O.d.R.; de Aguiar, D.S.; de Souza, C.C.; Oliveira-da-Costa, M. Risk Assessment of Mercury-Contaminated Fish Consumption in the Brazilian Amazon: An Ecological Study. *Toxics* **2023**, *11*, 800. [CrossRef]
50. Rengifo, P.D.; Reyes, L.W. Presencia de Mercurio En La Amazonía Peruana, Río Napo. In *Memoria del Primer Encuentro de Investigadores Ambientales*; Ministerio del Ambiente, Dirección General de Investigación e Información Ambiental: Iquitos, Peru, 2012; pp. 1–6.

51. National Research Council (US). *Subcommittee on the Tenth Edition of the Recommended Dietary Allowances*, 10th ed.; National Academies Press (US): Washington, DC, USA, 1989.
52. da Silva Costa, M.; Viana, L.F.; Lima Cardoso, C.A.; Gonar Silva Isacksson, E.D.; Silva, J.C.; Florentino, A.C. Landscape Composition and Inorganic Contaminants in Water and Muscle Tissue of Plagioscion Squamosissimus in the Araguari River (Amazon, Brazil). *Environ. Res.* **2022**, *208*, 112691. [CrossRef] [PubMed]
53. Souza-Araujo, J.; Souza-Junior, O.G.; Guimarães-Costa, A.; Hussey, N.E.; Lima, M.O.; Giarrizzo, T. The Consumption of Shark Meat in the Amazon Region and Its Implications for Human Health and the Marine Ecosystem. *Chemosphere* **2021**, *265*, 129132. [CrossRef] [PubMed]
54. Instituto Geológico, Minero y Metalúrgico (INGEMMET). *Mapa Metalogenético del oro del Perú: Operaciones y Proyectos Mineros;* Instituto Geológico, Minero y Metalúrgico (INGEMMET): Lima, Peru, 2023; Available online: https://hdl.handle.net/20.500.12544/3839 (accessed on 19 July 2024).
55. Mestanza-Ramón, C.; Jiménez-Oyola, S.; Montoya, A.V.G.; Vizuete, D.D.C.; D'Orio, G.; Cedeño-Laje, J.; Straface, S. Assessment of Hg Pollution in Stream Waters and Human Health Risk in Areas Impacted by Mining Activities in the Ecuadorian Amazon. *Environ. Geochem. Health* **2023**, *45*, 7183–7197. [CrossRef] [PubMed]

toxics

MDPI

Article

Associations between Ethylene Oxide Exposure and Liver Function in the US Adult Population

Shanshan Li [1,†], Jinzhou Wang [2,†], Dengliang Lei [1], Dadi Peng [1], Kezhen Zong [1], Kaili Li [1], Zhongjun Wu [1], Yanyao Liu [1,*] and Zuotian Huang [1,*]

1 First Affiliated Hospital of Chongqing Medical University, Chongqing 400000, China; 2022110196@stu.cqmu.edu.cn (S.L.); ldldoctor@126.com (D.L.); dadi_peng@163.com (D.P.); zongkezhen23@163.com (K.Z.); 2019110257@stu.cqmu.edu.cn (K.L.); wzjtcy@126.com (Z.W.)

2 Affiliated Hospital of North Sichuan Medical College, Nanchong 637000, China; wjz19990819@163.com

* Correspondence: liuyanyao147@sina.com (Y.L.); huangzuotian@cqu.edu.cn (Z.H.)

† These authors contributed equally to this work.

Abstract: Background: Ethylene oxide, a reactive epoxy compound, has been widely used in various industries for many years. However, evidence of the combined toxic effects of ethylene oxide exposure on the liver is still lacking. Methods: We analyzed the merged data from the National Health and Nutrition Examination Survey (NHANES) from 2013 to 2016. Ultimately, 4141 adults aged 18 and over were selected as the sample. We used linear regression to explore the association between blood ethylene oxide and LFT indicators. Results: The weighted linear regression model showed that HbEO is positively correlated with ALP (β = 2.61, 95% CI 1.97, 3.24, $p < 0.0001$), GGT (β = 5.75, 95% CI 4.46, 7/05, $p < 0.0001$), ALT (β = 0.50, 95% CI 0.09, 0.90, p = 0.0158), and AST (β = 0.71, 95% CI 0.44, 0.98, $p < 0.0001$) and negatively correlated with TBIL (β = −0.30, 95% CI −0.43, −0.16, $p < 0.0001$). Conclusions: Ethylene oxide exposure is significantly associated with changes in liver function indicators among adults in the United States. Future work should further examine these relationships.

Keywords: ethylene oxide; NHANES; liver function test

1. Introduction

As the largest synthetic organ in the human body, the liver participates in physiological functions such as plasma protein synthesis, gluconeogenesis and glycogen storage, cholesterol metabolism, bile acid synthesis, and detoxification [1,2]. In recent decades, liver diseases, such as non-alcoholic fatty liver disease, alcoholic liver disease, and viral hepatitis, have become one of the leading causes of death and illness worldwide, with approximately 2 million people dying from these diseases each year [3,4]. Since the last century, liver function tests (LFTs) have been the primary means of diagnosing liver disease [5]. During the progression of liver diseases, when hepatocyte necrosis or liver cell membrane damage occurs, the serum levels of alanine aminotransferase (ALT), aspartate aminotransferase (AST), and total bilirubin (TBIL) often increase [6,7]. Alkaline phosphotase (ALP) and gamma-glutamyl transferase (GGT) are commonly used to identify cholestasis in medical research [8,9]. Increasing evidence suggests that many pollutants and chemical contaminants in the environment may cause liver damage and increase the risk of liver disease [10–12].

Ethylene oxide (EO), a reactive epoxy compound, is widely utilized in the production of plastics and surfactants and in the sterilization of fragrances, cosmetics, and medical devices. The primary marker for EO exposure is the ethylene oxide adduct in hemoglobin (HbEO), measured using a modified Edman reaction. EO exposure predominantly occurs through exogenous pathways, including inhalation and ingestion, impacting occupational, environmental, and consumer health. Additionally, EO is endogenously produced in the body via cytochrome P450 2E1-mediated oxidation of ethylene [13–15]. However, despite its widespread use, EO has associated health risks that have garnered significant attention. Existing animal studies have revealed that high-dose EO exposure leads to damage across multiple systems, including the respiratory, hematological, nervous, reproductive, and renal systems [16–19]. More alarmingly, the International Agency for Research on Cancer has classified the alkylating agent EO as a Group 1 human carcinogen [20]. In recent years, beyond the aforementioned health risks, large-scale cross-sectional studies have also suggested potential links between EO and chronic kidney disease, asthma, dyslipidemia, and hypertension [21–24]. However, the relationship between EO exposure and liver damage remains unclear.

We conducted a cross-sectional study using data from the NHANES 2013–2016 to investigate the relationship between ethylene oxide exposure and liver function damage among adults in the United States. Initially, 20,146 participants were enrolled. A total of 4141 participants were included in our final analysis after excluding individuals with missing data on liver function tests (n = 7338) and those with missing data on ethylene oxide (n = 8667).

2. Materials and Methods

2.1. Study Population

Data were obtained from NHANES, a national population-based cross-sectional survey to collect information about the potential health risk factors and nutrition status of non-institutionalized US civilians, which was conducted by the National Center for Health Statistics (NCHS) [25]. A complex, stratified, multistage probability cluster sampling design was employed to recruit a representative sample of the whole US population. The specific research method is as follows: Counties are stratified into 15 distinct clusters based on shared characteristics for the purposes of the NHANES. From each cluster, one representative county is selected annually to participate in the survey. Subsequently, within each selected county, 20 to 24 neighborhoods are identified as smaller sampling units. Comprehensive lists of all residential units within these neighborhoods are compiled, from which approximately 30 households per neighborhood are randomly chosen for inclusion in the study. NHANES personnel initiate contact with these selected households to administer a preliminary questionnaire, which gathers essential demographic data including the age, race, and gender of all household members. A computerized random selection algorithm is then employed to determine the final inclusion of individuals from these households into the survey cohort, with the selection process potentially including some, all, or none of the household members. All NHANES participants provided informed signed agreement, and approval was obtained from the Research Ethics Committee of the National Centre for Health Statistics. The detailed NHANES study design and data are publicly available at https://www.cdc.gov/nchs/nhanes/ (accessed on 25 June 2024). Participants received a standardized in-home interview and health examination at mobile examination centers to assess their medical and physiological status, and laboratory tests were conducted to collect their laboratory data. Our study was based on two NHANES survey cycles from 2013 to 2014 and from 2015 to 2016, knowing these two cycles include data on both HbEO and liver function tests. The inclusion criteria for the participants were as follows: (1) individuals over 18 years old, (2) individuals with comprehensive demographic information, and (3) individuals with complete ethylene oxide and liver function tests. The exclusion criteria were as follows: (1) individuals lacking ethylene oxide laboratory data, (2) individuals without liver function test data, (3) individuals younger than 18 years old. A total of 20,146 participants were enrolled at first. Individuals missing data on liver function tests (n = 7338) and ethylene oxide (n = 8667) were then excluded, and 4141 participants were included in our final analysis (Figure 1).

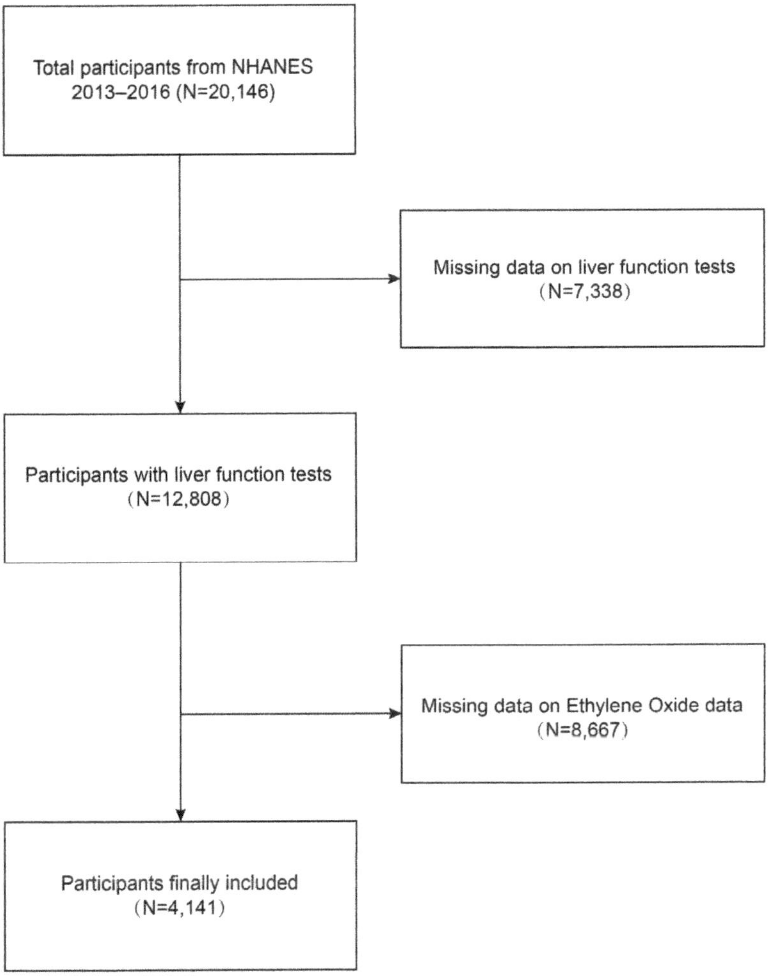

Figure 1. Process map for sample collection from NHANES.

2.2. Assessment of Hemoglobin Ethylene Oxide Levels

The measurement of HbEO in this investigation was conducted according to the NHANES Laboratory/Medical Technologist Procedures Manual, which may be found at https://wwwn.cdc.gov/Nchs/Nhanes/2013-2014/ETHOX_H.htm (accessed on 25 June 2024). The collection, processing, and transportation of specimens were conducted in accordance with established protocols.

The Division of Laboratory Sciences of the National Center for Environmental Health (NCEH) has been assigned the responsibility of measuring HbEO. Detailed information about the laboratory analysis techniques can be found on the corresponding webpage. The researchers utilized the modified Edman reaction and high-performance liquid chromatography coupled with tandem mass spectrometry to identify the presence of ethylene oxide (EO) adducts in hemoglobin. Specifically, they focused on detecting two types of adducts: N-(2-carbamoyl-ethyl) valine EO adducts (CEVs) and N-(2-hydroxycarbamoyl-ethyl) valine EO adducts (HEVs). The levels of HbEO were quantified and expressed in picomoles per gram of hemoglobin (pmol/g Hb). The assays' accuracy and precision were in line with the quality control and quality assurance standards set by the NCEH Laboratory Science Division (CDC 2023).

2.3. Measurement of Liver Function

Serum LFTs were measured using various methods utilizing a Beckman Coulter UniCel DxC800 Synchron Clinical System (Beckman Coulter, Inc., Brea, CA, USA). The activities of both ALT and ALP were determined using the kinetic rate method commonly employed in medical research. The enzymatic rate method was used to determine the activities of AST and GGT. The TBIL serum level was measured using a timed-endpoint Diazo method.

2.4. Covariates

Potential covariates that might confound the association between HbEO and LFTs were summarized in the multivariable-adjusted models. Covariates in our study included gender (male/female), age (<50 and ≥50 years), race, education level, poverty-to-income ratio (PIR), total cholesterol level (mg/dL), HDL level (mmol/L), body mass index (BMI), smoking status (smoking or not), diabetes, aspirin, alcohol, acetaminophen, statins, hepatitis B, and hepatitis C.

PIR was estimated as the ratio of family income to the poverty threshold, and participants were divided into low-income (PIR < 1.3), middle-income (PIR = 1.30–3.50), and high-income (PIR ≥ 3.50) groups. BMI was categorized as <25, 25–29.9, and ≥30 kg/m^2, which correspond to normal weight, overweight, and obese population for all participants. All detailed measurement processes for study variables are publicly available at www.cdc.gov/nchs/nhanes/ (accessed on 25 June 2024).

2.5. Statistical Analysis

All statistical analyses were conducted according to Centers for Disease Control and Prevention (CDC) guidelines, and an appropriate NHANES sampling weight was applied, accounting for the complex multistage cluster survey design in the analysis. Continuous variables are presented as means with standard deviation, and categorical variables are presented as a percentage. Either a weighted Student's *t*-test (for continuous variables) or weighted chi-square test (for categorical variables) was used to evaluate the differences in groups divided by HbEO (quartiles). Multivariate logistic regression models were employed to explore the independent relationship between HbEO and liver function tests in three different models. In model 1, no covariates were adjusted. Model 2 was adjusted for gender, age, and race. Model 3 was adjusted for gender, age, race, education level, poverty-to-income ratio, HDL, total cholesterol, BMI, smoking status, diabetes, aspirin, alcohol, statins, hepatitis B, and hepatitis C. Smooth curve fitting (penalized spline method) and weighted generalized additive model (GAM) regression were conducted to further assess the nonlinear relationship between HbEO and liver function tests. Subgroup analysis stratified by gender, age, BMI, diabetes, and education level was also performed via stratified multivariate regression analysis. In addition, an interaction term was added to test the heterogeneity of associations between the subgroups using the log likelihood ratio test model. $p < 0.05$ was considered statistically significant. All analyses were performed using Empower version 4.1 (www.empowerstats.com; X&Y solutions, Inc., Boston, MA, USA) and R version 3.4.3 (http://www.R-project.org, The R Foundation, Vienna, Austria).

3. Results

3.1. Baseline Characteristics of Participants

Weighted demographic baseline characteristics of included participants are shown in Table 1. A total of 4141 participants were included in our study, of whom 50.02% were male and 49.98% were female, with the average age of 43.68 ± 18.99 years. The mean of log2 HbEO was 4.74 ± 1.47, and the ranges of log2 HbEO for quartiles 1–4 were 2.54–3.91, 3.91–4.37, 4.37–5.18, and 5.18–10.35, respectively. In total, compared to those in quartile 1, participants in quartile 4 had lower rates of ALP and TBIL and a higher rate of GGT. In addition, we found statistically significant differences by age, gender, race, education level, PIR, BMI, diabetes, smoking, serum HDL, serum cholesterol, alcohol, acetaminophen, statins, hepatitis B, and hepatitis C (all $p < 0.05$) among log2 HbEO quartiles. Similarly, the results in the population baseline table remained consistent across quartiles of HbEO that had not undergone logarithmic transformation (Supplement Table S1).

Table 1. Baseline characteristics of the study population.

Characteristic	Q1 N = 1029	Q2 N = 1035	Q3 N = 1041	Q4 N = 1036	p-Value
Age (years)	18.98	19.75	20.71	16.32	<0.0001
<50	44.54	42.19	38.76	51.47	
≥50	55.46	57.81	61.24	48.53	
Gender					<0.0001
Male	42.87	45.57	56.95	49.52	
Female	57.13	54.43	43.05	50.48	
Race, n (%)					<0.0001
Mexican American	7.29	8.95	8.88	5.70	
Other Hispanic	5.01	4.69	5.09	4.02	
Non-Hispanic White	76.60	69.60	62.78	69.20	
Non-Hispanic Black	6.43	9.78	11.76	14.43	
Other Race	4.68	6.98	11.49	6.66	
Education Level, n (%)					<0.0001
Less than high school	10.62	13.01	12.31	22.16	
High school	19.41	19.07	31.87	28.20	
More than high school	69.97	67.92	55.82	49.64	
PIR					<0.0001
<1.3	14.94	18.22	27.42	41.25	
1.3–3.5	40.32	38.11	35.15	36.26	
≥3.5	44.74	43.66	37.42	22.49	
BMI (kg/m^2)					<0.0001
<25	26.52	21.58	28.92	31.37	
>25	73.18	78.42	71.08	68.63	
Smoking, n (%)					<0.0001
Yes	33.75	31.00	45.25	88.25	
No	66.25	69.00	54.75	11.75	
Diabetes, n (%)					<0.0001
Yes	12.36	18.95	27.76	15.29	
No	87.64	81.05	72.21	84.71	
Alcohol, n (%)					<0.0001
Yes	78.24	66.57	78.18	83.37	
No	21.76	33.43	21.82	16.63	
Aspirin, n (%)					0.1284
Yes	68.58	73.78	74.05	59.80	
No	31.42	26.22	25.95	40.20	
Acetaminophen					0.0021
Yes	0.61	1.22	0.58	1.71	
No	99.39	98.78	99.42	98.29	
Statins, n (%)					0.0121
Yes	82.65	87.93	82.35	83.76	
No	17.35	12.07	17.65	16.24	
Hepatitis B, n (%)					<0.0001
Yes	1.25	1.80	1.64	3.55	
No	98.75	98.20	98.36	96.45	
Hepatitis C, n (%)					<0.0001
Yes	1.06	0.24	1.46	6.03	
No	98.94	99.76	98.54	93.97	
AST (U/L)	26.04 ± 10.41	25.38 ± 16.32	24.85 ± 10.15	30.09 ± 25.75	<0.0001
ALT (U/L)	24.82 ± 15.66	24.48 ± 14.54	24.93 ± 14.56	28.62 ± 26.88	<0.0001
GGT (U/L)	26.29 ± 27.69	25.53 ± 32.51	25.23 ± 21.24	46.95 ± 91.90	<0.0001
ALP (U/L)	69.11 ± 38.62	71.46 ± 40.62	72.11 ± 40.67	72.64 ± 30.06	0.0242
TBIL (μmol/L)	10.81 ± 6.88	10.44 ± 4.99	10.53 ± 4.48	9.38 ± 4.14	<0.0001
HDL (mmol/L)	54.77 ± 18.00	52.29 ± 14.52	51.35 ± 15.36	50.23 ± 15.83	<0.0001
Total cholesterol (mmol/L)	186.89 ± 40.65	181.75 ± 43.00	179.66 ± 40.33	187.98 ± 42.82	<0.0001

Continuous variables are presented as means ± standard deviation, and the p value was calculated using the weighted linear regression model. Categorical variables are displayed as a percentage.

3.2. Multiple Linear Regression Associations of Ethylene Oxide with LFTs in Adults

Table 2 shows the association between ethylene oxide and LFTs. Firstly, the log2-transformed HbEO was utilized as a continuous variable to investigate its correlation with liver function. In model 1, we found that ALT (β 0.69, 95% CI 0.40, 0.99, $p < 0.0001$), AST (β 0.71, 95% CI 0.44, 0.98, $p < 0.0001$), and GGT (β 1.63, 95% CI 0.80, 2.45, $p < 0.001$) were positively related to HbEO. In contrast, TBIL (β −0.42, 95% CI −0.50, −0.34, $p < 0.0001$) was negatively linked with HbEO. In model 2, we found that ALP ($\beta = 2.61$, 95% CI 1.97, 3.24, $p < 0.0001$), GGT ($\beta = 5.75$, 95% CI 4.46, 7/05, $p < 0.0001$), and ALT ($\beta = 0.50$, 95% CI 0.09, 0.90, $p = 0.0158$) had a positive relationship with HbEO. However, TBIL ($\beta = -0.30$, 95% CI −0.43, −0.16, $p < 0.0001$) was negatively linked with HbEO. Then, sensitivity analysis was conducted, treating log2-transformed HbEO as a categorical variable (quartiles). In the fully adjusted model (model 2), compared with the lowest HbEO quartile (quartile 1), participants in the top HbEO quartile had 8.48 IU/L higher ALP, 15.06 IU/L higher GGT, 2.60 IU/L lower AST, and 1.19 IU/L lower TBIL than those in the HbEO quartile, and the P values for trends were <0.0001, <0.0001, 0.0695, <0.0001, correspondingly. However, the association between ALT (β −2.41, 95% CI −7.83, 3.01, $p = 0.3853$) and HbEO quartiles met statistical significance only in model 1. Moreover, smooth curve fitting exhibited a non-linear relationship between LFTs and HbEO (Figure 2). We further calculated the inflection points for ALP, ALT, AST, and GGT to be 6.73, 6.58, 6.62, and 6.08, respectively. To the left of the inflection point, a positive relationship between ALT, AST, GGT, and HbEO ($\beta = -0.41$, 95% CI: −1.16, 0.35, $p = 0.2884$; $\beta = -1.82$, 95% CI: −2.67, −0.97, $p < 0.0001$; $\beta = -2.10$, 95% CI: −4.42, 0.23, $p = 0.0769$) was detected. Conversely, to the right of the inflection point, a negative relationship between ALT, AST, GGT, and HbEO ($\beta = 3.43$, 95% CI: 1.83, 5.03, $p < 0.0001$; $\beta = 4.02$, 95% CI: 2.16, 5.89, $p < 0.0001$; $\beta = 17.81$, 95% CI: 14.38, 21.23, $p < 0.0001$) was observed. After the adjustment of covariates, the logarithmic likelihood ratio test P value was <0.001 (Supplement Table S2). However, in the quartiles of HbEO without Log2 transformation, the linear regression results did not exhibit statistically significant differences (Supplement Table S3).

Table 2. The association between log2-transform HbEO and the liver function test.

LFTs	Model	Continuous log2-Transformed EO	Quartile 1 β (95% CI)	Quartile 2 β (95% CI)	Quartile 3 β (95% CI)	Quartile 4 β (95% CI)	p for Trend
ALP	Crude	1.00 (0.40, 1.60) 0.0012	0.00 (Ref.)	2.35 (−0.06, 4.75) 0.0556	3.00 (0.47, 5.53) 0.0201	3.53 (1.06, 6.00) 0.0051	0.0179
	Model 1	0.47 (−0.12, 1.06) 0.1169	0.00 (Ref.)	1.98 (−0.36, 4.31) 0.0974	2.97 (0.48, 5.46) 0.0194	1.68 (−0.73, 4.10) 0.1722	0.4080
	Model 2	2.61 (1.97, 3.24) <0.0001	0.00 (Ref.)	0.48 (−1.78, 2.74) 0.6760	3.75 (1.30, 6.20) 0.0027	8.48 (5.75, 11.22) <0.0001	<0.0001
ALT	Crude	0.72 (0.42, 1.01) <0.0001	0.00 (Ref.)	−0.34 (−1.51, 0.84) 0.5754	0.11 (−1.12, 1.35) 0.8573	3.80 (2.59, 5.01) <0.0001	<0.0001
	Model 1	0.69 (0.40, 0.99) <0.0001	0.00 (Ref.)	−0.42 (−1.57, 0.73) 0.4747	−0.73 (−1.96, 0.49) 0.2398	3.65 (2.46, 4.83) <0.0001	<0.0001
	Model 2	0.50 (0.09, 0.90) 0.0158	0.00 (Ref.)	−1.65 (−3.07, −0.24) 0.0223	−0.25 (−1.79, 1.29) 0.7517	0.36 (−1.36, 2.07) 0.6846	0.3020
AST	Crude	0.67 (0.40, 0.94) <0.0001	0.00 (Ref.)	−0.67 (−1.73, 0.40) 0.2187	−1.20 (−2.32, −0.08) 0.0358	4.05 (2.95, 5.14) <0.0001	<0.0001
	Model 1	0.71 (0.44, 0.98) <0.0001	0.00 (Ref.)	−0.67 (−1.72, 0.39) 0.2136	−1.71 (−2.84, −0.59) 0.0028	4.16 (3.07, 5.25) <0.0001	<0.0001
	Model 2	−0.39 (−0.89, 0.11) 0.1242	0.00 (Ref.)	−2.54 (−4.29, −0.78) 0.0047	−3.17 (−5.07, −1.26) 0.0011	−2.60 (−4.73, −0.48) 0.0165	0.0695
GGT	Crude	4.53 (3.72, 5.35) <0.0001	0.00 (Ref.)	−0.75 (−3.98, 2.48) 0.6476	−1.06 (−4.46, 2.35) 0.5430	20.66 (17.34,23.98) <0.0001	<0.0001
	Model 1	4.62 (3.80, 5.44) <0.0001	0.00 (Ref.)	−1.09 (−4.31, 2.12) 0.5049	−2.70 (−6.13, 0.72) 0.1222	20.81 (17.49,24.14) <0.0001	<0.0001
	Model 2	5.75 (4.46, 7.05) <0.0001	0.00 (Ref.)	−3.84 (−8.43, 0.76) 0.1018	−1.33 (−6.32, 3.66) 0.6016	15.06 (9.50, 20.63) <0.0001	<0.0001
TBIL	Crude	−0.39 (−0.48, −0.31) <0.0001	0.00 (Ref.)	−0.38 (−0.71, −0.04) 0.0302	−0.29 (−0.64, 0.07) 0.1150	−1.43 (−1.78, −1.08) <0.0001	<0.0001
	Model 1	−0.42 (−0.50, −0.34) <0.0001	0.00 (Ref.)	−0.42 (−0.75, −0.09) 0.0125	−0.62 (−0.98, −0.27) 0.0005	−1.55 (−1.89, −1.21) <0.0001	<0.0001
	Model 2	−0.30 (−0.43, −0.16) <0.0001	0.00 (Ref.)	0.18 (−0.29, 0.65) 0.4593	0.10 (−0.41, 0.61) 0.7009	−1.19 (−1.76, −0.62) <0.0001	<0.0001

Crude model: no covariates were adjusted. Model 1: age, gender, and race were adjusted. Model 2: age, gender, race, educational level, BMI, family income-to-poverty ratio, moderate activities, diabetes status, aspirin, acetaminophen, alcohol, statins, hepatitis B, hepatitis C, smoking, HDL level, and total cholesterol were adjusted.

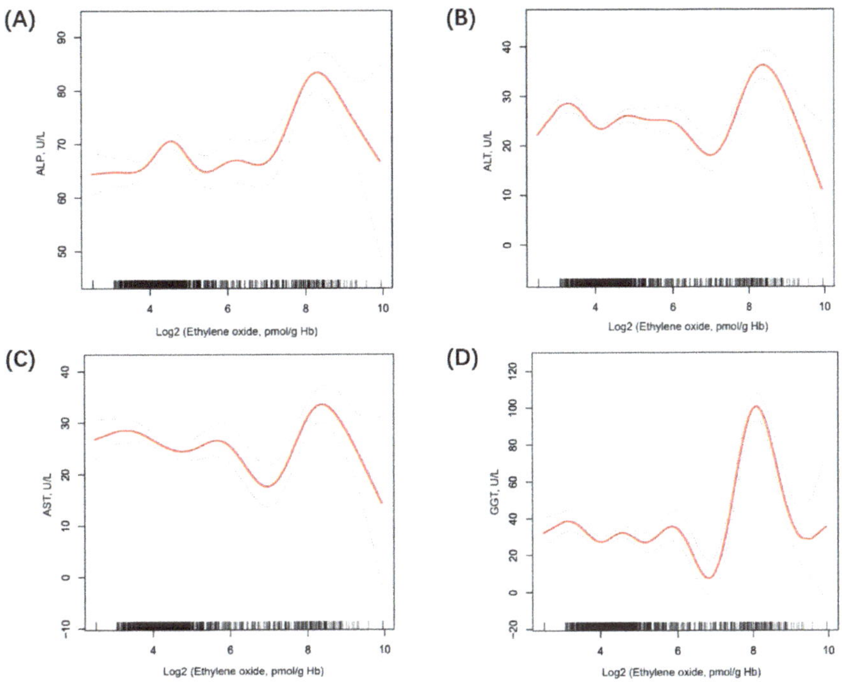

Figure 2. The nonlinear relationship between LFTs and log2-HbEO. (**A**) The association between ALP and HbEO; (**B**) The association between ALT and HbEO; (**C**) The association between AST and HbEO; (**D**) The association between GGT and HbEO. The solid line and dashed lines represent the fitted line and 95% confidence interval, respectively.

3.3. Subgroup Analysis

In order to evaluate whether the association between ethylene oxide and LFTs was consistent in the overall population and find the potential different population settings, we conducted subgroup analysis and an interaction test stratified by gender, age, education level, BMI, diabetes, and smoking (Table 3). In the male group, there was a negative correlation between ALT and GGT ($\beta = -0.75$, 95% CI -1.35, -0.14, $p < 0.0001$; $\beta = -0.70$, 95% CI -2.59, 1.19, $p < 0.0001$) and a robust positive correlation between ALP and HbEO concentrations ($\beta = 3.81$, 95%CI 2.86, 4.76, $p < 0.0001$). In the younger subgroup stratified by age, ALP and TBIL exhibited positive correlation with HbEO ($\beta = 5.56$, 95% CI 3.78, 7.33, $p = 0.0002$; $\beta = 0.05$, 95% CI -0.21, 0.30, $p = 0.0036$), while ALT and GGT showed negative association (all $p < 0.05$). Regarding subgroup analyses stratified by education level, ALT, GGT, and HbEO in the high school groups showed a negative connection ($\beta = -1.10$, 95% CI -2.05, -0.16, $p = 0.0245$; $\beta = -0.41$, 95% CI 3.35, 2.52, $p = 0.0007$). With regard to subgroup analyses stratified by BMI, GGT was strongly positive linked with HbEO in the high BMI group ($\beta = 2.32$, 95% CI 1.20, 3.44, $p = 0.0227$), while AST and GGT showed negative association ($\beta = -0.88$, 95% CI -1.42, -0.34, $p = 0.0016$). With reference to diabetes-stratified subgroup analyses, there was a positive correlation between ALT and HbEO in the diabetes groups ($\beta = 1.49$, 95% CI 0.81, 2.18, $p < 0.0001$). Furthermore, GGT showed positive correlation with HbEO in smokers compared with non-smokers ($\beta = 5.51$, 95% CI 4.09, 6.94, $p < 0.0001$). Taken together, the substantial connection with the p for interaction suggested that this association between liver function and HbEO showed dependence on gender, age, education level, BMI, diabetes, and smoking (p for interaction < 0.05).

Table 3. Subgroup analysis of the association between log2-HbEO and LFTs.

Subgroup	ALP [β (95% CI)]	*p* for Interaction	ALT [β (95% CI)]	*p* for Interaction	AST [β (95% CI)]	*p* for Interaction	GGT [β (95% CI)]	*p* for Interaction	TBIL [β (95% CI)]	*p* for Interaction
Gender		<0.0001		<0.0001		0.2503		<0.0001		0.7400
Male	3.81 (2.86, 4.76)		−0.75 (−1.35, −0.14)		−0.36 (−1.12, 0.40)		−0.70 (−2.59, 1.19)		−0.22 (−0.43, −0.02)	
Female	0.87 (0.00, 1.74)		1.23 (0.68, 1.78)		−0.96 (−1.65, −0.27)		8.83 (7.11, 10.56)		−0.27 (−0.45, −0.09)	
Age		0.0002		0.0086		0.5331		0.0002		0.0036
<50	5.56 (3.78, 7.33)		−0.86 (−1.98, 0.27)		−0.91 (−2.30, 0.49)		−0.47 (−4.11, 3.17)		0.05 (−0.21, 0.30)	
≥50	1.97 (1.26, 2.67)		0.75 (0.30, 1.19)		−0.44 (−0.99, 0.12)		7.04 (5.59, 8.48)		−0.38 (−0.53, −0.23)	
Education level		0.0403		0.0245		0.5037		0.0007		<0.0001
Less than high school	1.95 (0.56, 3.34)		0.03 (−0.87, 0.92)		−1.68 (−2.80, −0.56)		4.70 (1.92, 7.48)		−0.97 (−1.26, −0.67)	
High school	3.47 (2.01, 4.94)		−1.10 (−2.05, −0.16)		−1.18 (−2.36, −0.00)		−0.41 (−3.35, 2.52)		0.14 (−0.18, 0.45)	
More than high school	1.33 (0.49, 2.16)		0.39 (−0.15, 0.93)		−0.92 (−1.59, −0.24)		6.04 (4.37, 7.71)		−0.18 (−0.36, 0.00)	
BMI		0.2370		0.2795		0.0016		0.0039		0.9680
<25	1.14 (−0.69, 2.97)		−0.06 (−1.21, 1.09)		1.56 (0.13, 3.00)		0.44 (−3.26, 4.14)		−0.29 (−0.67, 0.10)	
≥25	2.31 (1.62, 2.99)		0.61 (0.18, 1.04)		−0.88 (−1.42, −0.34)		6.22 (4.83, 7.61)		−0.29 (−0.44, −0.15)	
Diabetes status		<0.0001		<0.0001		0.0253		0.0597		0.7444
Yes	0.21 (−0.85, 1.28)		1.49 (0.81, 2.18)		−1.35 (−2.20, −0.51)		6.85 (4.65, 9.05)		−0.37 (−0.60, −0.14)	
No	3.53 (2.74, 4.32)		−0.37 (−0.88, 0.13)		−0.16 (−0.79, 0.47)		4.25 (2.62, 5.88)		−0.32 (−0.49, −0.15)	
Smoking		0.3743		0.2015		0.9654		<0.0001		0.0048
Yes	1.89 (1.17, 2.60)		0.40 (−0.06, 0.86)		−0.68 (−1.25, −0.11)		5.51 (4.09, 6.94)		−0.46 (−0.61, −0.31)	
No	2.83 (0.86, 4.79)		−0.46 (−1.71, 0.79)		−0.72 (−2.29, 0.85)		−4.05 (−7.96, −0.15)		0.15 (−0.25, 0.55)	

Adjusted for age, gender, race, educational level, BMI, family income-to-poverty ratio, moderate activities, diabetes status, aspirin, acetaminophen, alcohol, statins, hepatitis B, hepatitis C, smoking, HDL level, and total cholesterol.

4. Discussion

In this nationally representative study, we primarily examined the impact of ethylene oxide (HbEO) on liver function tests (LFTs) in adults, revealing significant associations between HbEO levels and GGT, TBIL, and ALP. Specifically, elevated EtO exposure was correlated with increasing ALP, ALT, and GGT, while, intriguingly, negative correlation emerged with TBIL. Additionally, the non-linear relationship between HbEO and ALP, ALT, AST, and GGT changes direction significantly beyond the identified inflection points of 6.73, 6.58, 6.62, and 6.08 pmol/g Hb. These findings provide new insights into the potential impact of ethylene oxide on liver function, underscoring the necessity of further research into the links between environmental exposure and liver health.

To our knowledge, this is the first study to examine the association between ethylene oxide and liver function indexes in US adults. Ethylene oxide, a reactive epoxy compound, is commonly used for sterilizing materials such as food, spices, and medical devices [26]. Previous studies have found that the health impacts of ethylene oxide are primarily due to its carcinogenicity, mutagenicity, and toxic effects [27–29]. Although the health impacts of ethylene oxide mainly affect workers in medical device sterilization, the general population's risk of exposure increases through activities such as renovations, smoking, and living near facilities that use ethylene oxide [30,31]. Several cross-sectional surveys based in the United States have discovered a significant correlation between exposure to ethylene oxide and conditions such as kidney stones, depression, asthma, and chronic kidney disease in the general population [22,32,33]. However, no reports on its impact on the liver have been published. In this study, we utilized multiple LFTs to quantitatively assess the liver damage in participants. The results indicate a positive correlation between exposure to ethylene oxide and liver function markers GGT and ALP and a negative correlation with TBIL and ALT, consistent with recent studies on the impact of environmental toxins on liver function [34,35]. The nonlinear relationship between liver function tests (LFTs) and hemoglobin-bound ethylene oxide (HbEO) exhibits a threshold effect: when the HbEO concentration is below the inflection point, ALP, ALT, AST, and GGT levels increase with the rise in HbEO levels. However, when HbEO concentration exceeds the inflection point, ALP, ALT, AST, and GGT levels begin to decrease. This observed threshold effect suggests that at lower HbEO levels, the liver mitigates oxidative stress by augmenting liver metabolite production, thereby promoting glutathione turnover to manage the elevated oxidative load. Nonetheless, when HbEO concentrations surpass the liver's oxidative stress management capacity, the ability of HbEO to produce liver metabolites and regulate oxidative stress becomes overwhelmed, leading to a decline in ALP, ALT, AST, and GGT levels. This pattern underscores the liver's adaptive response to oxidative stress, with glutathione acting as a biomarker for liver metabolism and oxidative stress levels. Subgroup analysis revealed that the impact of ethylene oxide exposure on liver function remains consistent across various subgroups. Further, subgroup analysis underscored the interaction between HbEO exposure and conditions such as diabetes and obesity, observing different impacts on liver enzyme levels. These interactions highlight the complex interplay between metabolic health and exposure to environmental toxins, suggesting that individuals with metabolic disorders might be more sensitive to the hepatotoxic effects of HbEO [36]. The variation in TBIL levels between smokers and non-smokers exposed to HbEO also suggests a potential modulatory effect of smoking on liver function and its response to environmental toxins [37].

The potential mechanisms linking ethylene oxide exposure to liver damage remain unclear and warrant further investigation. Our study findings indicate a positive correlation between ethylene oxide exposure and certain liver injuries, suggesting that increased exposure could potentially adversely affect liver health. Several possible mechanisms and genes could underpin these associations. Firstly, EO generates reactive oxygen species (ROS), resulting in oxidative stress and DNA damage. This oxidative stress disrupts cellular functions and leads to hepatotoxicity [38]. Additionally, EO can cause epigenetic modifications such as DNA methylation and histone modification, which alter gene expression patterns and contribute to liver dysfunction [39]. EO exposure induces an inflammatory response in the liver, characterized by immune cell activation and pro-inflammatory cytokine release, which exacerbates liver damage [40]. Moreover, EO disrupts the hepatic metabolic pathways crucial for detoxification, leading to the accumulation of toxic intermediates and further liver damage [41]. The exposure also activates apoptotic and necrotic pathways in liver cells, causing significant tissue damage and functional decline [38]. The key genes affected by EO include TP53, vital for DNA repair and apoptosis regulation, and cytochrome P450 enzymes such as CYP2E1 and CYP3A4, which are involved in EO metabolism [42,43]. EO impacts the Nrf2 signaling pathway, reducing antioxidant capacity and increasing oxidative stress. Additionally, genes encoding pro-inflammatory cytokines IL-6 and TNF-α and apoptosis regulators BAX and BCL-2 are modulated by EO, promoting chronic inflammation and apoptotic cell death [44]. Molecular biomarkers associated with EO exposure and liver function include 8-hydroxy-2′-deoxyguanosine (8-OHdG), indicating oxidative DNA damage, and reduced glutathione (GSH) levels, reflecting oxidative stress. Elevated liver enzymes ALT and AST signify liver damage, while increased serum levels of IL-6 and TNF-α indicate inflammation. Dysregulated microRNAs, such as miR-122 and miR-192, serve as biomarkers for EO-induced liver toxicity [45,46].

Our study boasts several advantages. Firstly, by utilizing nationwide representative data and a robust statistical framework, we provide insights into the exposure to ethylene oxide and its association with liver function, especially by identifying the inflection point in the ALP/ALT/AST/GGT–HbEO relationship. This offers a new dose–response understanding of the hepatotoxic effects of EtO. However, certain limitations must be considered. The cross-sectional design limits the ability to infer causality between HbEO exposure and changes in liver function tests. Additionally, relying on self-reported data for certain demographic and lifestyle factors could introduce bias. Future research should focus on longitudinal designs to better elucidate the temporal dynamics between HbEO exposure and liver function, as well as mechanistic studies to understand the underlying biological pathways.

5. Conclusions

In summary, our study demonstrates a significant association between high levels of HbEO exposure and liver function tests (LFTs). Moreover, our data suggest that exposure to ethylene oxide may be linked to liver damage. Given the potential limitations of the current study, further longitudinal research is needed to validate the hepatotoxicity of ethylene oxide exposure and explore potential mechanisms.

Supplementary Materials: The following supporting information can be downloaded at: https://www.mdpi.com/article/10.3390/toxics12080551/s1, Table S1: Baseline characteristics of the study population, Table S2: The threshold effect of log2-HbEO on LFTs using a two-stage phased regression model, Table S3: The association between HbEO and the liver function test.

Author Contributions: Conceptualization, Z.H. and Y.L.; methodology, S.L. and J.W.; formal analysis, Z.W., K.Z. and K.L.; data curation, D.L. and D.P.; writing—original draft preparation, S.L. and J.W.; writing—review and editing, Z.H. and Y.L.; supervision, Z.H. and Y.L.; funding acquisition, Z.W. and Z.H. All authors have read and agreed to the published version of the manuscript.

Funding: This study was supported by Chongqing Technology Innovation and Application Development Key Project (cstc2021jscx-gksbX0060, Zhongjun Wu), Chongqing Science and Health Joint Project (2024GGXM005, Zhongjun Wu), and Chongqing Research Performance Incentive and Guidance Project (cstc2022jxjl120032, Zuotian Huang).

Institutional Review Board Statement: The study was conducted in accordance with the Declaration of Helsinki and approved by the U.S. National Center for Health Statistics Research Ethics Review Board. No further ethical approval is required.

Informed Consent Statement: Informed consent was obtained from all subjects involved in the study.

Data Availability Statement: The original data presented in this study are openly available in the National Health and Nutrition Examination Survey at https://www.cdc.gov/nchs/nhanes/index.htm (accessed on 25 June 2024).

Conflicts of Interest: The authors declare no conflicts of interest.

References

1. Trefts, E.; Gannon, M.; Wasserman, D.H. The liver. *Curr. Biol.* **2017**, *27*, R1147–R1151. [CrossRef] [PubMed]
2. Hu, C.; Zhao, L.; Li, L. Current understanding of adipose-derived mesenchymal stem cell-based therapies in liver diseases. *Stem Cell Res. Ther.* **2019**, *10*, 199. [CrossRef] [PubMed]
3. Xiao, J.; Guo, R.; Fung, M.L.; Liong, E.C.; Tipoe, G.L. Therapeutic approaches to non-alcoholic fatty liver disease: Past achievements and future challenges. *Hepatobiliary Pancreat. Dis. Int.* **2013**, *12*, 125–135. [CrossRef] [PubMed]
4. Xiao, J.; Wang, F.; Wong, N.K.; He, J.; Zhang, R.; Sun, R.; Xu, Y.; Liu, Y.; Li, W.; Koike, K.; et al. Global liver disease burdens and research trends: Analysis from a Chinese perspective. *J. Hepatol.* **2019**, *71*, 212–221. [CrossRef] [PubMed]
5. Newsome, P.N.; Cramb, R.; Davison, S.M.; Dillon, J.F.; Foulerton, M.; Godfrey, E.M.; Hall, R.; Harrower, U.; Hudson, M.; Langford, A.; et al. Guidelines on the management of abnormal liver blood tests. *Gut* **2018**, *67*, 6–19. [CrossRef] [PubMed]
6. Abeysekera, K.W.M.; Macpherson, I.; Glyn-Owen, K.; McPherson, S.; Parker, R.; Harris, R.; Yeoman, A.; Rowe, I.A.; Dillon, J.F. Community pathways for the early detection and risk stratification of chronic liver disease: A narrative systematic review. *Lancet Gastroenterol. Hepatol.* **2022**, *7*, 770–780. [CrossRef] [PubMed]
7. Yu, L.; Yang, M.; Cheng, M.; Fan, L.; Wang, X.; Xu, T.; Wang, B.; Chen, W. Associations between urinary phthalate metabolite concentrations and markers of liver injury in the US adult population. *Environ. Int.* **2021**, *155*, 106608. [CrossRef] [PubMed]
8. Lee, S.; Song, D.; Shin, S.; Hong, N.; Rhee, Y. Elevated serum γ-glutamyl transferase is associated with low muscle function in adults independent of muscle mass. *Nutrition* **2022**, *103–104*, 111813. [CrossRef] [PubMed]
9. Robles-Diaz, M.; Garcia-Cortes, M.; Medina-Caliz, I.; Gonzalez-Jimenez, A.; Gonzalez-Grande, R.; Navarro, J.M.; Castiella, A.; Zapata, E.M.; Romero-Gomez, M.; Blanco, S.; et al. The value of serum aspartate aminotransferase and gamma-glutamyl transpetidase as biomarkers in hepatotoxicity. *Liver Int.* **2015**, *35*, 2474–2482. [CrossRef] [PubMed]
10. Park, E.; Kim, J.; Kim, B.; Park, E.Y. Association between environmental exposure to cadmium and risk of suspected non-alcoholic fatty liver disease. *Chemosphere* **2021**, *266*, 128947. [CrossRef]
11. Sen, P.; Qadri, S.; Luukkonen, P.K.; Ragnarsdottir, O.; McGlinchey, A.; Jäntti, S.; Juuti, A.; Arola, J.; Schlezinger, J.J.; Webster, T.F.; et al. Exposure to environmental contaminants is associated with altered hepatic lipid metabolism in non-alcoholic fatty liver disease. *J. Hepatol.* **2022**, *76*, 283–293. [CrossRef] [PubMed]
12. Yi, W.; Ji, Y.; Gao, H.; Pan, R.; Wei, Q.; Cheng, J.; Song, J.; He, Y.; Tang, C.; Liu, X.; et al. Does the gut microbiome partially mediate the impact of air pollutants exposure on liver function? Evidence based on schizophrenia patients. *Environ. Pollut.* **2021**, *291*, 118135. [CrossRef] [PubMed]
13. Kirman, C.R.; Li, A.A.; Sheehan, P.J.; Bus, J.S.; Lewis, R.C.; Hays, S.M. Ethylene oxide review: Characterization of total exposure via endogenous and exogenous pathways and their implications to risk assessment and risk management. *J. Toxicol. Environ. Health B Crit. Rev.* **2021**, *24*, 1–29. [CrossRef] [PubMed]
14. Lynch, H.N.; Kozal, J.S.; Russell, A.J.; Thompson, W.J.; Divis, H.R.; Freid, R.D.; Calabrese, E.J.; Mundt, K.A. Systematic review of the scientific evidence on ethylene oxide as a human carcinogen. *Chem. Biol. Interact.* **2022**, *364*, 110031. [CrossRef]
15. Vincent, M.J.; Kozal, J.S.; Thompson, W.J.; Maier, A.; Dotson, G.S.; Best, E.A.; Mundt, K.A. Ethylene Oxide: Cancer Evidence Integration and Dose-Response Implications. *Dose Response* **2019**, *17*, 1559325819888317. [CrossRef] [PubMed]
16. Xie, R.; Liu, L.; Liu, C.; Xie, S.; Huang, X.; Zhang, Y. Associations of ethylene oxide exposure and "Life's Essential 8". *Environ. Sci. Pollut. Res. Int.* **2023**, *30*, 121150–121160. [CrossRef] [PubMed]
17. Filser, J.G.; Kessler, W.; Artati, A.; Erbach, E.; Faller, T.; Kreuzer, P.E.; Li, Q.; Lichtmannegger, J.; Numtip, W.; Klein, D.; et al. Ethylene oxide in blood of ethylene-exposed B6C3F1 mice, Fischer 344 rats, and humans. *Toxicol. Sci.* **2013**, *136*, 344–358. [CrossRef] [PubMed]
18. Kamalov, M.I.; Lavrov, I.A.; Yergeshov, A.A.; Siraeva, Z.Y.; Baltin, M.E.; Rizvanov, A.A.; Kuznetcova, S.V.; Petrova, N.V.; Savina, I.N.; Abdullin, T.I. Non-invasive topical drug delivery to spinal cord with carboxyl-modified trifunctional copolymer of ethylene oxide and propylene oxide. *Colloids Surf. B Biointerfaces* **2016**, *140*, 196–203. [CrossRef] [PubMed]
19. Grosse, Y.; Baan, R.; Straif, K.; Secretan, B.; El Ghissassi, F.; Bouvard, V.; Altieri, A.; Cogliano, V. Carcinogenicity of 1,3-butadiene, ethylene oxide, vinyl chloride, vinyl fluoride, and vinyl bromide. *Lancet Oncol.* **2007**, *8*, 679–680. [CrossRef]
20. Teta, M.J.; Sielken, R.L., Jr.; Valdez-Flores, C. Ethylene oxide cancer risk assessment based on epidemiological data: Application of revised regulatory guidelines. *Risk Anal.* **1999**, *19*, 1135–1155. [CrossRef]
21. Wu, S.; Yang, Y.M.; Zhu, J.; Wang, L.L.; Xu, W.; Lyu, S.Q.; Wang, J.; Shao, X.H.; Zhang, H. Impact of hemoglobin adducts of ethylene oxide on the prevalence and prognosis of chronic kidney disease in US adults: An analysis from NHANES 2013–2016. *Environ. Sci. Pollut. Res. Int.* **2024**, *31*, 2802–2812. [CrossRef] [PubMed]

22. Li, Z.; Shi, P.; Chen, Z.; Zhang, W.; Lin, S.; Zheng, T.; Li, M.; Fan, L. The association between ethylene oxide exposure and asthma risk: A population-based study. *Environ. Sci. Pollut. Res. Int.* **2023**, *30*, 24154–24167. [CrossRef] [PubMed]
23. Zhou, W.; Zhao, Y.; Jin, J.; Cheng, M.; Bai, Y.; Xu, J. The association of hemoglobin ethylene oxide levels with albuminuria in US adults: Analysis of NHANES 2013–2016. *Environ. Sci. Pollut. Res. Int.* **2024**, *31*, 4130–4139. [CrossRef] [PubMed]
24. Wu, N.; Cao, W.; Wang, Y.; Liu, X. Association between blood ethylene oxide levels and the prevalence of hypertension. *Environ. Sci. Pollut. Res. Int.* **2022**, *29*, 76937–76943. [CrossRef] [PubMed]
25. Tang, M.; Liu, M.; Zhang, Y.; Xie, R. Association of family income to poverty ratio and vibration-controlled transient elastography quantified degree of hepatic steatosis in U.S. adolescents. *Front. Endocrinol.* **2023**, *14*, 1160625. [CrossRef] [PubMed]
26. Jinot, J.; Fritz, J.M.; Vulimiri, S.V.; Keshava, N. Carcinogenicity of ethylene oxide: Key findings and scientific issues. *Toxicol. Mech. Methods* **2018**, *28*, 386–396. [CrossRef] [PubMed]
27. Marsh, G.M.; Keeton, K.A.; Riordan, A.S.; Best, E.A.; Benson, S.M. Ethylene oxide and risk of lympho-hematopoietic cancer and breast cancer: A systematic literature review and meta-analysis. *Int. Arch. Occup. Environ. Health* **2019**, *92*, 919–939. [CrossRef] [PubMed]
28. Jones, R.R.; Fisher, J.A.; Medgyesi, D.N.; Buller, I.D.; Liao, L.M.; Gierach, G.; Ward, M.H.; Silverman, D.T. Ethylene oxide emissions and incident breast cancer and non-Hodgkin lymphoma in a US cohort. *J. Natl. Cancer Inst.* **2023**, *115*, 405–412. [CrossRef] [PubMed]
29. Thier, R.; Bolt, H.M. Carcinogenicity and genotoxicity of ethylene oxide: New aspects and recent advances. *Crit. Rev. Toxicol.* **2000**, *30*, 595–608. [CrossRef]
30. Jain, R.B. Associations between observed concentrations of ethylene oxide in whole blood and smoking, exposure to environmental tobacco smoke, and cancers including breast cancer: Data for US children, adolescents, and adults. *Environ. Sci. Pollut. Res. Int.* **2020**, *27*, 20912–20919. [CrossRef]
31. St Helen, G.; Jacob, P., 3rd; Peng, M.; Dempsey, D.A.; Hammond, S.K.; Benowitz, N.L. Intake of toxic and carcinogenic volatile organic compounds from secondhand smoke in motor vehicles. *Cancer Epidemiol. Biomark. Prev.* **2014**, *23*, 2774–2782. [CrossRef] [PubMed]
32. Song, W.; Hu, H.; Ni, J.; Zhang, H.; Zhang, H.; Yang, G.; Wang, Y.; Zhang, Y.; Peng, B. The relationship between ethylene oxide levels in hemoglobin and the prevalence of kidney stones in US adults: An exposure-response analysis from NHANES 2013–2016. *Environ. Sci. Pollut. Res. Int.* **2023**, *30*, 26357–26366. [CrossRef] [PubMed]
33. Wang, H.; Chen, X.; Lin, F.; Zheng, J.; Chen, K.; Wang, X.; Lin, X.; Chen, X.; Ye, Q.; Wang, Y.; et al. Association between ethylene oxide levels and depressive symptoms: A cross-sectional study based on NHANES 2013–2018 database. *J. Affect. Disord.* **2024**, *348*, 135–142. [CrossRef] [PubMed]
34. Chen, X.; Hu, G.; He, B.; Cao, Z.; He, J.; Luo, H.; Li, Y.; Yu, Q. Effect of brominated flame retardants exposure on liver function and the risk of non-alcoholic fatty liver disease in the US population. *Ecotoxicol. Environ. Saf.* **2024**, *273*, 116142. [CrossRef] [PubMed]
35. Yun, J.; Kwon, S.C. The Association of Perfluoroalkyl Substance Exposure and a Serum Liver Function Marker in Korean Adults. *Toxics* **2023**, *11*, 965. [CrossRef] [PubMed]
36. Guo, J.; Wan, Z.; Cui, G.; Pan, A.; Liu, G. Association of exposure to ethylene oxide with risk of diabetes mellitus: Results from NHANES 2013–2016. *Environ. Sci. Pollut. Res. Int.* **2021**, *28*, 68551–68559. [CrossRef] [PubMed]
37. Szwiec, E.; Friedman, L.; Buchanan, S. Levels of Ethylene Oxide Biomarker in an Exposed Residential Community. *Int. J. Environ. Res. Public Health* **2020**, *17*, 8646. [CrossRef] [PubMed]
38. Villeneuve, D.L.; Crump, D.; Garcia-Reyero, N.; Hecker, M.; Hutchinson, T.H.; LaLone, C.A.; Landesmann, B.; Lettieri, T.; Munn, S.; Nepelska, M.; et al. Adverse outcome pathway (AOP) development I: Strategies and principles. *Toxicol. Sci.* **2014**, *142*, 312–320. [CrossRef] [PubMed]
39. Boobis, A.R.; Doe, J.E.; Heinrich-Hirsch, B.; Meek, M.E.; Munn, S.; Ruchirawat, M.; Schlatter, J.; Seed, J.; Vickers, C. IPCS framework for analyzing the relevance of a noncancer mode of action for humans. *Crit. Rev. Toxicol.* **2008**, *38*, 87–96. [CrossRef]
40. Meek, M.E.; Boobis, A.; Cote, I.; Dellarco, V.; Fotakis, G.; Munn, S.; Seed, J.; Vickers, C. New developments in the evolution and application of the WHO/IPCS framework on mode of action/species concordance analysis. *J. Appl. Toxicol.* **2014**, *34*, 1–18. [CrossRef]
41. Vinken, M.; Landesmann, B.; Goumenou, M.; Vinken, S.; Shah, I.; Jaeschke, H.; Willett, C.; Whelan, M.; Rogiers, V. Development of an adverse outcome pathway from drug-mediated bile salt export pump inhibition to cholestatic liver injury. *Toxicol. Sci.* **2013**, *136*, 97–106. [CrossRef] [PubMed]
42. Houle, C.D.; Ton, T.V.; Clayton, N.; Huff, J.; Hong, H.H.; Sills, R.C. Frequent p53 and H-ras mutations in benzene- and ethylene oxide-induced mammary gland carcinomas from B6C3F1 mice. *Toxicol. Pathol.* **2006**, *34*, 752–762. [CrossRef] [PubMed]
43. Mori, K.; Inoue, N.; Fujishiro, K.; Kikuchi, M.; Chiba, S. Biochemical changes in rat erythrocytes caused by ethylene oxide exposure. *Fundam. Appl. Toxicol.* **1990**, *15*, 441–447. [CrossRef] [PubMed]
44. Crabtree, A.A.; Boehnke, N.; Bates, F.S.; Hackel, B.J. Consequences of poly(ethylene oxide) and poloxamer P188 on transcription in healthy and stressed myoblasts. *Proc. Natl. Acad. Sci. USA* **2023**, *120*, e2219885120. [CrossRef] [PubMed]

45. Katoh, T.; Higashi, K.; Inoue, N.; Tanaka, I. Effects of chronic inhalation of ethylene oxide on lipid peroxidation and glutathione redox cycle in rat liver. *Res. Commun. Chem. Pathol. Pharmacol.* **1988**, *61*, 281–284. [PubMed]
46. Zhu, X.; Kong, X.; Chen, M.; Shi, S.; Cheang, I.; Zhu, Q.; Lu, X.; Yue, X.; Tang, Y.; Liao, S.; et al. Blood ethylene oxide, systemic inflammation, and serum lipid profiles: Results from NHANES 2013–2016. *Chemosphere* **2022**, *299*, 134336. [CrossRef]

toxics

MDPI

Article

Effects of 6PPD-Quinone on Human Liver Cell Lines as Revealed with Cell Viability Assay and Metabolomics Analysis

Yunqing Qi, Aiqing Qiu, Xinyue Wei, Yiting Huang, Qing Huang and Wei Huang *

Guangdong Key Laboratory of Environmental Pollution and Health, College of Environment and Climate, Jinan University, Guangzhou 510632, China
* Correspondence: huangwei@jnu.edu.cn

Abstract: *N*-(1,3-Dimethyl butyl)-*N′*-phenyl-phenylenediamine-quinone (6PPD-Q) is a derivative of the widely used rubber tire antioxidant 6PPD, which was first found to be acutely toxic to coho salmon. Subsequent studies showed that 6PPD-Q had species-specific acute toxicity in fishes and potential hepatotoxicity in mice. In addition, 6PPD-Q has been reported in human urine, demonstrating the potential widespread exposure of humans to this chemical. However, whether 6PPD-Q poses a higher risk to humans than its parent compound, 6PPD, and could cause adverse effects in humans is still unclear. In this study, we utilized two human liver cell models (the human proto-hepatocyte model L02 and the human hepatocellular carcinoma cell line HepG2) to investigate the potentially differential effects of these two chemicals. Cell viability curve analysis showed that 6PPD-Q had lower IC_{50} values than 6PPD for both liver cell lines, suggesting higher toxicity of 6PPD-Q to human liver cells than 6PPD. In addition, L02 cells are more sensitive to 6PPD-Q exposure, which might be derived from its weaker metabolic transformation of 6PPD-Q, since significantly lower levels of phase I and phase II metabolites were detected in 6PPD-Q-exposed L02 cell culture medium. Furthermore, pathway analysis showed that 6PPD-Q exposure induced changes in phenylalanine, tyrosine, and tryptophan biosynthesis and tyrosine metabolism pathways in L02 cells, which might be the mechanism underlying its liver cell toxicity. Gene expression analysis revealed that exposure to 6PPD-Q induced excessive ROS production in L02 cells. Our results further supported the higher risk of 6PPD-Q than 6PPD and provided insights for understanding the effects of 6PPD-Q on human health.

Keywords: 6PPD-Q; human liver cells; cytotoxicity; transformation products; metabolomics

1. Introduction

N-(1,3-dimethylbutyl)-*N′*-phenyl-p-phenylenediamine (6PPD) is widely used as an antioxidant in the rubber industry, which raised significant concerns due to its ozonized transformation product, 6PPD-quinone (6PPD-Q), identified to be of acute toxicity on several aquatic species at environmentally relevant concentrations in recent years [1]. Since the hydrolysis half-life of 6PPD-Q is significantly longer than that of 6PPD [2], subsequent studies reported the detection of 6PPD-Q in various environmental matrices, such as dust, soil, water, sediments, and atmospheric particles [3,4]. The widespread occurrence of 6PPD-Q in the environmental matrices has raised concerns about its effects on environmental and human health. Especially, the finding of 6PPD-Q in the atmosphere and human urine implied that humans might also be generally exposed to 6PPD-Q, which raises an urgent need for its toxicity assessment.

To date, the toxicity assessment of 6PPD-Q has mainly been conducted on aquatic species. Research has shown that 6PPD-Q can cause acute mortality in silver salmon by disrupting the blood–brain barrier or affecting the mitochondrial electron transport chain [5,6]. Additionally, a study found that both 6PPD and 6PPD-Q can enter the circulatory system and affect the nervous system of zebrafish larvae, leading to developmental and behavioral changes as well as cardiotoxicity at high concentrations [7]. As for toxicity to mammalians, knowledge is still very limited, especially for humans. Fang et al. found that 6PPD-Q oral administration caused damage to the liver tissue of mice via activated inflammation and disturbed glycolipid metabolism [8], revealing that 6PPD-Q might also pose the potential to cause adverse effects on the human liver.

However, there are still no human-relevant studies about the effects of 6PPD-Q on the liver. The liver is an important organ for maintaining normal physiological functions and plays an important role in metabolism and detoxification [9] and, therefore, might be the target organ of many xenobiotics. In vitro liver cell models have been widely used in toxicology for the screening of cytotoxic and genotoxic compounds and the determination of characteristic liver lesions and associated biochemical mechanisms induced by toxic compounds [10]. With the development of molecular toxicology, multiple omics techniques have been applied for toxicity assessment. Metabolomics is the systematic identification and quantification of all metabolites in a given biological sample to directly reflect the dynamics of metabolic levels under toxicant exposure or disease states to identify altered metabolic pathways resulting from an exposure factor or pathophysiological perturbation [11].

In the present study, using the human liver cell lines HepG2 and L02 as models, we systematically assessed the cytotoxicity of 6PPD-Q on human liver cells and investigated the potential metabolic perturbance via metabolomic profiling, aiming to illustrate the potential toxicity of this emerging chemical on humans.

2. Materials and Methods

2.1. Chemicals and Materials

The standards of 6PPD-Q and 6PPD were purchased from DR. EHRENSTORFER (>99% purity, LGC, Luckenwalde, Germany). Dimethyl sulfoxide (DMSO, >99.9%) and 4-chloro-phenylalanine (4-Cl-Phe) were purchased from Sigma-Aldrich (St. Louis, MO, USA). Dulbecco's modified Eagle's medium (DMEM), RPMI-1640 medium, fetal bovine serum (FBS), penicillin-streptomycin, 0.25% trypsin-EDTA, and phosphate-buffered saline (PBS) were from Gibco (Thermo Fisher Scientific, Waltham, MA, USA). Cell culture bottles and plates were bought from Corning (Corning Incorporated, Corning, NY, USA). All other chemicals used, including water (H_2O), methanol (MeOH), acetonitrile (ACN), and isopropanol (IPA), were of high-performance liquid chromatography (HPLC)-grade (Merck & Co., Billerica, MA, USA). Human normal hepatocyte cell line L02 and human hepatocellular carcinoma cell line HepG2 were obtained from the American Type Culture Collection (ATCC, Manassas, VA, USA).

2.2. Cell Culture

As recommended by ATCC, HepG2 cells were cultured in DMEM supplemented with 10% FBS and 1% penicillin-streptomycin, and L02 cells were cultured in RPMI-1640 medium supplemented with 20% FBS and 1% penicillin-streptomycin. Both cell lines were maintained at 37 °C in a humidified environment with 5% carbon dioxide. The cells were passaged for three generations before inoculating into 96-well or 6-well plates for subsequent experiments. The 6PPD-Q and 6PPD standard solutions were prepared with DMSO to achieve a stock concentration of 1000 mg/L.

2.3. MTT Assay

The cells were initially plated into a 25 cm^2 culture bottle and harvested via trypsin digestion at 37 °C for 5 min when reaching 80% confluence. Afterward, cells were inoculated into 96-well plates at a density of 20,000 per well and further incubated for 24 h. The medium in the 96-well plate was then replaced with the FBS-free medium containing 6PPD or 6PPD-Q at a final exposure concentrations of 1–1000 μg/L, and the medium containing 0.1% DMSO was used as a vehicle control. For each exposure concentration, six replicates were set up and cultured for 48 h. At the end of exposure, cell viability was assessed using the MTT Cell Proliferation and Cytotoxicity Assay Kit (Leagene, Beijing, China) following the manufacturer's instructions. Briefly, the medium was carefully aspirated, 100 μL of fresh serum-free medium and 10 μL of MTT solution (5 mg/mL in PBS) were added to each well, and the incubation was continued for 4 h at 37 °C. Then, 100 μL of SDS-HCl solution (1 g of SDS dissolved in 10 mL of 0.01 M HCl) was added to each well. The plate was incubated in a 37 °C humidified chamber for 4 h followed by low-speed oscillation for 10 min on a shaking table to fully dissolve the purple formazan. Finally, the absorbance of each well was measured at 570 nm using an enzyme marker, and the results were expressed as a percentage of cell viability normalized to the control. As the viability curves were non-monotonic functions, we employed nonlinear fitting of the cell viability data using the dose–response inhibition function in GraphPad Prism software (version 9, GraphPad Software, Inc., La Jolla, CA, USA) after logarithmic transformation of the concentrations. This yielded the corresponding IC_{50} values, which were then assessed for quality via the R-squared values generated after fitting the curves.

2.4. Analysis of Transformation Products in Cell Culture Medium

The L02 and HepG2 cells were inoculated at 1×10^6 cells/well in a six-well plate and cultured in complete medium to 60% confluence, followed by changing the medium to FBS-free medium with different 6PPD-Q concentrations (0 and 50 μg/L). Six duplicates were prepared for each treatment. After exposure for another 48 h, the medium was carefully collected. The cell culture medium (1 mL) collected from 0 and 50 μg/L 6PPD-Q exposure was spiked with 4-Cl-Phe as an internal standard and acidified with 400 μL of 10% formic acid/H_2O (v/v), followed by the addition of 1.2 g of sodium sulfate and 0.6 g of sodium chloride. The samples were then extracted twice with 4 mL and 3 mL of ACN, respectively, and the extracts were combined, nitrogen-blown to near dryness, and re-dissolved in 200 μL of ACN/H_2O (15:85, v/v) for analysis.

2.5. Sample Preparation for Metabolomics Analysis

The sample preparation for metabolomics was conducted as previously reported [12]. The L02 cells were inoculated at 1×10^6 cells/well in a six-well plate and cultured in complete medium to 60% confluence, followed by changing the medium to FBS-free medium with different 6PPD-Q concentrations (0, 1, and 50 μg/L). Six duplicates were prepared for each treatment. After exposure for another 48 h, the medium was carefully removed, and the cells were rapidly washed with PBS and collected using a cell scraper. The cell pellet was quickly quenched by adding 600 μL of frozen MeOH/H_2O (4:1, v/v), while 4-Cl-Phe was added as an internal standard. Three repetitive freeze–thaw cycles with liquid nitrogen were conducted for cell lysis. The samples were then centrifuged at 16,000× g for 10 min at 4 °C. Finally, 350 μL of the upper layer was collected for metabolomics analysis. The samples were vacuum-dried, redissolved in 100 μL of 50% MeOH/H_2O (v/v), vortexed for 3 min, and then centrifuged at 16,000× g for 8 min at 4 °C. The supernatants were collected and subjected to LC-MS analysis. The proteins were retained and measured for data correction.

2.6. Instrumental Analysis

The metabolomics analysis and semi-quantification of the transformation products were conducted on an ultra-high-performance liquid chromatography system (UHPLC) coupled to an Orbitrap Exploris™ 240 mass spectrometer (MS) (Thermo Scientific, Waltham, MA, USA). Five microliters of each sample were injected for analysis. Detailed chromatographic conditions and MS parameters are summarized in Table S1. Samples from the control and exposure groups were randomly analyzed, with solvent blanks and QC samples inserted every six samples. The samples were analyzed under both positive ionization and negative ionization modes.

2.7. Data Processing and Analysis

For metabolomics raw data, deconvolution, peak extraction, peak alignment, and compound identification were conducted using Compound Discoverer 3.3 (Thermo Scientific, Waltham, MA, USA). The parameters are set as follows: MS1 tolerance, 5 ppm; MS2 tolerance, 5 ppm; alignment model, adaptive curve; maximum shift, 2 min; intensity tolerance, 30%; S/N threshold, 3; and minimum peak height, 20,000. The adduct ions in positive ionization mode include $[M + H]^+$, $[M + K]^+$, $[M + NH_4]^+$, $[M + H - H_2O]^+$, $[M + Na]^+$, $[M + ACN + H]^+$, $[M + ACN + Na]^+$, $[2M + H]^+$, $[2M + Na]^+$, $[2M + K]^+$, $[2M + NH4]^+$, $[2M + ACN + H]^+$, and $[M + ACN + Na]^+$. The adduct ions in negative ionization mode include $[M - H]^-$, $[M + Cl]^-$, $[M + FA - H]^-$, $[M - H_2O - H]^-$, $[2M - H]^-$, and $[2M + Hac - H]^-$. The compounds were annotated with accurate mass-to-charge ratios (m/z) of the precursor ion and matching of the MS/MS profiles in accordance with the mzCloud and mzVault databases. Compounds that were annotated were manually identified as plausible compounds when at least three fragment ions were matched to compounds in the above libraries. The ultimate peak area of the identified compounds was corrected with the peak area of the internal standard (4-Cl-Phe for both the positive and negative ionization modes) and the protein amount of the corresponding sample. The online platform MetaboAnalyst 5.0 (https://www.metaboanalyst.ca/, accessed on 25 December 2023) was implemented to perform partial least squares discriminant analysis (PLS-DA). Differential metabolites between the exposure and control groups were filtered by p-value (<0.05) and multiplicity of fold change (FC, >1.20 or <0.83). The differential metabolites were then subjected to metabolic pathway and enrichment analyses using MetaboAnalyst 5.0 (https://www.metaboanalyst.ca/, accessed on 25 December 2023) according to the Kyoto Encyclopedia of Genes and Genomes (KEGG) pathway database (www.genome.jp/kegg/, accessed on 25 December 2023).

In processing of transformation product data, potential transformation products from the literature were confirmed with accurate MS1 mass and MS2 fragments using Freestyle software 1.5 (Thermo Scientific, Waltham, MA, USA). The relative peak area was used for comparison between the two cell lines.

2.8. RNA Extraction and Quantitative Reverse Transcription PCR

The cell treatment and collection were identical to that utilized in preparation of samples for metabolomics analysis. In brief, 1×10^6 L02 cells/well were inoculated in six-well culture plates and cultured in a complete medium until 60% confluence was reached. Thereafter, the medium was changed to an FBS-free medium with different concentrations of 6PPD-Q (0, 1, and 50 μg/L). Six replicates were prepared for each concentration and each treatment was repeated three times. Following a further 48 h of exposure, the medium was carefully removed, the cells were rapidly washed with PBS, and they were collected using a cell scraper. Total RNA was extracted from the treated cells with TRIzol reagent (Invitrogen, Carlsbad, CA, USA) as per the supplied instructions. The concentration and purity of the RNA samples were detected with a NanoDrop spectrophotometer (Thermo Fisher Scientific, Waltham, MA, USA). The expression level of specific genes was assessed via quantitative reverse transcription PCR (RT-qPCR). cDNA was synthesized with reverse-transcribed total RNA using the Evo M-MLV RT Mix kit with gDNA clean for qPCR (Accurate Biology, Beijing, China) in a total volume of 20 μL according to the manufacturer's instructions. All the primers were obtained from the Beijing Genomics Institute (Shenzhen, China) and the primer sequences were listed in Table S2. The gene expression level was calculated using the comparative Ct method and normalized against GAPDH.

2.9. Quantitative Analysis of Cellular Reactive Oxygen Species (ROS) Level

Cells were first inoculated into all-black 96-well cell culture plates (Corning, Corning, NY, USA) at a density of 20,000 cells per well and incubated for an additional 24 h. Subsequently, the medium in the 96-well plates was replaced with an FBS-free medium containing 6PPD-Q at concentrations of 0, 1, and 50 μg/L. Six replicates were set up for each exposure concentration, and the plates were incubated for 48 h. At the end of exposure, the cellular ROS level was assessed using the ROS Assay Kit (Beyotime, Shanghai, China) according to the manufacturer's instructions. Briefly, at the end of the exposure, the solution was meticulously absorbed, 100 µL of a diluted 2′,7′-dichlorofluorescin diacetate (DCFH-DA) solution (10 µM) was added to each well, and the plates were incubated in an incubator for 20 min. This was followed by three washes with serum-free medium, which effectively removed the non-internalized DCFH-DA. Using a Multi-Function Measuring Instrument (Bio-Tek, Winooski, VT, USA), the fluorescence intensity was measured at 488 nm excitation wavelength and 525 emission wavelengths, and the results were expressed as normalized to the amount of ROS produced in the control group. Six replicates were set up for each concentration and each treatment was repeated three times.

2.10. Statistical Analysis

Statistical analyses of the metabolomics data were performed using GraphPad Prism version 9.0 for Windows (GraphPad Software, San Diego, CA, USA), OriginPro 2021 (OriginLab Corp., Armonk, NY, USA), and the online data processing website MetaboAnalyst 5 (http://www.metaboAnalyst.ca/, accessed on 25 December 2023). Comparisons between two groups were conducted with the Student's t-test, while comparisons among groups were conducted with one-way ANOVAs followed by Tukey's post hoc test. Two-sided $p < 0.05$ was thought to be of significance.

3. Results

3.1. 6PPD-Q Induced Differential Effects on Liver Cell Viability

The MTT assay revealed that after exposure to 6PPD-Q for 48 h, no significant change in cell viability was observed when the concentrations were less than 1 µg/L for both cell lines. The cell viability under 6PPD-Q exposure for both cell lines was significantly reduced when the exposure time was 48 h. However, the viability of L02 cells was significantly reduced in a dose-dependent manner when the concentration of 6PPD-Q exceeded 1 µg/L. More interestingly, we found that the L02 cell viability at exposure concentrations of 5 µg/L and 20 µg/L was lower than some of the higher exposures (Figure 1A). For HepG2 cells, a significant decrease in cell viability was observed at concentrations of 6PPD-Q exceeding 50 µg/L (Figure 1B). While for 6PPD exposure, concentrations that resulted in significant changes in cell viability were not consistent with 6PPD-Q. As shown in Figure 1C, the viability of the L02 cell did not undergo a significant decrease when exposed to any concentrations of 6PPD ranging from 0 to 5000 µg/L. For HepG2 cells, when the concentration of 6PPD was less than 300 µg/L, no significant change was observed in the cells, whereas when it was greater than 300 µg/L, the cells showed a significant increase compared with the control group (Figure 1D).

After fitting the viability curve (Figure S1), the calculated 48 h exposure IC_{50} values of 6PPD-Q for HepG2 cells and L02 cells were 127.50 µg/L and 22.51 µg/L, respectively, while the 48 h exposure IC_{50} of 6PPD exceeded the testing concentration range. These results indicated that 6PPD and 6PPD-Q induced differential liver cell toxicity while exhibiting cell line specificity, suggesting that 6PPD-Q is more toxic compared to 6PPD. Although the R-squared value derived from the IC_{50} curve fit did not demonstrate a high-quality fit, it is evident that L02 cells exhibited a heightened sensitivity to 6PPD-Q exposure.

3.2. Differences in the Transformation of 6PPD-Q between HepG2 and L02 Cells

Through literature research and data analysis, two transformation products of 6PPD-Q were identified in the cell culture medium, which were its phase I metabolite hydroxylated 6PPD-Q (6PPD-Q-OH) and phase II metabolite 6PPD-Q-O-glucuronide (6PPD-Q-O-Gluc) (Table S3 and Figures S2–S4). By comparing the relative peak area of 6PPD-Q and its transformation products in the two cell culture media, we found that the residual 6PPD-Q content in the L02 cell culture medium was much higher than that in HepG2 cells (Figure 2A). The 6PPD-Q-OH content in the HepG2 cell culture medium was significantly higher than that in the L02 cell culture medium, whereas no 6PPD-Q-O-Gluc was detected in the 6PPD-Q-exposed L02 cell culture medium (Figure 2B).

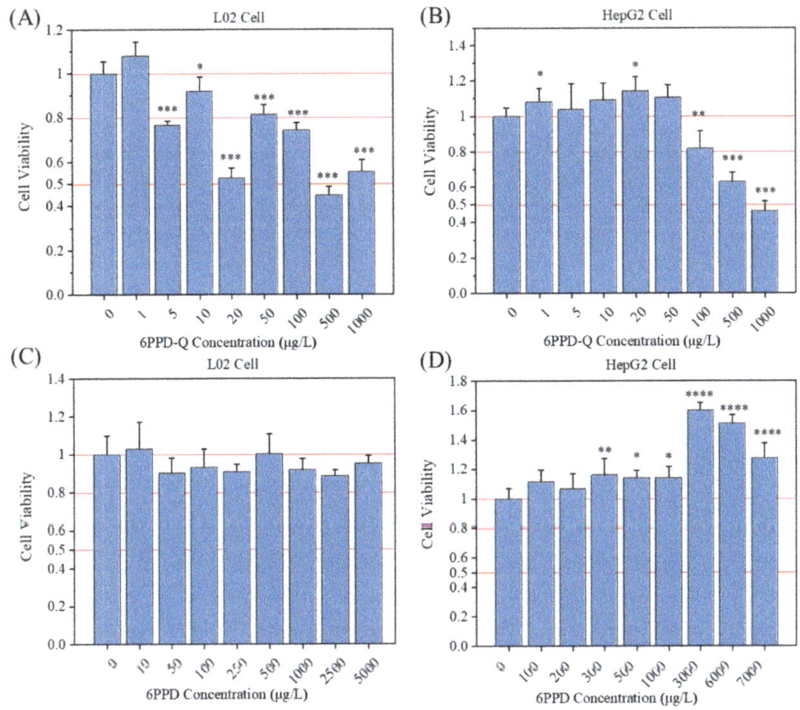

Figure 1. Results of cytotoxicity assay for both cells after 6PPD-Q and 6PPD exposure for 48 h. (**A**) 6PPD-Q-exposed L02 cells; (**B**) 6PPD-Q-exposed HepG2 cells; (**C**) 6PPD-exposed L02 cells; and (**D**) 6PPD-exposed HepG2 cells. Data are expressed as mean ± standard error of the mean ($n = 6$). * $p < 0.05$, ** $p < 0.01$, *** $p < 0.001$, and **** $p < 0.0001$ indicate significant differences between the exposure group and the control group.

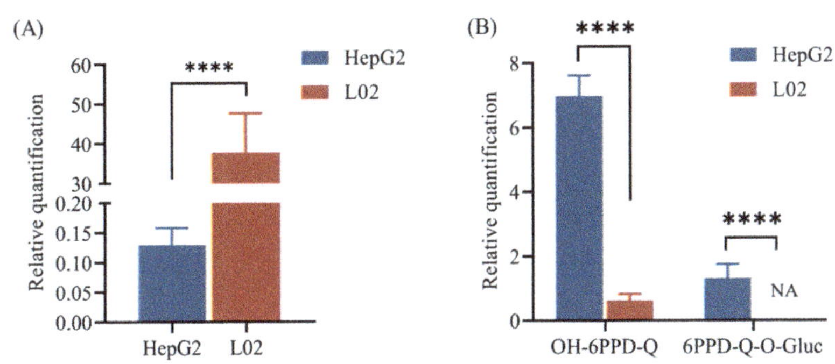

Figure 2. Transformation products in 50 μg/L of 6PPD-Q-exposed cell culture medium. (**A**) The residual 6PPD-Q in the two cell culture media and (**B**) 6PPD-Q biotransformation products in the two cell culture media. Data are expressed as mean ± standard error of the mean ($n = 6$). **** $p < 0.0001$ indicates significant differences between the two cell culture media. NA, not detected.

3.3. Mechanistic Insights into the Effects of 6PPD-Q on Liver Cells

As a newly identified chemical of concern, the pathways that underlie the effects of 6PPD-Q on human liver cells are still unknown. Since L02 cells were more sensitive to 6PPD-Q exposure, we further conducted pathway enrichment analysis with the differential metabolites in 6PPD-Q-exposed L02 cells to investigate the potential metabolic mechanism underlying the toxicity. Metabolomic analysis showed that exposure to 6PPD-Q induced metabolic perturbation in the liver cells. PLS-DA score plots showed the obvious separation of the controls from the exposure groups (Figure 3A). Using $p < 0.05$ and FC > 1.20 or <0.83 as the criteria, we found that 20 and 31 metabolites were significantly changed in L02 cells with 1 μg/L and 50 μg/L of 6PPD-Q exposure, respectively (Figure 3B,C).

Further pathway enrichment analysis results showed that the differential metabolites in the 1 μg/L exposure group were enriched in the phenylalanine, tyrosine, and tryptophan biosynthesis; pantothenic acid and CoA biosynthesis; alanine metabolism; cysteine metabolism; and tyrosine metabolism pathways (Figure 3D), while the differential metabolites of 50 μg/L were found to be enriched in the biosynthetic pathways of phenylalanine, tyrosine, and tryptophan, as well as in the biosynthesis in tyrosine metabolism and propanoate metabolism (Figure 3E). Particularly, 13 metabolites were simultaneously and consistently changed at both 1 μg/L and 50 μg/L exposure concentrations compared with the control group (Table 1), and were enriched in phenylalanine, tyrosine, and tryptophan biosynthesis and tyrosine metabolism pathways, indicating that 6PPD-Q exposure induced disruption of these amino acid metabolism pathways.

Table 1. Common differential metabolites in 1 and 50 μg/L of 6PPD-Q exposure of L02 cells [a].

Differential Metabolites	HMDB ID	FC [b] (1 μg/L vs. Control)	FC (50 μg/L vs. Control)
1-(4-Bromophenyl)-2-(7H-purin-6-ylsulfanyl) ethanol	HMDB0258663	0.73	0.67
beta-Ala-Phe	HMDB0304795	0.69	0.59
N-[[3-(b-D-Glucopyranosyloxy)-2,3-dihydro-2-oxo-1H-Indol-3-yl]acetyl]aspartic acid	HMDB0039409	0.70	0.71
3-[2-[[2-[[2-Acetamido-3-(4-Hydroxyphenyl)propanoyl]amino]-3-Methylbutanoyl]amino]propanoylamino]-4-oxobutanoic acid	HMDB0247776	0.51	0.48
2-Hydroxy-3-(4-methoxyphenyl) propanoic acid	HMDB0039427	0.51	0.45
2-Aminonicotinic acid	HMDB0061680	0.70	0.68
6-Amino-1-benzyl-5-methylamino-1H-pyrimidine-2,4-dione	HMDB0258564	0.72	0.66
Trigonelline	HMDB0000875	0.55	0.36
Fulvic acid	HMDB0252514	0.49	0.42
L-Tyrosine	HMDB0000158	0.71	0.65
7-hydroxy-3-(hydroxymethyl)-octahydropyrrolo[1,2-a]pyrazine-1,4-dione	HMDB0253728	0.71	0.65
Secologanin	HMDB0304482	0.48	0.38
Methyl dihydrophaseate	HMDB0039376	0.70	0.64

[a] The differential metabolites were filtered by using $p < 0.05$ and FC > 1.20 or <0.83 as the criteria; [b] FC, fold change.

3.4. PPD-Q Exposure Induced Oxidative Stress on Liver Cells

RT-qPCR analysis showed that oxidative stress-related genes were generally significantly upregulated in L02 cells after exposure to different concentrations of 6PPD-Q compared to controls. As shown in Figure 4, the expression of catalase (*CAT*), nuclear factor erythroid 2-related factor 2 (*Nrf2*), and mammalian selenoprotein thioredoxin reductase 1 (*TrxR1*) increased in a significant dose-dependent manner. The expression of superoxide dismutase (*SOD-1*), heme hydroxylase-1 (*HO-1*), and glutathione peroxidase 1 (*GPX1*) showed an inverted U-shape distribution with increasing concentration. These results demonstrated that 6PPD-Q exposure significantly induces oxidative damage responses in L02 cells. We further quantified the intracellular ROS levels. As seen in Figure 4G, the cellular ROS level exhibited a dose-dependent increase under 6PPD-Q exposure. When exposed to 50 μg/mL of 6PPD-Q, the ROS level was significantly higher than the control group. These results further indicated that 6PPD-Q exposure induced the production of cellular ROS.

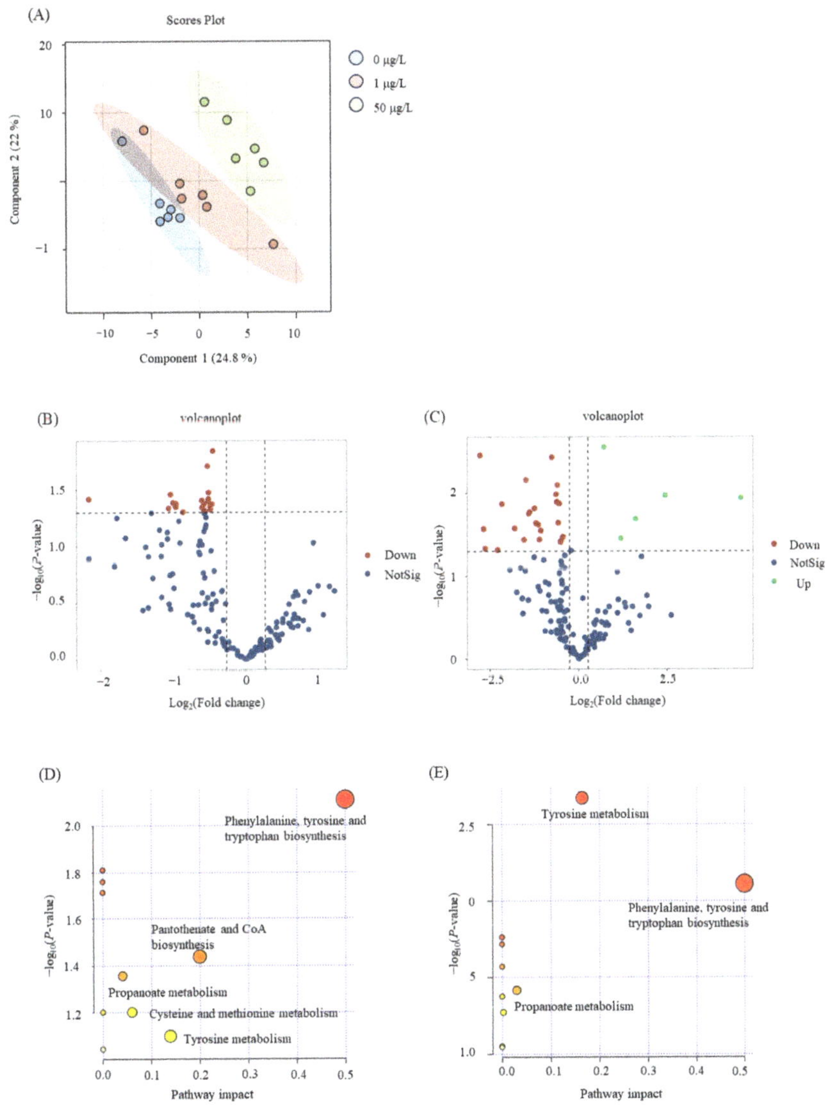

Figure 3. Non-targeted metabolomics analysis of the 6PPD-Q-exposed L02 cells. (**A**) PLS-DA score plots of L02 cells exposed to 6PPD-Q; (**B**) volcano plots of the metabolites between 1 μg/L of 6PPD-Q exposure and control group; (**C**) volcano plots of the metabolites between 50 μg/L of 6PPD-Q exposure and control group; (**D**) KEGG pathway analysis of the differential metabolites in 1 μg/L of 6PPD-Q-exposed L02 cells; and (**E**) KEGG pathway analysis of the differential metabolites in 50 μg/L of 6PPD-Q-exposed L02 cells.

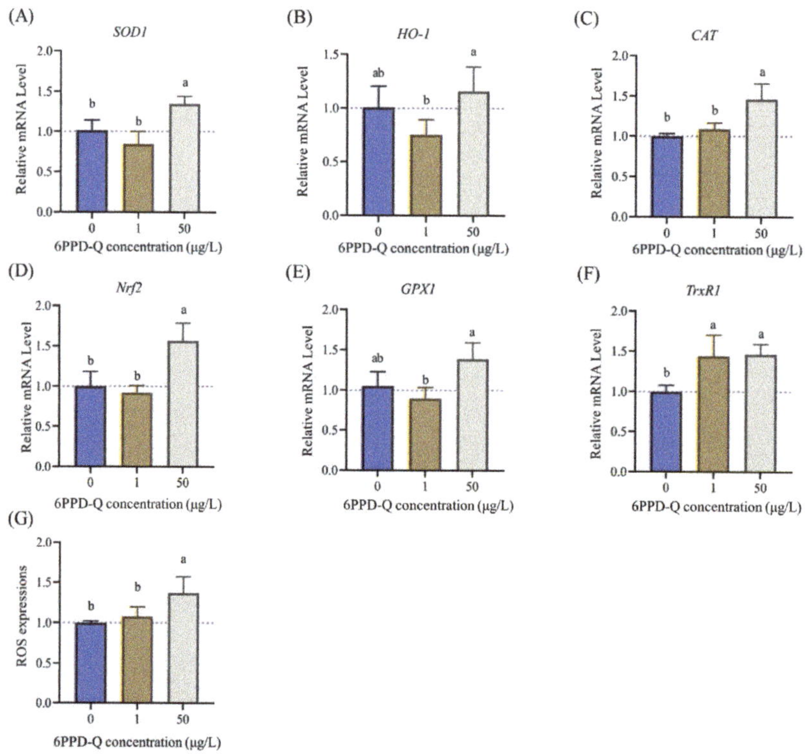

Figure 4. Expression of L02 cells with oxidative stress response-related genes with increasing concentration of 6PPD-Q exposure. (**A**) Superoxide dismutase (*SOD1*); (**B**) heme oxygenase-1 (*HO-1*); (**C**) catalase (*CAT*); (**D**) nuclear factor erythroid 2-related factor 2 (*Nrf2*); (**E**) glutathione peroxidase (*GPx1*); and (**F**) the mammalian selenoprotein thioredoxin reductase 1 (*TrxR1*). (**G**) Quantitative analysis of ROS expression based on DCF fluorescence intensity. Data are expressed as mean ± standard error of the mean (n = 6). Different letters above the columns indicate significant differences at $p < 0.05$, as determined via one-way ANOVA with Tukey's post hoc test.

4. Discussion

In this study, we investigated the potential toxic effects and mechanism of action of 6PPD-Q on human hepatocytes based on in vitro liver cell exposure models. The viability curve showed that the 48 h IC_{50} values of 6PPD-Q on the two human liver cell lines were significantly different, in which L02 cells were more sensitive to 6PPD-Q exposure. In addition, 6PPD-Q exhibited higher toxicity to the two liver cells in comparison with its precursor compound 6PPD. This result is consistent with that found in juvenile coho salmon, that 6PPD-Q exhibited high toxicity while 6PPD did not [1]. Zhao et al. treated mice with 6PPD and 6PPD-Q, finding that 6PPD-Q showed ~1.5–8-times higher bioaccumulation than 6PPD in all tissue types, and the liver appeared to be the major target organ for both 6PPD and 6PPD-Q after oral ingestion [13]. Di et al. found that 6PPD-Q was more stable in water solutions than 6PPD, indicating that the toxic effects of 6PPD-Q on sensitive species could be persistent in water [2]. These results also support our finding of differences in the toxicity of 6PPD and 6PPD-Q on the liver cell lines.

The viability analysis showed that L02 cells exhibited more severe cytotoxicity at low 6PPD-Q exposure compared to higher exposure, indicating that the dose–response curve is not a monotonic function, but rather a non-monotonic one. A considerable number of toxicological dose–response curves have been reported to exhibit a U-shaped, inverted

U-shaped, or even a wavy pattern. As the research on 6PPD-Q is still in progress and there are still many uncharted territories awaiting investigation, we will adjust the research on 6PPD-Q toxicity at a later date to delve more deeply into the issues related to the effects produced by the 6PPD-Q dose. We also found that L02 cells are more sensitive to 6PPD-Q exposure since its 48 h IC_{50} value was lower than that of HepG2. The toxicity of 6PPD-Q to fish appears to be highly species-specific, and many of the tested fish species to date do not show any abnormal physiological responses or acute mortality, even after exposure to much greater, nonenvironmentally relevant concentrations. Montgomery et al. suggested that differences in species sensitivity to 6PPD-Q are a result of differences in basal expression of the biotransformation enzymes across various fish species since they found that tolerant species might detoxify 6PPD-Q more effectively [14]. Indeed, our semi-quantitative results of 6PPD-Q and its biotransformation products in the two cell culture media showed that HepG2 cells could metabolize 6PPD-Q into 6PPD-Q-OH (phase I) and 6PPD-Q-O-Gluc (phase II) metabolite more efficiently. Similar to fish species, this phenomenon might also arise from differences in the enzymes associated with the uptake and metabolism of 6PPD-Q in L02 and HepG2 cells. Consistent with our results, in the study of biotransformation of triclosan in L02 cells versus HepG2 cells, Zhang et al. observed that triclosan underwent a more rapid transformation in HepG2 cells [12].

The application of metabolomics further revealed that 6PPD-Q exposure affected cellular tyrosine metabolism and phenylalanine, tyrosine, and tryptophan biosynthesis in L02 cells, suggesting that 6PPD-Q may lead to liver cell toxicity by interfering with these amino acid metabolism pathways. H.C. et al. demonstrated that phenylalanine, tyrosine, and tryptophan may be involved in the pathogenesis of liver failure and hepatic encephalopathy [15]. Lower levels of tryptophan have been associated with increased metabolic inflammation and fibrosis, which may lead to non-alcoholic fatty liver disease (NAFLD) [16]. Teunis et al. have demonstrated that NAFLD-associated inflammation can be reduced by modulating tryptophan metabolism [17]. In our study, we observed that the biosynthetic pathways of phenylalanine, tyrosine, and tryptophan were disrupted in the exposure groups following 6PPD-Q exposure. It has been demonstrated that certain pollutants may cause NAFLD by affecting tyrosine metabolism [18]. The L-tyrosine content in L02 cells decreased 0.71-fold and 0.65-fold, respectively, in the 1 and 50 μg/L exposure groups. These results indicated that 6PPD-Q exposure may potentially lead to hepatotoxicity by influencing metabolic pathways such as tyrosine metabolism and tryptophan biosynthesis.

In addition, several typical oxidative stress-related genes were significantly upregulated upon 6PPD-Q exposure, suggesting that 6PPD-Q might trigger ROS production in liver cells. Previous mouse studies have shown that 6PPD-Q exposure caused partial oxidative damage and an inflammatory response in the liver of the mice [8]. In addition, Wang et al. have demonstrated that 6PPD-Q in $PM_{2.5}$ exhibit moderate oxidative potential assessed via the acellular dithiothreitol assay [19]. The overproduction of ROS has been demonstrated to have an inescapable detrimental effect on liver function. It is well documented in the medical literature that oxidative stress plays a significant role in the pathogenesis of inflammatory chronic liver disease. Oxidative stress has been shown to trigger hepatocyte-associated emergency pathways, which in turn lead to the development of inflammation and steatosis [20]. In the same vein as above, it is well documented that ROS are involved in the formation of liver fibers leading to hyperfibrosis [21], causing liver injury [22]. Chen et al. demonstrated that antioxidants associated with oxidative stress were present in the majority of clinical samples of NAFLD, indicating a robust correlation between oxidative stress and NAFLD [23]. Therefore, our results suggested that 6PPD-Q may result in substantial damage to the human liver by inducing excessive oxidative stress.

5. Conclusions

In this study, the potential toxicity of 6PPD-Q on human liver cells was evaluated for the first time with in vitro cell models, finding that 6PPD-Q exhibited higher toxicity to liver cells than its precursor compound 6PPD, with differing 48 h IC_{50} values for the two human liver cell lines. HepG2 cells showed higher tolerance to 6PPD-Q exposure, which might be due to its higher metabolic detoxification capacity. Further analysis showed that 6PPD-Q may potentially lead to hepatotoxicity by inducing perturbations in phenylalanine, tyrosine, and tryptophan biosynthesis and tyrosine metabolism pathways, as well as excessive oxidative stress. This study provides basic data for future studies on the population health effects and risk assessment of 6PPD-Q.

Supplementary Materials: The following supporting information can be downloaded at: https://www.mdpi.com/article/10.3390/toxics12060389/s1, Figure S1: Fitted viability curves and calculated IC_{50} values of human liver cell lines exposed to 6PPD-Q for 48 h; Figure S2: Transformation products detected in cell culture media exposed to 6PPD-Q and the predicted potential transformation pathways based on chemical structure and known enzymatic reactions; Figure S3: LC-MS spectra for the identification of the phase I metabolite OH-6PPD-Q; Figure S4: LC-MS spectra for the identification of the phase II metabolite 6PPD-Q-O-Gluc; Table S1: Instrumental method for metabolomic analysis by UHPLC-Orbitrap MS; Table S2: Primer sequences of the oxidative-stress related genes for RT-qPCR; Table S3: Abbreviation, structure, molecular weight (MW), and transformation pathway of 6PPD-Q metabolic transformation products.

Author Contributions: Conceptualization, W.H. and Y.Q.; methodology, Y.Q. and A.Q.; data curation, X.W. and Y.H.; writing—review and editing, W.H., Y.Q. and Q.H. All authors have read and agreed to the published version of the manuscript.

Funding: This research was funded by the National Natural Science Foundation of China (No. 42277417), the Guangdong basic and applied basic research foundation (No. 2024A1515012525) and the Major Talent Program of Guangdong Provincial (No. 2021QN02Y944). And the APC was funded by National Natural Science Foundation of China (No. 42277417).

Institutional Review Board Statement: Not applicable.

Informed Consent Statement: Not applicable.

Data Availability Statement: The raw data supporting the conclusions of this article will be made available by the authors on request.

Conflicts of Interest: The authors declare they have no actual or potential competing financial interests.

References

1. Tian, Z.; Zhao, H.; Peter, K.T.; Gonzalez, M.; Wetzel, J.; Wu, C.; Hu, X.; Prat, J.; Mudrock, E.; Hettinger, R.; et al. A ubiquitous tire rubber-derived chemical induces acute mortality in coho salmon. *Science* **2021**, *371*, 185–189. [CrossRef] [PubMed]
2. Di, S.; Liu, Z.; Zhao, H.; Li, Y.; Qi, P.; Wang, Z.; Xu, H.; Jin, Y.; Wang, X. Chiral perspective evaluations: Enantioselective hydrolysis of 6PPD and 6PPD-quinone in water and enantioselective toxicity to *Gobiocypris rarus* and *Oncorhynchus mykiss*. *Environ. Int.* **2022**, *166*, 107374. [CrossRef] [PubMed]
3. Huang, W.; Shi, Y.; Huang, J.; Deng, C.; Tang, S.; Liu, X.; Chen, D. Occurrence of Substituted p-Phenylenediamine Antioxidants in Dusts. *Environ. Sci. Technol. Lett.* **2021**, *8*, 381–385. [CrossRef]
4. Cao, G.; Wang, W.; Zhang, J.; Wu, P.; Zhao, X.; Yang, Z.; Hu, D.; Cai, Z. New Evidence of Rubber-Derived Quinones in Water, Air, and Soil. *Environ. Sci. Technol.* **2022**, *56*, 4142–4150. [CrossRef] [PubMed]
5. Cataldo, F.; Faucette, B.; Huang, S.; Ebenezer, W. On the early reaction stages of ozone with N,N′-substituted p-phenylenediamines (6PPD, 77PD) and N,N′,N″-substituted-1,3,5-triazine "Durazone®": An electron spin resonance (ESR) and electronic absorption spectroscopy study. *Polym. Degrad. Stab.* **2015**, *111*, 223–231. [CrossRef]
6. Varshney, S.; Gora, A.H.; Siriyappagouder, P.; Kiron, V.; Olsvik, P.A. Toxicological effects of 6PPD and 6PPD quinone in zebrafish larvae. *J. Hazard. Mater.* **2022**, *424*, 127623. [CrossRef] [PubMed]
7. Ricarte, M.; Prats, E.; Montemurro, N.; Bedrossiantz, J.; Bellot, M.; Gómez-Canela, C.; Raldúa, D. Environmental concentrations of tire rubber-derived 6PPD-quinone alter CNS function in zebrafish larvae. *Sci. Total Environ.* **2023**, *896*, 165240. [CrossRef]
8. Fang, L.; Fang, C.; Di, S.; Yu, Y.; Wang, C.; Wang, X.; Jin, Y. Oral exposure to tire rubber-derived contaminant 6PPD and 6PPD-quinone induce hepatotoxicity in mice. *Sci. Total Environ.* **2023**, *869*, 161836. [CrossRef] [PubMed]
9. Han, H.-S.; Kang, G.; Kim, J.S.; Choi, B.H.; Koo, S.-H. Regulation of glucose metabolism from a liver-centric perspective. *Exp. Mol. Med.* **2016**, *48*, e218. [CrossRef]
10. Guillouzo, A. Liver cell models in in vitro toxicology. *Environ. Health Perspect.* **1998**, *106*, 511–532. [CrossRef]
11. Wang, R.; Li, B.; Lam, S.M.; Shui, G. Integration of lipidomics and metabolomics for in-depth understanding of cellular mechanism and disease progression. *J. Genet. Genomics* **2020**, *47*, 69–83. [CrossRef]

12. Zhang, H.; Shao, X.; Zhao, H.; Li, X.; Wei, J.; Yang, C.; Cai, Z. Integration of metabolomics and lipidomics reveals metabolic mechanisms of triclosan-induced toxicity in human hepatocytes. *Environ. Sci. Technol.* **2019**, *53*, 5406–5415. [CrossRef]
13. Zhao, H.N.; Thomas, S.P.; Zylka, M.J.; Dorrestein, P.C.; Hu, W. Urine Excretion, Organ Distribution, and Placental Transfer of 6PPD and 6PPD-Quinone in Mice and Potential Developmental Toxicity through Nuclear Receptor Pathways. *Environ. Sci. Technol.* **2023**, *57*, 13429–13438. [CrossRef]
14. Montgomery, D.; Ji, X.; Cantin, J.; Philibert, D.; Foster, G.; Selinger, S.; Jain, N.; Miller, J.; McIntyre, J.; de Jourdan, B.; et al. Interspecies Differences in 6PPD-Quinone Toxicity Across Seven Fish Species: Metabolite Identification and Semiquantification. *Environ. Sci. Technol.* **2023**, *57*, 21071–21079. [CrossRef]
15. Dejong, C.H.; van de Poll, M.C.; Soeters, P.B.; Jalan, R.; Damink, S.W.O. Aromatic amino acid metabolism during liver failure. *J. Nutr.* **2007**, *137*, 1579S–1585S. [CrossRef]
16. Ji, Y.; Yin, Y.; Li, Z.; Zhang, W. Gut microbiota-derived components and metabolites in the progression of non-alcoholic fatty liver disease (NAFLD). *Nutrients* **2019**, *11*, 1712. [CrossRef]
17. Teunis, C.; Nieuwdorp, M.; Hanssen, N. Interactions between tryptophan metabolism, the gut microbiome and the immune system as potential drivers of non-alcoholic fatty liver disease (NAFLD) and metabolic diseases. *Metabolites* **2022**, *12*, 514. [CrossRef]
18. Holme, E.; Mitchell, G.A. Tyrosine metabolism. In *Physician's Guide to the Diagnosis, Treatment, and Follow-Up of Inherited Metabolic Diseases*; Springer: Berlin/Heidelberg, Germany, 2013; pp. 23–31.
19. Wang, W.; Cao, G.; Zhang, J.; Chen, Z.; Dong, C.; Chen, J.; Cai, Z. p-Phenylenediamine-Derived Quinones as New Contributors to the Oxidative Potential of Fine Particulate Matter. *Environ. Sci. Technol. Lett.* **2022**, *9*, 712–717. [CrossRef]
20. Arroyave-Ospina, J.C.; Wu, Z.; Geng, Y.; Moshage, H. Role of oxidative stress in the pathogenesis of non-alcoholic fatty liver disease: Implications for prevention and therapy. *Antioxidants* **2021**, *10*, 174. [CrossRef]
21. Ivanov, A.V.; Bartosch, B.; Smirnova, O.A.; Isaguliants, M.G.; Kochetkov, S.N. HCV and oxidative stress in the liver. *Viruses* **2013**, *5*, 439–469. [CrossRef]
22. Wu, D.; Cederbaum, A.I. Oxidative stress and alcoholic liver disease. In *Seminars in Liver Disease*; Thieme Medical Publishers: New York, NY, USA, 2009; pp. 141–154.
23. Chen, Z.; Tian, R.; She, Z.; Cai, J.; Li, H. Role of oxidative stress in the pathogenesis of nonalcoholic fatty liver disease. *Free. Radic. Biol. Med.* **2020**, *152*, 116–141. [CrossRef] [PubMed]

toxics

MDPI

Review

Challenges in Ultra-Trace Beryllium Analysis: Utilizing Recent Extraction Techniques in Combination with Spectrometric Detection

Lucia Nemček * and Ingrid Hagarová

Institute of Laboratory Research on Geomaterials, Faculty of Natural Sciences, Comenius University in Bratislava, Mlynská dolina, Ilkovičova 6, 842 15 Bratislava, Slovakia; ingrid.hagarova@uniba.sk

* Correspondence: lucia.nemcek@uniba.sk

Abstract: Beryllium (Be) is one of the most toxic non-radioactive elements on the periodic table, and its presence or intake can negatively impact both the environment and human health. Classified as a carcinogen, Be is dangerous even at trace concentrations, stressing the necessity of developing reliable methods for quantifying it at very low levels. Spectrometric techniques for quantifying Be vary in sensitivity and applicability, with inductively coupled plasma mass spectrometry (ICP-MS) being the most sensitive for ultra-trace analysis. Flame atomic absorption spectrometry (FAAS) is suitable for higher Be concentrations, but preconcentration techniques can significantly lower detection limits. Electrothermal atomic absorption spectrometry (ETAAS) provides enhanced sensitivity for low-level Be quantification, further optimized using pyrolytically coated graphite tubes and chemical modifiers such as $Mg(NO_3)_2$ or $Pd(NO_3)_2$. Effective separation and preconcentration techniques are essential for reliable Be quantification in complex matrices. Liquid-liquid extraction (LLE), including single-drop microextraction (SDME) and dispersive liquid-liquid microextraction (DLLME), have evolved to reduce the use of hazardous solvents. When combined with ETAAS, surfactant-assisted DLLME using agents like cetylpyridinium ammonium bromide (CPAB) and dioctyl sodium sulfosuccinate (AOT) achieves preconcentration factors of approximately 25, reducing LOD to 1 ng/L. Vesicle-mediated DLLME coupled with ETAAS further enhances sensitivity, allowing detection limits as low as 0.01 ng/L in seawater. Cloud-point extraction (CPE), often employing Triton X-114, facilitates Be extraction using complexing agents or nanomaterials like graphene oxide. These advancements are critical for accurately quantifying Be at ultra-trace levels in diverse environmental and biological samples, overcoming challenges posed by low analyte concentrations and matrix interferences.

Keywords: beryllium; spectrometric quantification; liquid-liquid extraction (LLE); cloud-point extraction (CPE); solid-phase extraction (SPE)

1. Introduction

Beryllium (Be), a Group IIA element in the periodic table, is present in the Earth's crust at an estimated concentration of 2.8–5 mg/kg [1]. This lightweight metal has a high melting point of 1287 °C and exceptional properties: it is lighter than aluminum, about 40% stronger, and approximately one-third more flexible than steel [2]. These unique physicochemical characteristics make beryllium invaluable in various alloys, where it enhances strength, increases electrical and thermal conductivity, and improves resistance to corrosion and wear. For this reason, beryllium is widely used in electrical devices, electronic instruments, telecommunications equipment, and structural components for airplanes, rockets, satellites, and nuclear reactors [3]. However, these applications contribute to the release of beryllium into the environment. Furthermore, activities such as fossil fuel combustion and ore smelting and mining generate industrial effluents that contaminate air, soil, and water bodies [4]. As a result, global beryllium contamination is rising, posing significant risks to both the environment and human health.

Beryllium is recognized as a toxic element, with reports of its toxicity dating back to the 1930s, when numerous cases of beryllium poisoning emerged in the rapidly expanding industries of that time [5]. Beryllium and its compounds can cause various skin issues, including inflammation, ulcer formation, and granulomas. One of the most serious conditions associated with beryllium exposure is berylliosis, also known as Chronic Beryllium Disease (CBD), which is characterized by chronic inflammation and granuloma formation in the lung tissues [6]. Inhalation of beryllium, particularly in the form of smoke, mist, or fine dust particles under 10 μm, can result in acute lung diseases such as bronchitis, pneumonia, and alveolar edema [7]. Moreover, animal studies have shown that beryllium and its compounds can be carcinogenic, teratogenic, and mutagenic [8]. With accumulating evidence of its carcinogenicity, beryllium-containing substances have been classified as carcinogenic to humans [5]. The International Agency for Research on Cancer (IARC) in Lyon has designated beryllium as a Group 1 carcinogen, a category reserved for agents with strong evidence of carcinogenic effects in humans [9].

To address the potential risks associated with even ultra-trace levels of beryllium, which can enter the food chain and pose significant health hazards, the ability to accurately measure such exceedingly low concentrations in environmental samples is crucial. To meet these concerns, advanced methods have been developed for the separation, preconcentration, and precise quantification of beryllium at ultra-trace levels.

While beryllium's unique properties have made it the subject of thousands of scientific publications, only a small fraction focus on developing analytical methods for its reliable quantification. Among the available approaches, spectrometry stands out for its effectiveness in detecting this element. This article explores the widely used spectrometric techniques combined with recent extraction strategies for accurately quantifying ultra-trace concentrations of beryllium in diverse real-world samples.

2. Spectrometric Methods for Beryllium Quantification

Quantification of beryllium can be performed using several spectrometric techniques, each offering different levels of sensitivity and applicability depending on the matrix and analytical objectives. This section briefly reviews the most common spectrometric techniques employed for beryllium quantification.

Flame atomic absorption spectrometry (FAAS) operates on the principle that free atoms in the gas phase absorb light at specific wavelengths. In this approach, a sample solution is introduced into a flame, where it is vaporized and converted into free atoms. A light source, typically a hollow cathode lamp, emits light at a wavelength specific to the element being analyzed, such as beryllium. As this light passes through the flame, the free atoms absorb part of it at the element-specific wavelength. A detector positioned after the flame measures the amount of absorbed light, which is directly proportional to the concentration of the element in the sample. Although FAAS is less frequently used for direct ultra-trace quantification of beryllium due to its relatively low sensitivity, it is effective for samples with higher beryllium concentrations or when combined with an efficient separation and preconcentration procedure for samples with very low beryllium concentrations [10]. The instrumental parameters for FAAS-based beryllium quantification are typically configured according to the manufacturer's guidelines. Studies often report the use of a hollow cathode lamp set to 234.9 nm and an N_2O–acetylene flame, while a deuterium lamp is typically used for background correction [10–12].

Electrothermal atomic absorption spectrometry (ETAAS) works on a similar principle to that of FAAS, with key differences in the atomization process. In ETAAS, a small volume of the sample (typically a few microliters) is introduced into a graphite furnace, which heats the sample in a controlled sequence of four stages: drying, ashing, atomization, and cleaning. A light source, usually a hollow cathode lamp, emits light at a wavelength specific to the element under analysis. As the light passes through the graphite furnace, free atoms within absorb a portion of it at the specific wavelength. The detector then measures the amount of light absorbed, which is directly proportional to the element's concentration in the sample. ETAAS offers significantly higher sensitivity than FAAS, making it the preferred method for quantifying beryllium at low levels across various sample types. However, certain limitations still exist, and to address these, adjustments such as pyrolytically coated graphite tubes [13] or metal atomizers [14] have been implemented. These modifications improve signal reproducibility and minimize memory effects compared to uncoated graphite tubes [15]. Using the Stabilized Temperature Platform Furnace (STPF) concept, which incorporates a suitable chemical modifier, no undesirable effects were observed in the quantification of beryllium in both synthetic mixtures and real-world samples [13]. Chemical modification may involve various agents, including $Mg(NO_3)_2$ [16–19], $La(NO_3)_3$ [20], $Pd(NO_3)_2$ [21], $ZrOCl_2$ [22], $Al(NO_3)_3$ [23], acetylacetone in ammonium acetate buffer [24], a mixture of ammonium phosphomolybdate and ascorbic acid [25], and lutetium [26,27]. These chemical modifiers primarily serve to stabilize beryllium, enabling higher thermal decomposition (ashing) temperatures without analyte loss, reducing matrix interferences, and enhancing sensitivity.

In the analysis of natural waters and wastewater, $Mg(NO_3)_2$ allowed for an ashing temperature of 1300 °C, improving both sensitivity and accuracy compared to measurements conducted without a chemical modifier [16]. For biological samples, specifically blood and blood serum, $Mg(NO_3)_2$ was effective only in blood analysis, where it increased sensitivity. In this case, an ashing temperature was set to 800 °C [18]. $La(NO_3)_3$ was employed in the determination of beryllium in Chinese yellow rice samples after its separation and concentration on a TiO_2@SiO_2 flexible nanofiber membrane. Reliable results were achieved with an ashing temperature of 1100 °C [20]. The highest thermal decomposition temperature, 1500 °C, was used with $Pd(NO_3)_2$. It is important to note that this measurement was conducted using graphite tubes with inserted zirconium-coated platforms, which served as a permanent chemical modifier [21]. $Pd(NO_3)_2$ was also one of the three chemical modifiers tested by Shimizu et al. [28], along with $Mg(NO_3)_2$ and $Ni(NO_3)_2$. Among these, $Pd(NO_3)_2$ provided the highest sensitivity for beryllium. At an ashing temperature of 1000 °C, its use enhanced sensitivity by 3.7 times compared to measurements without a chemical modifier. When zirconium was used as a chemical modifier, pyrolysis was performed in two steps at 900 °C and 1000 °C. Additionally, using a tungsten platform in a pyrolytically coated graphite tube enhanced sensitivity by 2.5 times compared to a pyrolytic graphite platform [22].

Based on our experimental work, we designed a figure illustrating the optimization of the temperature program for trace beryllium quantification in fungi using ETAAS. It visually outlines the process from sample collection to temperature optimization and measurement, demonstrating the use of $Mg(NO_3)_2$ and $Pd(NO_3)_2$ as chemical modifiers (Figure 1).

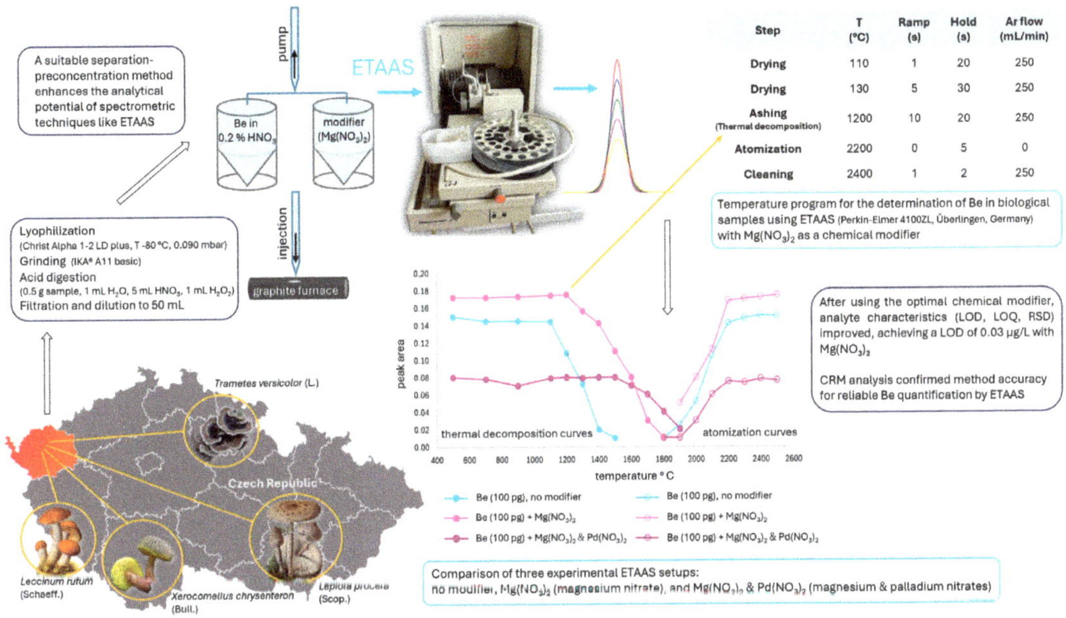

Figure 1. Optimization of the temperature program for trace beryllium quantification in fungi using electrothermal atomic absorption spectrometry (ETAAS). Thermal decomposition and atomization curves were compared for three setups: no modifier, $Mg(NO_3)_2$, and $Mg(NO_3)_2$ + $Pd(NO_3)_2$. The optimal thermal decomposition temperatures were 1100 °C (no modifier), 1200 °C ($Mg(NO_3)_2$), and 1500 °C ($Mg(NO_3)_2$ + $Pd(NO_3)_2$), with a consistent atomization temperature of 2200 °C. The lowest limit of detection (LOD) of 0.03 µg/L and the results of the analysis using certified reference material (CRM) confirmed $Mg(NO_3)_2$ as the most suitable modifier for reliable beryllium quantification.

Inductively coupled plasma optical emission spectrometry (ICP-OES) detects the light emitted by atoms and ions excited in a high-temperature plasma, typically ranging from 6000 to 10,000 K. When these excited species return to lower energy states, they emit light at wavelengths specific to each element. This emitted light is collected and separated by a spectrometer, with the intensity at each wavelength measured by a detector. The intensity of the emitted light is directly proportional to the concentration of each element in the sample, enabling accurate quantification. ICP-OES can simultaneously analyze multiple elements with relatively high sensitivity, making it a widely adopted method for analyzing a variety of samples. Its ability to handle multiple elements at once makes it particularly valuable in laboratories that need to monitor numerous samples and elements in parallel. For beryllium, ICP-OES is effective for quantifying moderate to high concentrations [29], or low levels when coupled with an appropriate separation and preconcentration procedure [30–32].

Inductively coupled plasma mass spectrometry (ICP-MS) is a powerful technique used to detect and quantify trace elements and isotopes in a sample. In ICP-MS, a liquid sample is first converted into an aerosol and introduced into a high-temperature plasma (typically around 6000–10,000 K), where it is atomized and ionized. The resulting ions are extracted into a mass spectrometer, where they are separated based on their mass-to-charge ratio (m/z). These ions are then detected, and their intensities are measured to determine the element concentration in the sample. ICP-MS is known for its high sensitivity and multi-elemental capability, allowing it to detect elements at extremely low concentrations.

Among spectrometric techniques, it is one of the most sensitive for quantifying beryllium. ICP-MS can detect ultra-trace levels of beryllium across a variety of matrices, making it ideal for environmental [33,34], biological [35–41], and occupational health monitoring [42].

While ICP-MS offers excellent detection capabilities, it is highly susceptible to matrix effects (e.g., interferences caused by sample components, space-charge effects, ion suppression, and changes in plasma conditions), which can limit its performance [43]. Beryllium, with its low mass, is particularly prone to being affected by space-charge effects, where heavier elements in the sample displace lighter ones from the ion beam, resulting in reduced sensitivity [44]. Matrix effects are more pronounced in inorganic samples (e.g., geological and environmental samples with high salt content) due to the presence of high concentrations of dissolved solids, which interfere with ionization efficiency and transmission in the mass spectrometer. In contrast, biological samples (e.g., blood, urine, and tissues) typically contain lower levels of dissolved salts, making matrix effects generally less severe. Additionally, modern ICP-MS instruments can be specifically tuned for low-mass measurements (e.g., Be at $m/z = 9$), where m/z refers to the mass-to-charge ratio of Be ions detected in ICP-MS. Since beryllium's most abundant isotope is ^{9}Be (with a mass of approximately 9 amu) and it typically forms a singly charged ion (Be^{+}, with $z = 1$), its m/z ratio is $9/1 = 9$. Optimizing ICP-MS conditions for low-mass measurements helps minimize space-charge effects. However, this does not mean that biological samples are completely free from matrix effects—proteins, lipids, and other organic components can still contribute to ionization suppression, though to a lesser extent than in highly mineralized samples. The severity of matrix effects depends on sample composition, preparation steps, and the tuning parameters of the ICP-MS instrument. Therefore, developing effective separation and preconcentration techniques is essential for the reliable quantification of beryllium in complex matrices, especially those with high salt concentrations [45].

X-ray fluorescence (XRF) spectrometry is a technique used to determine the elemental composition of materials. In XRF, a sample is exposed to high-energy X-rays, which cause the atoms within the material to emit secondary X-rays (fluorescent X-rays) that are characteristic of the elements present. These emitted X-rays are then detected, and their energies are used to identify the elements, while their intensities provide information about the concentration of each element in the sample. XRF is a non-destructive method widely used for the rapid screening of various elements in solid samples, such as soils, dust, or metal alloys. It is typically applied to determine elemental composition at ppm or percent levels but is not suitable for trace or ultra-trace analysis. Although XRF is less sensitive than some other analytical techniques, it remains valuable for quick, on-site analysis. Moreover, XRF encounters significant challenges when detecting elements with an atomic number of 9 or lower. These limitations become increasingly pronounced as the atomic number decreases, making direct quantification of beryllium (atomic number 4) nearly impossible. To overcome these issues, indirect methods for beryllium quantification with XRF have been proposed [46]. Alternatively, employing specialized instrumentation and/or using specific sample preparation techniques can improve the accuracy of beryllium quantification.

Laser-induced breakdown spectroscopy (LIBS) is an analytical technique used to determine the elemental composition of materials by focusing a high-powered pulsed laser at a target (material to be analyzed), generating a plasma from the target material within the surrounding medium (ambient air, a vacuum, or some other controlled atmosphere), enabling the spectral analysis of the emitted light. The resulting plasma, reaching temperatures between 10,000 and 25,000 K in less than 10 microseconds, is hot enough to break down molecules into atoms or ions and to excite electrons in both neutral atoms and ions from their ground state to higher energy levels. As these excited species return to their ground states, they emit characteristic radiation across a broad spectral range, from the infrared (IR) to the X-ray region. The identification of atoms or ions within the sample is achieved using well-established emission lines, and elemental concentrations are determined by measuring the intensity of these lines. LIBS is a rapid and versatile technique that requires minimal sample preparation and is capable of analyzing various materials, though it faces challenges like matrix effects and spectral overlap. For beryllium quantification at higher concentration levels, LIBS commonly and effectively uses the ionic Be II emission doublet lines at 313.04 and 313.11 nm [47]. However, determining beryllium concentrations in the range of 0.1–5 wt% with this doublet is challenging due to its resonance nature, which leads to strong self-absorption [48]. Several studies have confirmed that at higher beryllium concentrations, reduced sensitivity due to self-absorption in the plasma occurs [49–51], highlighting the need for careful calibration and spectral analysis. One solution to this problem is to use LIBS to detect the BeO diatomic molecular emission, a technique known as molecular LIBS (MLIBS) [51,52].

Fluorescence spectroscopy (FS) is an analytical technique used to examine the fluorescent properties of substances by measuring the light they emit after absorbing light or other forms of electromagnetic radiation. During this process, a sample is exposed to light, typically in the ultraviolet or visible range, which excites the electrons in the molecules to a higher energy state. As the electrons relax, they release energy and eventually return to their ground state by emitting light with a longer wavelength, known as fluorescence. This emitted light is detected and analyzed, providing valuable information about the sample's composition, concentration, and molecular environment. When FS is used for quantifying an element, it involves the formation of a fluorescent complex with the element of interest, typically by reacting it with specific reagents. The fluorescence intensity of the resulting complex is then measured. For beryllium ions, the reagent is usually a fluorescent dye or molecule that forms a stable complex with beryllium, exhibiting fluorescence. Common reagents include hydroxybenzoquinoline sulfonate (HBQS) [53–55], beryllon II [56], and morin [57,58], all of which form highly fluorescent complexes with beryllium ions. Although less common, this method is used in specialized applications.

UV-Vis spectrophotometry (UV-Vis) measures light absorption by a substance at specific wavelengths within the ultraviolet and visible regions of the electromagnetic spectrum. A light source emits light across these regions, and a monochromator selects particular wavelengths to pass through the sample, which is usually contained in a cuvette in liquid form. As light interacts with the sample, certain wavelengths are absorbed depending on the concentration of the absorbing molecules. The remaining light passes through the sample and is detected by a photodetector, which measures the intensity of the transmitted light. Absorbance is calculated by comparing the intensity of incident light to that of transmitted light. This absorbance value is then plotted against wavelength to generate an absorption spectrum, which reveals information about the sample's molecular structure and concentration based on the wavelengths at which absorption occurs.

The quantification of beryllium by UV-Vis spectrophotometry requires the formation of colored complexes using specific reagents, which are then analyzed by measuring absorbance in the UV-Vis range. The development and application of spectrophotometric techniques for beryllium analysis have been extensively researched over several decades, resulting in the identification of numerous organic reagents capable of forming vividly colored beryllium complexes with high molar absorptivities. Important photometric reagents include hydroxy acids, chromotropic acids, β-diketones, azo dyes, and derivatives of hydroxyquinone and triphenylmethane. Among the spectrophotometric reagents suitable for beryllium analysis, chrome azurol S (CAS) is one of the most widely used [59–63].

Other important reagents worth mentioning are anthralin [64] and hematoxylin [65]. This method is particularly suitable for simple matrices with high beryllium concentrations. Beryllium's tendency to form stable complexes affects its quantification in UV-Vis and FS, where chelation with organic reagents is necessary but adds complexity to the analysis. In ICP-MS, ICP-OES, and FAAS, beryllium complexation with strong ligands can lead to signal suppression due to incomplete dissociation during atomization or ionization.

Among the techniques mentioned above, only ICP-MS is suitable for quantifying very low levels of beryllium in natural samples. Most other methods require integration with an appropriate separation/preconcentration procedure to reliably measure ultra-trace concentrations of this element. Later in the text, we will discuss various effective separation techniques combined with spectrophotometry, flame atomic absorption spectrometry, electrothermal atomic absorption spectrometry, and inductively coupled plasma optical emission spectrometry in more detail.

Comparison of Spectroanalytical Techniques for Beryllium Quantification

When selecting an analytical technique for beryllium quantification, factors such as sensitivity, specificity, susceptibility to matrix interferences, and practical considerations like cost and sample preparation must be weighed (Table 1).

Table 1. Comparison of spectroanalytical techniques for beryllium quantification based on sensitivity, specificity, and susceptibility to interferences. The techniques are roughly ordered by their typical detection ranges, though actual performance may vary due to element-specific factors, matrix effects, and analytical conditions.

Technique	Typical Detection Range	Sensitivity	Specificity	Matrix Interference Susceptibility	Advantages	Disadvantages
ICP-MS	ppt to % levels	very high	very high	low	extreme sensitivity (ppt range), isobaric interferences for Be are generally low, multi-element detection	expensive instrumentation, high maintenance, Be's high ionization potential (9.3 eV) → ~70–75% ionization in Ar plasma, space-charge effects within the ion beam
ETAAS	ppb levels	high	high	moderate	high sensitivity (ppb range) for Be, small sample volume required	longer analysis time than FAAS, requires precise temperature control to avoid Be loss, more complex sample preparation
FS	ppb to ppm levels	moderate	low	high	high sensitivity when Be forms fluorescent complexes with organic reagents	highly susceptible to matrix effects, requires derivatization
ICP-OES	ppb to % levels	high	high	moderate to low	multi-element analysis, high throughput	relatively costly (although less than ICP-MS), susceptible to matrix effects
FAAS	ppm levels	moderate	moderate	moderate	simple, cost-effective	limited sensitivity for Be (ppm range), matrix effects

Table 1. *Cont.*

Technique	Typical Detection Range	Sensitivity	Specificity	Matrix Interference Susceptibility	Advantages	Disadvantages
UV-Vis	ppm levels	low to moderate	low	high	inexpensive, simple operation	limited sensitivity for Be, requires complexation with organic ligands for Be detection, strong matrix effects
LIBS	ppm to % levels	moderate	moderate	moderate	fast, minimal sample preparation	limited sensitivity for Be due to low emission intensity, susceptible to matrix effects
XRF	ppm to % levels	moderate	moderate to high	low	minimal sample preparation, non-destructive	poor sensitivity for Be due to its low atomic number, less effective for light elements like Be

ICP-MS: inductively coupled plasma mass spectrometry; ETAAS: electrothermal atomic absorption spectrometry; FS: fluorescence spectroscopy; ICP-OES: inductively coupled plasma optical emission spectrometry; FAAS: flame atomic absorption spectrometry; UV-Vis: UV-Vis spectrophotometry; LIBS: laser-induced breakdown spectroscopy; XRF: X-ray fluorescence.

FAAS and ETAAS are generally more affordable compared to ICP-based techniques, with FAAS being the simpler option. FAAS is commonly used for routine analysis due to its straightforward operation, minimal expertise requirements, and lower cost. However, it is limited to higher concentration levels (typically in the mg/L range) and is more susceptible to matrix interferences such as spectral overlaps or chemical interactions with co-existing ions (e.g., Al^{3+}, Fe^{3+}). On the other hand, the interferences in FAAS are typically more predictable and less complex compared to those in some other methods, allowing easier correction via background subtraction or matrix modifiers [66]. In contrast, ETAAS offers higher sensitivity, enabling the detection of beryllium at trace concentrations (ng/L to μg/L levels), but it involves intricate sample preparation and optimization. Beryllium forms refractory compounds, such as the stable oxide BeO, which require high atomization temperatures for complete dissociation into free atoms. Inadequate heating during the atomization step fails to break Be-O bonds, reducing sensitivity, while excessive temperatures (overheating) during the ashing step risk the premature volatilization of beryllium, leading to analyte loss [67]. ETAAS thus relies on precise temperature programming across three critical phases to effectively remove the matrix and atomize the analyte. First, *drying* eliminates solvents without splattering. Next, *ashing* removes organic and inorganic matrix components at controlled temperatures (<1500 °C for Be [e.g., 16,20–24,28]) to prevent analyte loss (Be vaporizing before measurement). Finally, the *atomization* involves rapid heating to ~2300–2900 °C [16,22,24,68,69], ensuring the release of beryllium atoms for accurate quantification. Each phase is crucial for maintaining sensitivity and precision in ETAAS analysis. Complex matrices, such as environmental or biological samples, may require optimized thermal profiles to prevent the co-volatilization of beryllium with interfering substances. Additionally, these samples may require chemical modifiers (e.g., $Mg(NO_3)_2$, [16,18], $Pd(NO_3)_2$ [21,28]) to stabilize beryllium during ashing. ETAAS demands specialized graphite furnaces, meticulous temperature control, and operator expertise to balance these factors, making it more complex and costly than FAAS.

For applications requiring higher sensitivity and multi-element analysis, ICP-based techniques are more suitable. ICP-OES is suitable for routine analysis, particularly for elements like beryllium. It offers reliable sensitivity at the ppb level and supports high-throughput analysis, making it ideal for regular monitoring, especially when analyzing multiple elements simultaneously. However, matrix interferences may require optimization to ensure accurate results, depending on the sample's complexity. ICP-MS offers the highest sensitivity, detecting beryllium at ultra-trace levels with excellent specificity. Isobaric interferences for beryllium in ICP-MS analysis are generally low due to its monoisotopic nature (^{9}Be) and low m/z, which avoids common polyatomic overlaps prevalent at higher masses. However, quantification challenges arise from its high first ionization potential (9.3 eV), resulting in only 70–75% of beryllium being ionized in a standard argon plasma. Additionally, being a very light element (9 amu), beryllium analysis is further complicated by space-charge effects within the ion beam. These shortcomings can be addressed by increasing the plasma power and optimizing the ion optics specifically for beryllium analysis [70,71]. While high matrix complexity could theoretically introduce rare polyatomic species, modern instrumentation effectively mitigates such interferences, leaving ionization efficiency and ion beam dynamics as the primary analytical constraints.

These limitations in solution-based ICP-MS have led to the development of alternative approaches, such as laser ablation ICP-MS (LA-ICP-MS), which bypasses the need for sample digestion and enables direct solid sample analysis. LA-ICP-MS offers high sensitivity, low detection limits, and the ability to detect elements lighter than sodium, including beryllium [72]. This technology enables in situ, real-time, rapid, and simultaneous multi-element detection along with isotopic ratio analysis [73]. It is widely used in gemological laboratories for identifying beryllium in gemstones [72].

To further improve the precision of ^{9}Be analysis in geological reference materials, Sproson et al. [33] introduced a new analytical procedure using high-resolution HR-ICP-MS. Their approach significantly reduced the error associated with ^{9}Be reactive phase measurements, achieving a precision range of 0.1 to 1.4%, whereas previous methods, such as AAS, ICP-OES, and ICP-MS, typically achieved a precision of 2 to 5%. This advancement has important implications for Earth Sciences, as it minimizes uncertainty in ^{10}Be/^{9}Be ratios and allows for a reduced sample size or leaching solution strength without compromising accuracy.

Spectroscopic techniques like FS and UV-Vis are lower-cost alternatives for beryllium quantification but come with significant limitations, including high susceptibility to matrix interferences and generally lower specificity. FS can achieve good sensitivity in the ppb to ppm range under certain conditions, particularly when fluorescence-based derivatization is applied. However, its effectiveness is highly dependent on the chemical environment [74–76]. Since beryllium itself is not fluorescent, its detection via FS requires complexation (a form of derivatization) with suitable organic reagents (e.g., morin, beryllon II, or hydroxyquinoline derivatives), which form highly fluorescent compounds. These complexes enhance detectability by significantly increasing fluorescence intensity, allowing detection at very low concentrations in optimal conditions. This is because fluorescence detection relies on emitted light, which, under ideal conditions, can provide a stronger [77–79] and more selective [80] signal than the absorbed light in techniques like FAAS. Some studies report detection limits in the ng/L to sub-ppb (<1 μg/L) range [55,81], making FS competitive with other trace beryllium detection techniques. Unlike absorption-based methods such as UV-Vis, FS benefits from a lower background signal (interference), which can improve sensitivity when ideal conditions are met. However, FS is highly prone to matrix interferences, as real-world samples (e.g., environmental, biological, or industrial) often contain substances that (1) quench fluorescence by interacting with sample components and reducing signal intensity, (2) scatter or absorb excitation/emission light, leading to signal loss or distortion, and/or (3) compete with Be for complexation, reducing the formation of the desired fluorescent Be complex. FS also typically has lower specificity compared to techniques like ICP-MS or ETAAS. The fluorescence response depends on the reagent used, and some organic ligands (e.g., morin and beryllon II) can form complexes with other metal ions [82,83], potentially leading to false positives or requiring additional masking agents for selective beryllium detection.

UV-Vis, while simple and inexpensive, lacks the sensitivity and specificity needed for reliable beryllium quantification, particularly at low concentrations. Nonetheless, some colorimetric methods using UV-Vis spectrophotometry can achieve detection of beryllium in the low ppb range. For example, Taylor and Sauer [84] described a colorimetric technique capable of detecting beryllium on surfaces at concentrations as low as 0.2 micrograms per 100 cm^2, which is equivalent to 2 ppb. This demonstrates that, with appropriate reagents and conditions, UV-Vis spectrophotometry can achieve the sensitivity required for low-level beryllium detection. Since beryllium itself does not absorb significantly in the UV-Vis range, complexation with organic ligands (e.g., CAS [63], anthralin [64]) is necessary to form chromogenic complexes that create detectable absorption changes, thereby enhancing its detectability.

For solid sample analysis, XRF and LIBS provide the advantage of minimal sample preparation and rapid analysis. XRF is non-destructive and offers moderate sensitivity, though it is less effective for detecting light elements like beryllium, due to their weak fluorescence signals. Beryllium's X-ray emissions are either too weak or absorbed by air or the detector window [85,86]. LIBS, on the other hand, is faster and offers superior spatial resolution, but Be's low emission intensity (due to its low atomic number) can limit sensitivity compared to heavier elements. According to published reports, LIBS sensitivity for light elements such as beryllium can be accurate down to the 1–10 ppm level [87]. Moreover, matrix effects in LIBS can further complicate ultra-trace detection, making it less reliable for applications that require high precision. Despite these limitations, both techniques remain valuable tools for the elemental analysis of solid samples, particularly when used complementarily.

Additionally, LA-ICP-MS, is also highly suitable for analyzing solid materials and offers greater analytical precision and significantly lower detection limits for all trace elements, including beryllium, compared to XRF and LIBS. While XRF detection limits range from ~1000 ppm for light elements to ~1 ppm for heavy elements, LA-ICP-MS typically achieves sub-ppm levels for most elements, reaching ppb for many heavy elements. Furthermore, LA-ICP-MS can detect light elements like beryllium, which XRF struggles with due to low-energy X-ray emission [72]. Another key advantage is its ability to analyze solid samples directly, making it useful for certain applications.

Ultimately, the choice of technique depends on the required detection limits, sample type, and available resources. While ICP-MS is the most powerful for ultra-trace level detection, methods like ETAAS or ICP-OES may be more practical in many laboratory settings. XRF, LIBS, and LA-ICP-MS offer advantages for direct solid analysis, while FS and UV-Vis remain useful for specific applications despite their limitations.

3. Extraction Techniques for the Separation and Preconcentration of Beryllium

Although higher concentrations of beryllium are commonly found in environments impacted by anthropogenic pollutants, such as those resulting from fossil fuel combustion for power generation and transport, or industrial processes like mining and smelting [3,34,88,89], many natural samples still contain only trace or ultra-trace amounts of this element. Given that even very low levels of beryllium can be toxic to living organisms, accurate quantification is essential for all types of samples.

Even though spectrometric methods offer relatively high sensitivity and selectivity, ultra-trace analysis remains a significant challenge. The two main issues are: (1) the analyte's concentration in the sample is often extremely low, complicating accurate measurement, and (2) the sample may contain numerous other components at much higher concentrations than the analyte, leading to potential interference. To address these challenges, employing an effective separation technique that separates and preconcentrates the analyte of interest is a practical solution.

Among separation techniques, extraction is one of the most widely used ones. In the analysis of liquid samples, extraction can occur either between a solid and a liquid phase or between two immiscible liquid phases, depending on the preferred technique. When the analyte is captured on a solid material, the process is referred to as solid-phase extraction (SPE). Alternatively, liquid-liquid extraction (LLE) involves the partitioning of the analyte between two unmixable liquid phases. Since their introduction, both extraction techniques have undergone numerous modifications, many of which align with the principles of green chemistry. The following discussion will explore some of the key modifications, both historical and recent.

3.1. *Liquid-Liquid Extraction*

Liquid-liquid extraction (LLE), also known as solvent extraction, operates on the principle that an analyte can partition itself between two immiscible solvents: typically, water (an aqueous phase) and an organic solvent (an organic phase) in a specific ratio. Initially, this technique involved the use of large volumes of hazardous organic solvents and sample solutions, often making the process both time-consuming and wasteful. Such practices generated substantial amounts of hazardous waste, which was not in line with the principles of green chemistry [90].

Modern analytical chemistry emphasizes eliminating hazardous solvents entirely and focuses on simplifying and miniaturizing sample preparation procedures. This approach reduces the consumption of samples, solvents, and reagents, leading to a significant decrease in laboratory waste. In this context, several modifications of traditional LLE have been developed, including single-drop microextraction (SDME), cloud-point extraction (CPE), dispersive liquid-liquid microextraction (DLLME), solidification of a floating organic droplet in dispersive liquid-liquid microextraction (SFO-DLLME), vortex-assisted liquid-liquid microextraction (VALLME), and others [91].

An earlier method for isolating beryllium from coal fly ash discharged by thermal power plants utilized a β-diketone liquid chelating exchange agent [92]. Among the various organic solvents tested, such as cyclohexane, isoamyl acetate, methyl isobutyl ketone, chloroform, carbon dioxide, and 1,2-dichloroethane, cyclohexane at pH 9.5 was the most effective for quantitatively extracting the Be-β-diketone complex. The extracted beryllium was then re-extracted into a 2 M HCl solution for quantification by ETAAS. Although relatively high concentrations of beryllium in the coal fly ash samples indicated that direct quantification might be feasible, this approach was not entirely reliable due to interference from other ions present in the samples. In the absence of the separation procedure, some measurements showed beryllium concentrations to be more than 300% higher than expected, likely due to interference from other ions. After applying the separation procedure, beryllium concentrations in the coal fly ash samples were found to range between 0.92 and 4.69 μg/g.

A liquid-liquid extraction paired with ICP-OES, where Be^{2+} ions were complexed with acetylacetone and extracted into p-xylene, achieved an impressive enhancement factor of 1300 [30]. The high flow rate ratio between the sample solution and p-xylene led to an enrichment factor of 75. Additionally, p-xylene (used as an organic solvent) contributed an extra enhancement of 10–20, making the observed factor of 1300 reasonable. The method achieved a limit of detection (LOD) of 8.0 ng/L for beryllium, a substantial improvement compared to the 3.1 µg/L LOD obtained via the conventional nebulization of an aqueous solution without liquid-liquid extraction. However, it is worth noting that this method was tested only on model solutions, with no real-world sample analysis conducted.

For the separation and preconcentration of ultra-trace levels of beryllium from effluents and natural water samples, two surfactant-assisted dispersive liquid-liquid microextraction (SA-DLLME) methods were developed [21,93]. In the first, cetylpyridinium ammonium bromide (CPAB), a cationic surfactant, served as both the ion-pairing and dispersing agent. The positively charged part of the CPAB molecule formed hydrophobic ion-pair complexes with the negatively charged beryllium-oxalate species, which were then extracted into chloroform [93]. In the second, dioctyl sodium sulfosuccinate (AOT), an anionic hydrophobic double-tailed surfactant, acted as the dispersing agent, forming vesicles that captured beryllium in the presence of salicylic acid, which were subsequently extracted into a small volume of chloroform [21]. For beryllium quantification, ETAAS was used. Both methods achieved a preconcentration factor of 25. Beryllium concentrations in drinking water and groundwater samples were below the LOD of 1 ng/L, while concentrations in effluent samples ranged from 9 to 92 µg/L. A highly sensitive vesicle-mediated dispersive liquid-liquid microextraction (VM-DLLME) procedure was developed for the quantification of beryllium at parts-per-quadrillion levels in seawater, air filter, and coal fly ash samples [94]. In this method, the anionic surfactant dioctyl sulfosuccinate (DOSS) serves as the dispersing agent, forming vesicle aggregates. After complexation with acetylacetonate, beryllium interacts with the hydrophobic solubilizing sites of the vesicles, enabling its extraction from the bulk aqueous phase into a small chloroform phase. The beryllium in chloroform is then back-extracted into diluted nitric acid, and this solution is used for beryllium quantification by ETAAS. Under optimized conditions, the method achieved an LOD of 0.01 ng/L for seawater, 0.15 ng/g for air filters, and 1.5 ng/g for coal fly ash samples.

3.2. Cloud-Point Extraction

Cloud-point extraction (CPE) is a specialized form of LLE that employs non-toxic surfactants as the extraction medium. It relies on non-ionic or zwitterionic surfactants, which form micelles in aqueous solutions when their concentrations exceed the critical micelle concentration (CMC). These micelles are spherical structures in which the hydrophobic tails of the surfactant molecules cluster together in the center, creating a non-polar core, while the hydrophilic heads remain oriented outward, interacting with the surrounding water. Micelle formation and the resulting turbidity occur spontaneously when the solution is heated to a specific temperature, referred to as the cloud-point temperature (CPT). Beyond this temperature, the initially uniform micellar solution separates into two distinct phases: a small-volume, surfactant-rich phase predominantly consisting of surfactant molecules, and a diluted aqueous phase where the surfactant concentration remains near the CMC.

In elemental analysis, the process typically begins with the addition of a complexing agent that forms hydrophobic complexes with the target element. These complexes are captured within the hydrophobic cores of the micelles and subsequently separate into the surfactant-rich phase, making their extraction easier. This process enhances both the extraction and concentration of the analyte, significantly improving the efficiency of the overall procedure [95,96].

Based on the information provided, it is evident that surfactants and complexing agents are crucial for developing effective extraction procedures. Among non-ionic surfactants, Triton X-114 (polyoxyethylene-7.5-octylphenoxy ether) stands out as the most commonly used agent in CPE procedures. Notably, over 80% of studies employing CPE for the separation, preconcentration, and speciation of inorganic analytes have utilized Triton X-114 [97]. In the context of beryllium analysis, Triton X-114 has been applied either on its own [17,32,98,99] or in combination with other surfactants such as cetylpyridinium chloride (CPC) [100,101] or cetyltrimethylammonium bromide (CTAB) [61]. When surfactants are combined, commonly by mixing non-ionic surfactants with ionic or zwitterionic ones, the procedure is referred to as mixed-micelle CPE (MM-CPE). This approach leads to the formation of mixed micelles with unique properties and often results in modifications to key parameters such as CMC and CPT.

In addition to surfactants, complexing agents play a vital role in extraction procedures. For beryllium analysis, a variety of complexing agents have been utilized, including chrome azurol S [60,61,98], 1,8-dihydroxyanthrone [64,101], 4-sulfamoylphenyl dithiocarbamate [99], and cupferron [17]. Recently, there has been a shift toward using nanomaterials as sorbents in various extraction procedures, including CPE. These materials facilitate the transport of analytes into the surfactant-rich phase, thereby minimizing the reliance on complexing agents. For instance, studies have demonstrated that beryllium can adsorb onto graphene oxide (GO) nanosheets, which are then preconcentrated using CPE [32]. This innovation represents a promising direction for improving extraction efficiency in analytical procedures.

Among spectrometric techniques, UV-Vis [60,61,64,98], ICP-OES [32,99,101], and ETAAS [17] have been employed for beryllium quantification following its separation and preconcentration by CPE. All studies that applied the CPE procedure reported an improved LOD. This parameter varies considerably across methods: for UV-Vis combined with CPE, the LOD ranges from 0.05 to 0.98 μg/L; for ICP-OES combined with CPE, it ranges from 0.001 to 0.005 μg/L; and for ETAAS combined with CPE, the reported LOD is 0.02 μg/L. The applicability of these methods was demonstrated through the analysis of real-world samples. Natural water samples of various origins and compositions were analyzed in all of the studies mentioned, with the exception of one that analyzed boron samples, including boron waste, boron ore, and processed boron ore [99]. Beryllium, quantified in several seawater samples, had reported mean concentrations of 0.13 μg/L [100], 4.93 μg/L and 5.61 μg/L [60], and 2.38 μg/L [101]. Additionally, wastewater samples were examined, revealing mean beryllium concentrations of 10.0 μg/L in influent and 1.00 μg/L in effluent samples [32]. The beryllium level in specific samples, such as boron, was below the LOD [99].

3.3. Solid-Phase Extraction

Solid-phase extraction (SPE) relies on a solid material to effectively retain the analyte of interest. A liquid sample is passed through a (mini)column, capillary, disk, cartridge, or syringe containing this material. The solid phase has a surface with specific chemical and/or physical properties that interact with the analyte based on its characteristics (e.g., polarity, charge, or hydrophobicity), allowing selective retention while other components pass through. However, column-based SPE often presents issues such as sorbent leaching, channeling, and cartridge clogging, which may extend the procedure beyond the desired timeframe. An alternative approach involves using the solid phase as a sorbent in a dispersion mode, characteristic of dispersive solid-phase extraction (DSPE) [102].

In DSPE, a small amount (typically tens of milligrams) of the solid phase is added directly to the liquid sample, and the mixture is stirred for a few minutes to promote analyte adsorption. Phase separation is then performed, usually by centrifugation, to remove the aqueous phase while retaining the solid phase with the adsorbed analyte. Depending on the detection technique used for further analysis, the next steps may include: (1) eluting the analyte from the solid phase with a small volume of a suitable eluent (typically hundreds of microliters to a few milliliters), (2) dissolving the solid phase containing the adsorbed analyte with a small volume of a suitable reagent, ensuring that the sorbent dissolves easily and does not introduce interferences, (3) drying the solid phase with the adsorbed analyte, followed by direct analysis (e.g., when using energy-dispersive X-ray fluorescence spectrometry (EDXRF) as a detection method), or (4) preparing a slurry by adding a small amount of a suitable reagent and directly analyzing the sample (e.g., for ETAAS in slurry sampling mode) [102].

A variety of sorbents for beryllium have been reported in the literature, including silica-based sorbents (both unmodified and modified), carbon-based sorbents (such as activated carbon, functionalized graphene, and graphene oxide), magnetic sorbents (e.g., MIIPs and magnetic MOFs), as well as specialized sorbents like oasis cartridges, strong-base anion-exchange resins, human hair, and TiO_2@SiO_2 flexible nanofiber membranes. These sorbents will be discussed in detail in the following sections.

3.3.1. Silica-Based Sorbents

Silica-based sorbents, primarily composed of silica (silicon dioxide, SiO_2), are materials widely used for adsorption in various separation and purification processes due to their excellent adsorptive properties, large surface area, and chemical stability. These materials are available in both unmodified and modified forms. Among the modified variants, octadecyl silica sorbents (C18) are the most common, with 'C18' referring to the length of the hydrocarbon chains chemically bonded to the silica surface. Other modifications, such as octadecyl silica gel treated with aluminon, octadecyl cartridges modified with quinalizarin, or silica gel bonded with benzenesulfonic acid, will be discussed later in the text.

As mentioned earlier, ICP-MS is known for its strong detection capabilities but can be limited by its sensitivity to matrix effects. Due to its low mass, beryllium is particularly vulnerable to space-charge effect (a specific type of matrix effect), where heavier elements can interfere with the ion beam, reducing sensitivity. Therefore, separation and preconcentration are essential for reliable quantification of beryllium in complex matrices, particularly those with high inorganic content, when using ICP-MS.

In seawater analysis, an effective approach involves using SPE technique with commercially available silica gel packed in a polypropylene column [45]. As seawater passes through the silica gel column, interfering matrix ions are removed by eluting with an EDTA solution, while beryllium remains bound to the silica gel. The beryllium is then quantitatively recovered by elution with HNO_3. This method was applied to analyze the vertical profile of beryllium in the eastern North Pacific Ocean, yielding interesting results. The beryllium concentration profile remained steady at depths of 10 to 200 m, with levels around 7 pmol/kg. It then rose with increasing depth from 200 to 3500 m, reaching approximately 30 pmol/kg before stabilizing between 3500 and 5000 m.

Among the elements quantified by ETAAS, beryllium has one of the lowest LODs. However, various preconcentration procedures have been developed to further improve its detection. One approach involves SPE using a custom-made C18 cartridge for the preconcentration of beryllium from hair samples [68] and marine organisms, such as fish, shrimp, octopus, lobster, oyster, and algae [69]. In both studies, beryllium was complexed with acetylacetone (acac) in the presence of an acetate buffer solution (pH 6.0). The procedures involved sample decomposition using a mixture of HNO_3 and H_2O_2 under microwave irradiation, followed by the addition of acetylacetone to form the $Be(acac)_2$ complex. This complex was retained on the C18 cartridge and subsequently eluted with methanol. The resulting methanolic solution was then introduced into a graphite furnace for ETAAS analysis. The reliability of the method was confirmed by analyzing certified reference materials (CRMs) of biological matrices and/or by applying the standard addition method. Beryllium concentrations in hair samples collected from healthy individuals ranged from 6.0 to 7.6 ng/g [68], while concentrations in marine organisms ranged from 7.1 to 24.7 ng/g [69].

A similar approach was applied to natural water samples (groundwater and spring water), utilizing a commercially available C18 cartridge (Sep-Pak C18) to capture the $Be(acac)_2$ complex, which was then eluted with methanol [103]. In this study, measurements were conducted using uncoated graphite cuvettes (tubes). Typically, pyrolytically coated tubes are preferred due to their lower porosity and greater resistance to high temperatures. Furthermore, the results were evaluated based on absorbance peak heights, which is a rather non-standard practice. Peak heights are generally not recommended for evaluation, as they are largely unreproducible and strongly depend on the quality of the graphite tube surface. Beryllium concentrations in the analyzed natural water samples were below the LOD (2.3 ng/L).

In another study, the adsorption of beryllium onto the surface of silica fibers from an alkaline medium (pH 9.5) was optimized for its separation and preconcentration from lake and seawater [104]. The results indicated that the adsorbed beryllium species were either $(\text{-SiO})Be(OH)_2^-$ or $(\text{-SiO})_2Be(OH)_2^{2-}$. These species were separated on three-layer filters containing silica fibers, and desorption was achieved using 0.5 M HCl prior to ETAAS measurements. After optimization, an impressive preconcentration factor of 300 was achieved. Despite this, beryllium concentrations in polluted lake water and unpolluted seawater samples were below the LOD (0.3 ng/L).

Farahmand [11] employed octadecyl silica gel modified with aurin tricarboxylic acid (aluminon) to separate and preconcentrate beryllium from tap water samples. The aluminon forms a complex with Be^{2+} ions. After passing the sample containing Be^{2+} through the cartridge, beryllium was extracted by rinsing with 0.1 M HNO_3. The amount of beryllium was then measured using FAAS. Following optimization, an enrichment factor of 330 was achieved, resulting in an LOD of 0.1 μg/L. However, the concentration of beryllium in the tap water samples was found to be below this detection limit.

An octadecyl silica cartridge modified with quinalizarin as a chelating agent was successfully used to extract beryllium from both simple matrices, such as tap and well water, and more complex matrices, such as Cu-Be alloy samples [105]. At a pH of 6–6.6, beryllium in the form of Be^{2+} was retained on the modified cartridge and then eluted with 0.5 M HNO_3 for quantification by FAAS. This method achieved an enrichment factor of 200 and an LOD of 0.2 μg/L. While beryllium concentrations in water samples were below the LOD, alloy samples contained beryllium at concentrations of 1.55% and 1.85%. Despite these relatively high percentages, the presence of other metals in significantly greater amounts posed a challenge for reliably quantifying beryllium even at concentrations this high. The use of an effective separation process, however, enhanced selectivity, demonstrating the method's applicability to complex matrices.

A functionalized nanosized mesoporous silica (MCM-41), modified with 2,4-dihydroxybenzaldehyde (4-OHsal), was used as an efficient sorbent for the extraction of Be^{2+} ions from aqueous solutions, followed by ICP-OES quantification [31]. SPE was carried out in batch mode, where 10 mg of the sorbent was added to a test tube containing the sample solution, followed by manual shaking and centrifugation. The aqueous phase was then decanted, beryllium was desorbed from the sorbent with 1.0 M HNO_3 and quantified by ICP-OES. This method was successfully applied for preconcentrating beryllium in water samples from various sources. Under optimal conditions, the method achieved an LOD of 0.3 ng/L. While beryllium concentrations in tap water were below the LOD, well water contained 0.028 µg/L and seawater 2.90 µg/L of beryllium. Additionally, the sorbent exhibited good reusability, as the modified MCM-41 was able to quantitatively extract Be^{2+} ions for more than six cycles.

Hasegawa utilized silica gel bonded with benzenesulfonic acid (SCX) in a column-based SPE setup for the determination of trace elements in pure molybdenum [106] and pure tungsten [107] samples using ICP-MS. The solid samples were decomposed with nitric acid for molybdenum and a mixture of HF, HNO_3, and H_2SO_4 for tungsten, followed by the addition of hydrogen peroxide to promote anionization. The cationic trace impurities were retained by the ion-exchange sorbent and then eluted with diluted nitric acid. Both methods were optimized to detect several trace elements, including beryllium. The LOD varied between the two analyses: 0.11 ng/g for tungsten [107] and 0.028 ng/g for molybdenum [106].

3.3.2. Carbon-Based Sorbents

Carbon-based materials are increasingly popular as sorbents in sample preparation due to their high surface area-to-volume ratios, high affinity for organic and inorganic molecules, metal ions, and gases, good physical and chemical stability, and low cost [108]. Among them, activated carbon, fullerenes, carbon nanotubes, graphene, and graphene oxide have been predominantly used in analytical applications.

Activated carbon (AC), composed of graphite crystallites, features a heterogeneous and irregular surface. It is produced through the pyrolysis or chemical treatment of materials such as nutshells, wood, and coal. The synthesis method and precursor material significantly influence its surface structure [109].

To separate and preconcentrate beryllium, AC suspensions have been applied to different matrices, including solid samples like coal, fly ash, and soil [110], as well as various water samples such as river, thermal, and freshwater [111], along with natural and flavored mineral water samples [12], prior to quantification by FAAS. Among the complexing agents tested—acetylacetone with morin, oxine, 1-(2-pyridylazo)-2-naphthol (PAN), and 4-(2-pyridylazo)resorcinol (PAR), the highest extraction recoveries (>85%) were achieved with a mixture of acetylacetone and morin [110]. This complexing agent was also used in studies by Avci [111] and Kılınç [12]. Procedure optimization led to excellent LOD of 0.010 µg/L [12] and 0.012 µg/L [111], resulting in a final preconcentration factor of 500. This improvement in detection allowed for the reliable quantification of ultra-trace beryllium concentrations in natural mineral water (0.05–0.94 µg/L), flavored mineral water (0.05–0.20 µg/L) [12], river water (0.07–0.183 µg/L), and freshwater (0.050–0.064 µg/L) [111]. Higher beryllium concentrations (0.815–1.687 µg/L) were detected in thermal water samples [111]. The method's LOD (0.12 µg/L), though somewhat higher, was still sufficient for the quantification of beryllium in solid samples, where beryllium concentrations ranged from 284 to 375 ng/g in soil, 2353 to 3947 ng/g in fly ash, and 417 to 845 ng/g in coal [110].

Graphene, a single layer of carbon atoms arranged in a two-dimensional honeycomb lattice, serves as the fundamental building block of other carbon-based materials like graphite, carbon nanotubes, and fullerenes. Its exceptional electrical and thermal conductivity, mechanical strength, flexibility, and transparency make it valuable in various applications, including electronics, sensors, and batteries. In analytical chemistry, graphene has recently been adopted more widely as a sorbent due to its large surface area, strong adsorption ability, and chemical stability. However, challenges such as aggregation and poor dispersibility limit its direct use in analytical extraction. To address these issues, graphene derivatives such as graphene oxide (GO), reduced graphene oxide (rGO), and functionalized reduced graphene oxide (frGO) have been developed [112]. Functionalized graphene enhances selectivity for specific applications. For instance, tannic acid-functionalized graphene (TAFG) was used in a vortex-assisted DSPE (VA-DSPE) for beryllium separation and preconcentration from water and street dust samples [19]. Using ETAAS detection, an LOD of 0.84 ng/L was achieved. While beryllium levels in water samples were below the LOD, street dust contained 37.6 ± 0.3 ng/g of beryllium.

A dispersive micro-solid-phase extraction (D-μSPE) using graphene oxide (GO) has been developed to extract trace amounts of beryllium, generated by beryllium processing plants, from wastewater [113]. In this approach, GO serves as a micro-sorbent, while 1-octanol acts as an extracting agent. GO nanosheets are dispersed in alkaline wastewater, where they efficiently capture Be^{2+} ions. To facilitate the separation and preconcentration of the beryllium-bound GO, sodium chloride is added, which neutralizes GO's surface charge, reducing its hydrophilicity and inducing aggregation. This allows GO to be easily extracted into a small volume of 1-octanol through hydrophobic interactions. Beryllium is then recovered from 1-octanol using ultrasonic extraction with diluted nitric acid and quantified via ETAAS. Under optimized conditions, this method achieves a preconcentration factor of 100 and an LOD of 2 ng/L.

3.3.3. Magnetic Sorbents

Magnetic solid-phase extraction (MSPE) is a variant of SPE conducted in dispersion mode using magnetic sorbents. This technique has gained considerable attention in sample pretreatment due to its unique magnetic features, ease of implementation, and cost-effectiveness. In MSPE, an external magnet is employed to isolate the magnetic sorbents loaded with target analytes, offering a simpler and more efficient alternative to conventional methods such as centrifugation or filtration.

A diverse range of magnetic sorbents has been developed for extracting various analytes from different matrices. Notable examples include Fe_3O_4-based materials such as metal–organic frameworks (Fe_3O_4@MOFs), covalent organic frameworks (Fe_3O_4@COFs), magnetic molecularly imprinted polymers (MMIPs), magnetic ion-imprinted polymers (MIIPs), and magnetic carbon materials (MCMs) [108]. Some of these materials have also been explored for the separation and preconcentration of beryllium.

One such application involved the synthesis of a magnetic metal–organic framework (MOF) using magnetite (Fe_3O_4) nanoparticles modified with 2-amino-5,8-dihydroxy-1,4-naphthoquinone (ADHNQ). These modified nanoparticles were then reacted with terephthalic acid and iron chloride to form a MIL-53(Fe)-type MOF (Fe_3O_4@SiO_2@ADHNQ/MIL-53(Fe)). This material was successfully employed for the extraction and preconcentration of beryllium ions, followed by quantification using FAAS [10]. Optimization of the procedure yielded an LOD of 0.07 μg/L and an LOQ of 0.20 μg/L. The method's analytical applicability was assessed through the analysis of seawater, well water, river water, and Cu–Be alloy samples. While beryllium concentrations in well water and river water were below the LOD, Caspian seawater contained 1.7 ± 0.05 μg/L of beryllium, and Cu–Be alloy samples had 0.64 ± 0.04%.

The use of magnetic ion-imprinted polymers (MIIPs) for the simultaneous separation and preconcentration of aluminum and beryllium from water samples was reported relatively recently [114]. Two new MIIPs were synthesized using chrome azurol S (CAS) as the ligand, (3-aminopropyl)triethoxysilane (APTES) as the functional monomer, tetraethyl orthosilicate (TEOS) as the cross-linker, with aluminum and beryllium ions serving as templates. These MIIPs functioned as magnetic sorbents. The optimized MSPE procedure was coupled with a spectrophotometric method using the mean centering of ratio (MCR) approach for quantification. For beryllium, an LOD of 0.90 μg/L was achieved. The method's performance was evaluated by applying it to tap and river water, though beryllium concentrations in these real-world samples were below the LOD. To assess accuracy, the samples were spiked with different beryllium concentrations, demonstrating the method's suitability for water analysis across varying compositions and sources.

3.3.4. Other Sorbents

This section will provide a discussion on traditional column-based SPE setups utilizing various sorbent materials, including Oasis HLB, strong-base anion-exchange resin, chelating ion exchangers, and human hair. Additionally, we will cover a specialized technique, a syringe membrane SPE (SMSPE), which employs a $TiO_2@SiO_2$ flexible nanofiber membrane.

A laboratory-prepared Oasis HLB cartridge was used to separate and preconcentrate beryllium from liver and muscle samples (bovine, chicken, and pork) after their decomposition with a mixture of HNO_3 and H_2O_2 [115]. Oasis HLB is a patented polymeric reversed-phase sorbent with both hydrophilic and lipophilic retention properties. 'HLB' stands for hydrophilic–lipophilic balance, referring to the sorbent's ability to (1) remain water-wettable and (2) retain a broad range of polar and non-polar compounds. In this method, beryllium was complexed with acetylacetone ($Be(acac)_2$), retained on the sorbent, and then eluted with methanol. A portion of the eluted solution was introduced into a graphite furnace for atomization using an optimized temperature program. This method achieved an LOD of 0.18 ng/g and an LOQ of 0.60 ng/g, enabling the detection of beryllium concentrations ranging from 2.3 to 4.7 ng/g in the analyzed samples.

For the selective binding of beryllium ions in mineral water, a specific type of ion-exchange resin with chelation properties (Ostsorb Salicyl) was used [116]. As part of the pretreatment process, EDTA was added to mask the interference of alkaline Earth metals and iron. The optimized extraction procedure was then combined with two detection techniques: ETAAS and ICP-OES, achieving LODs of 0.01 μg/L and 0.25 μg/L, respectively. These low LODs enabled the quantification of beryllium in natural mineral water samples from the Czech Republic, in a concentration range of 0.07 to 94.5 μg/L.

The preconcentration of beryllium ions using a strong-base anion-exchange resin is another example of an SPE technique based on a column setup [117]. After retaining the beryllium on the resin, it was eluted with 1.5 M HCl and measured using FAAS. After optimization, the method achieved an LOD of 0.045 μg/L and was successfully applied to spring, river, and wastewater samples. Interestingly, beryllium concentrations in spring and wastewater samples were similar, 0.17 and 0.15 μg/L, respectively, while river water contained higher levels (~0.35 μg/L). However, the study did not specify the sampling locations, leaving the source of these variations unclear.

An unconventional sorbent, human hair, was used to adsorb beryllium prior to its spectrophotometric quantification [62]. A custom-made column was filled with 1.0 g of human hair, which had been washed with synthetic detergent, then rinsed with deionized water and 0.5 M HNO_3. After optimization, the method enabled the detection of ultra-trace beryllium levels. In canal water samples, the mean concentration was 0.22 μg/L, while in tap water samples, it was 0.12 μg/L. The detection of these concentrations was made possible due to an enrichment factor of 50, leading to an LOD of 0.028 μg/L.

Recently, an efficient method for quantifying beryllium in Chinese yellow rice wines was reported by Wang [20]. In this approach, wine samples were first diluted with ultrapure water, then preconcentrated using syringe membrane SPE (SMSPE), followed by detection via ETAAS. The sorbent used in the SMSPE process was a TiO_2@SiO_2 flexible nanofiber membrane (TSFNFM), which effectively enriched beryllium while simultaneously removing interfering matrix components. With an LOD of 0.52 ng/L, this method was highly sensitive for detecting beryllium concentrations, which ranged from 0.09 to 0.41 μg/L in wine samples. Notably, the reusability of the sorbent was investigated, demonstrating that its extraction efficiency remained above 90% for at least 12 cycles, confirming TSFNFM's potential for repeated use without significant loss of performance (sorption ability).

4. Conclusions

The quantification of beryllium presents significant challenges due to the complexities associated with analyzing this element at trace levels, potential interferences from other components in the sample matrix, its tendency to form stable complexes, adsorption losses, and the limited sensitivity of certain analytical methods. This study has thoroughly examined various spectrometric techniques available for beryllium analysis, including flame atomic absorption spectrometry (FAAS), electrothermal atomic absorption spectrometry (ETAAS), inductively coupled plasma optical emission spectrometry (ICP-OES), inductively coupled plasma mass spectrometry (ICP-MS), X-ray fluorescence (XRF), laser-induced breakdown spectroscopy (LIBS), and UV-Vis spectrophotometry (UV-Vis). While these methods vary in sensitivity and applicability, they share common obstacles that must be addressed to ensure accurate quantification of beryllium in diverse matrices. Research on trace toxic element analysis often involves monitoring several toxic elements concurrently. This approach usually enables better characterization and correlation of data, making techniques like ICP-MS and ICP-OES particularly attractive due to their versatility and sensitivity. One of the primary challenges in quantifying beryllium using ICP-MS is managing matrix effects caused by variations in sample composition, which can impact ionization efficiency and signal stability. While beryllium's low mass minimizes isobaric interferences, polyatomic interferences such as $^{1}H^{8}O^{+}$ and matrix effects must be carefully addressed during analysis. The low atomic number of beryllium (4) makes it particularly susceptible to space-charge effects, where the presence of heavier elements in a sample can reduce the transmission efficiency of lighter elements like beryllium, leading to a significant reduction in sensitivity and accuracy. This phenomenon can complicate the reliable detection of beryllium, especially in complex natural samples where matrix interference is prevalent. For instance, while ICP-MS can achieve detection limits as low as 0.3 ng/L for beryllium, the presence of high salt concentrations or other competing species can drastically impair performance, necessitating effective separation and preconcentration techniques.

While ETAAS offers higher sensitivity than FAAS, with limits of detection (LOD) reaching approximately 0.02 μg/L when combined with cloud-point extraction (CPE), it still faces limitations related to reproducibility and memory effects. Modifications such as the use of pyrolytically coated graphite tubes can improve performance, but these solutions do not entirely eliminate the issues associated with method reliability.

Direct measurement of beryllium by X-ray fluorescence (XRF) is problematic due to beryllium's low atomic number, which results in reduced sensitivity compared to heavier elements. Indirect methods have been proposed to address this issue, but they often require specialized instrumentation and careful sample preparation to achieve acceptable accuracy. This challenge is further compounded by the fact that XRF generally offers lower sensitivity than other techniques, making it unsuitable for ultra-trace analysis.

Even in techniques like UV-Vis spectrophotometry, where the formation of colored complexes is essential for detection, the requirement for specific reagents and optimal conditions can complicate the process. For example, using chrome azurol S (CAS) as a reagent has been effective for high beryllium concentrations, but its applicability is limited to simpler matrices, and sample preparation can introduce variability in the results.

Liquid-liquid extraction (LLE) and solid-phase extraction (SPE) have proven effective in addressing these challenges. However, the classic LLE techniques that previously relied on large volumes of hazardous solvents have been phased out in favor of greener alternatives, such as dispersive liquid-liquid microextraction (DLLME) and single-drop microextraction (SDME). These modern techniques combined with spectrometric detection achieve impressive enhancement factors, with some methods reporting LODs as low as 8.0 ng/L for beryllium, but they still necessitate careful optimization and validation in real-world scenarios to ensure reliability.

Additionally, the quantification of beryllium in environmental samples, such as seawater, wastewater, and various solid matrices, is particularly challenging due to the trace concentrations typically encountered. For instance, beryllium concentrations in seawater have been reported as low as 0.13 μg/L, while effluent samples can vary significantly, ranging from 9 to 92 μg/L. The inherent variability in sample composition demands robust analytical protocols and an understanding of the potential interferences that may arise during analysis

As anthropogenic activities continue to impact the natural environment, the demand for reliable and sensitive methods to quantify beryllium is more urgent than ever. The synthesis and application of novel sorbents, such as those based on graphene oxide or magnetic materials, represent promising advancements in addressing the challenges of beryllium quantification. Nevertheless, the ongoing development of analytical methods must prioritize overcoming the limitations associated with matrix effects, detection sensitivity, and method reproducibility.

In summary, while significant progress has been made in the quantification of beryllium, the challenges presented by its low concentration, susceptibility to interference, and the complexities of sample matrices necessitate continued research and innovation in analytical methodologies. By enhancing the accuracy and reliability of beryllium measurement techniques, we can better assess the environmental and health risks associated with this toxic element, ultimately contributing to more effective regulatory measures and public health initiatives.

Author Contributions: Conceptualization, L.N. and I.H.; methodology, L.N. and I.H.; software, L.N. and I.H.; validation, L.N. and I.H.; formal analysis, L.N. and I.H.; investigation, L.N. and I.H.; resources, L.N. and I.H.; data curation, L.N. and I.H.; writing—original draft preparation, L.N. and I.H.; writing—review and editing, L.N. and I.H.; visualization, L.N. and I.H.; supervision, L.N. and I.H.; project administration, L.N. and I.H.; funding acquisition, I.H. All authors have read and agreed to the published version of the manuscript.

Funding: The work was supported by the Scientific Grant Agency of the Ministry of Education, Science, Research and Sport of the Slovak Republic and the Slovak Academy of Sciences under the contract VEGA 1/0135/22.

Institutional Review Board Statement: Not applicable.

Informed Consent Statement: Not applicable.

Data Availability Statement: The original contributions presented in this study are included in the article. Further inquiries can be directed to the corresponding author.

Acknowledgments: We thank Filip Polák from the Department of Soil Science and Soil Protection at the Czech University of Life Sciences in Prague for his assistance with sample collection and preparation, and Michal Miklovič for his help with the graphical abstract.

Conflicts of Interest: The authors declare no conflicts of interest.

References

1. Armiento, G.; Bellatreccia, F.; Cremisini, C.; Della Ventura, G.; Nardi, E.; Pacifico, R. Beryllium natural background concentration and mobility: A reappraisal examining the case of high Be-bearing pyroclastic rocks. *Environ. Monit. Assess.* **2013**, *185*, 559–572. [CrossRef]
2. Ryan, J.G. Beryllium. In *Encyclopedia of Geochemistry*; Encyclopedia of Earth Sciences Series; White, W.M., Ed.; Springer: Cham, Switzerland, 2018; pp. 93–95.
3. Tanveer, M.; Wang, L. Potential targets to reduce beryllium toxicity in plants: A review. *Plant Physiol. Biochem.* **2019**, *139*, 691–696. [CrossRef] [PubMed]
4. Shah, A.N.; Tanveer, M.; Hussain, S.; Yang, G.Z. Beryllium in the environment: Whether fatal for plant growth? *Rev. Environ. Sci. Bio-Technol.* **2016**, *15*, 549–561. [CrossRef]
5. Vaessen, H.; Szteke, B. Beryllium in food and drinking water—A summary of available knowledge. *Food Addit. Contam.* **2000**, *17*, 149–159. [CrossRef] [PubMed]
6. Elguero, J.; Alkorta, I. The dubious origin of beryllium toxicity. *Struct. Chem.* **2023**, *34*, 391–398. [CrossRef]
7. Taylor, T.P.; Ding, M.; Ehler, D.S.; Foreman, T.M.; Kaszuba, J.P.; Sauer, N.N. Beryllium in the environment: A review. *J. Environ. Sci. Health Part A-Toxic/Hazard. Subst. Environ. Eng.* **2003**, *38*, 439–469. [CrossRef]
8. Aller, A.J. The clinical significance of beryllium. *J. Trace Elem. Electrolytes Health Dis.* **1990**, *4*, 1–6.
9. IARC. *IARC Monographs on the Evaluation of Carcinogenic Risks to Humans*; IARC: Lyon, France, 1993; pp. 41–117.
10. Rezabeyk, S.; Manoochehri, M. Selective extraction and determination of beryllium in real samples using amino-5,8-dihydroxy-1,4-naphthoquinone functionalized magnetic MIL-53 as a novel nanoadsorbent. *Rsc Adv.* **2020**, *10*, 36897–36905. [CrossRef]
11. Farahmand, A.R.; Yousefi, S.R.; Fumani, N.S.; Mirza, S.; Shamsipur, M.; Hassan, J. Preconcentration of beryllium via octadecyl silica gel microparticles doped with aluminon, and its determination by flame atomic absorption spectrometry. *Microchim. Acta* **2009**, *166*, 89–94. [CrossRef]
12. Kilinç, E.; Bakirdere, S.; Yaman, M. Trace level determination of beryllium in natural and flavored mineral waters after pre-concentration using activated carbon. *Food Addit. Contam. Part A-Chem. Anal. Control Expo. Risk Assess.* **2011**, *28*, 455–460. [CrossRef]
13. Manning, D.C.; Slavin, W. The determination of trace elements in natural waters using the stabilized temperature platform furnace. *Appl. Spectrosc.* **1983**, *37*, 1–11. [CrossRef]
14. Černohorský, T.; Kotrlý, S. Determination of beryllium in drinking and waste-water by tungsten furnace atomic-absorption spectrometry. *J. Anal. At. Spectrom.* **1995**, *10*, 155–160. [CrossRef]
15. Shan, X.Q.; Yian, Z.; Ni, Z.M. Determination of beryllium in urine by graphite-furnace atomic-absorption spectrometry. *Anal. Chim. Acta* **1989**, *217*, 271–280.
16. Hagarová, I.; Macháčková, L.; Žemberyová, M.; Návojová, V. Determination of beryllium in various types of natural waters by electrothermal atomic absorption spectrometry. *Glob. Nest J.* **2012**, *14*, 40–47.
17. Macháčková, L.; Žemberyová, M. Cloud point extraction for preconcentration of trace beryllium and chromium in water samples prior to electrothermal atomic absorption spectrometry. *Anal. Methods* **2012**, *4*, 4042–4048. [CrossRef]
18. Stephan, C.H.; Fournier, M.; Brousseau, P.; Sauvé, S. Graphite furnace atomic absorption spectrometry as a routine method for the quantification of beryllium in blood and serum. *Chem. Cent. J.* **2008**, *2*, 14. [CrossRef]
19. Yavuz, E.; Tokalioglu, S.; Patat, S. Dispersive solid-phase extraction with tannic acid functionalized graphene adsorbent for the preconcentration of trace beryllium from water and street dust samples. *Talanta* **2018**, *190*, 397–402. [CrossRef]

20. Wang, Y.R.; Yan, J.T.; Wang, C.L.; Lu, D.B.; Chen, S.Z. TiO_2@SiO_2 flexible nanofiber membrane-based syringe membrane solid phase extraction for determination of beryllium in Chinese yellow rice wine samples by graphite furnace atomic absorption spectrometry. *J. Food Meas. Charact.* **2024**, *18*, 756–763. [CrossRef]
21. Meeravali, N.N.; Madhavi, K.; Kumar, S.J. A novel surfactant assisted dispersive liquid-liquid microextraction for the removal/recovery of beryllium from industrial effluents. *Desalination Water Treat.* **2018**, *101*, 283–290. [CrossRef]
22. Castro, M.A.; Robles, L.C.; Lumbreras, J.M.; de Celis, B.; Aller, A.J.; Littlejohn, D. Determination of beryllium by electrothermal atomic absorption spectrometry using tungsten surfaces and zirconium modifier. *Anal. Chim. Acta* **2009**, *636*, 158–162. [CrossRef]
23. Thorat, D.D.; Mahadevan, T.N.; Ghosh, D.K. Optimisation of GFAAS technique for beryllium determination in environmental samples. *Indian J. Chem. Technol.* **2003**, *10*, 67–71.
24. Wang, H.C.; Peng, H.W.; Kuo, M.S. Determination of beryllium and selenium in human urine and of selenium in human serum by graphite-furnace atomic absorption spectrophotometry. *Anal. Sci.* **2001**, *17*, 527–532. [CrossRef] [PubMed]
25. Horng, C.J.; Horng, P.H.; Lin, S.C.; Tsai, J.L.; Lin, S.R.; Tzeng, C.C. Determination of urinary beryllium, arsenic, and selenium in steel production workers. *Biol. Trace Elem. Res.* **2002**, *88*, 235–246. [CrossRef] [PubMed]
26. Burguera, J.L.; Burguera, M.; Rondón, C.; Carrero, P. Semi-permanent lutetium modifier for the determination of beryllium in urine by electrothermal atomic absorption spectrometry. *Spectrochim. Acta Part B-At. Spectrosc.* **1999**, *54*, 1743–1753. [CrossRef]
27. Burguera, J.L.; Burguera, M.; Rondón, C.; Carrero, P.; Brunetto, M.R.; de Peña, Y.P. Determination of beryllium in natural and waste waters using on-line flow-injection preconcentration by precipitation/dissolution for electrothermal atomic absorption spectrometry. *Talanta* **2000**, *52*, 27–37. [CrossRef]
28. Shimizu, T.; Ohya, K.; Kawaguchi, H.; Shijo, Y. Determination of ultratrace beryllium in natural water by electrothermal atomic absorption spectrometry after preconcentration with one-drop solvent. *Bull. Chem. Soc. Jpn.* **1999**, *72*, 249–252. [CrossRef]
29. Aslan, A.; Karapinar, H.S.; Kilicel, F.; Boyacioglu, T.; Pekin, C.; Toprak, S.S.; Cihan, M.; Yilmaz, B.S. Trace element levels in serum and gastric mucosa in patients with Helicobacter pylori positive and negative gastritis. *J. Trace Elem. Med. Biol.* **2023**, *75*, 127108. [CrossRef]
30. Okamoto, Y.; Nakata, F.; Obata, Y.; Takahashi, T.; Fujiwara, T.; Yamamoto, M. Optimisation of on-line liquid-liquid extraction for beryllium determination by inductively coupled plasma atomic emission spectrometry (ICP-AES). *J. Anal. At. Spectrom.* **2002**, *17*, 277–279. [CrossRef]
31. Yousefi, S.R.; Shemirani, F.; Jamali, M.R.; Salavati-Niasari, M. Extraction and preconcentration of ultra trace amounts of beryllium from aqueous samples by nanometer mesoporous silica functionalized by 2,4-dihydroxybenzaldehyde prior to ICP OES determination. *Microchim. Acta* **2010**, *169*, 241–248. [CrossRef]
32. Krishna, D.S.; Meeravali, N.N.; Kumar, S.J. Graphene oxide nanosheets in basic medium: A new potential adsorbent for microwave assisted cloud point extraction of beryllium from industrial effluents prior to ICP-OES determination. *Anal. Methods* **2019**, *11*, 2456–2464. [CrossRef]
33. Sproson, A.D.; Aze, T.; Behrens, B.; Yokoyama, Y. Initial measurement of beryllium-9 using high-resolution inductively coupled plasma mass spectrometry allows for more precise applications of the beryllium isotope system within the Earth Sciences. *Rapid Commun. Mass Spectrom.* **2021**, *35*, e9059. [CrossRef] [PubMed]
34. Goddard, S.L.; Brown, R.J.C.; Ghatora, B.K. Determination of beryllium concentrations in UK ambient air. *Atmos. Environ.* **2016**, *147*, 320–329. [CrossRef]
35. de Oliveira, M.; Gianeti, T.M.R.; da Rocha, F.C.G.; Lisboa, P.N.; Piacenti-Silva, M. A preliminary study of the concentration of metallic elements in the blood of patients with multiple sclerosis as measured by ICP-MS. *Sci. Rep.* **2020**, *10*, 13112. [CrossRef]
36. Nawi, A.M.; Chin, S.F.; Jamal, R. Simultaneous analysis of 25 trace elements in micro volume of human serum by inductively coupled plasma mass spectrometry (ICP-MS). *Pract. Lab. Med.* **2020**, *18*, e00142. [CrossRef]
37. Lavanya, R.D.; Reddy, B.S.; Sattar, S.A.; Rao, A.D.P. Trace element imbalances in blood serum of Alzheimer's disease patients. *Spectrosc. Lett.* **2021**, *54*, 458–471. [CrossRef]
38. Tajchman, K.; Ukalska-Jaruga, A.; Bogdaszewski, M.; Pecio, M.; Dziki-Michalska, K. Accumulation of toxic elements in bone and bone marrow of deer living in various ecosystems. A case study of farmed and wild-living deer. *Animals* **2020**, *10*, 2151. [CrossRef] [PubMed]
39. Barrientos, G.; Alves, J.; Toro, V.; Robles, M.C.; Muñoz, D.; Maynar, M. Association between trace elements and body composition parameters in endurance runners. *Int. J. Environ. Res. Public Health* **2020**, *17*, 6563. [CrossRef]
40. Muñoz, D.; Grijota, F.J.; Bartolomé, I.; Siquier-Coll, J.; Toro-Román, V.; Maynar, M. Serum and urinary concentrations of arsenic, beryllium, cadmium and lead after an aerobic training period of six months in aerobic athletes and sedentary people. *J. Int. Soc. Sports Nutr.* **2020**, *17*, 43. [CrossRef]
41. Saribal, D. ICP-MS analysis of trace element concentrations in cow's milk samples from supermarkets in Istanbul, Turkey. *Biol. Trace Elem. Res.* **2020**, *193*, 166–173. [CrossRef]

42. Bena, A.; Orengia, M.; Gandini, M.; Bocca, B.; Ruggieri, F.; Pino, A.; Alimonti, A.; Ghione, F.; Farina, E. Human biomonitoring of metals in workers at the waste-to-energy incinerator of Turin: An Italian longitudinal study. *Int. J. Hyg. Environ. Health* **2020**, *225*, 113454. [CrossRef]
43. Sohrin, Y.; Bruland, K.W. Global status of trace elements in the ocean. *Trac-Trends Anal. Chem.* **2011**, *30*, 1291–1307. [CrossRef]
44. Tan, S.H.; Horlick, G. Matrix-effect observations in inductively coupled plasma mass-spectrometry. *J. Anal. At. Spectrom.* **1987**, *2*, 745–763. [CrossRef]
45. Tazoe, H.; Yamagata, T.; Obata, H.; Nagai, H. Determination of picomolar beryllium levels in seawater with inductively coupled plasma mass spectrometry following silica-gel preconcentration. *Anal. Chim. Acta* **2014**, *852*, 74–81. [CrossRef]
46. Zawisza, B. Determination of beryllium by using X-ray fluorescence spectrometry. *Anal. Chem.* **2008**, *80*, 1696–1701. [CrossRef]
47. Khater, M.A. Trace detection of light elements by laser-induced breakdown spectroscopy (LIBS): Applications to non-conducting materials. *Opt. Spectrosc.* **2013**, *115*, 574–590. [CrossRef]
48. Cremers, D.; Radziemski, L. *Handbook of Laser-Induced Breakdown Spectroscopy*; John Wiley & Sons Inc.: Chichester, UK, 2015.
49. Janovszky, P.; Jancsek, K.; Palásti, D.J.; Kopniczky, J.; Hopp, B.; Tóth, T.M.; Galbács, G. Classification of minerals and the assessment of lithium and beryllium content in granitoid rocks by laser-induced breakdown spectroscopy. *J. Anal. At. Spectrom.* **2021**, *36*, 813–823. [CrossRef]
50. Cremers, D.A.; Radziemski, L.J. Direct detection of beryllium on filters using the laser spark. *Appl. Spectrosc.* **1985**, *39*, 57–63. [CrossRef]
51. Gaft, M.; Nagli, L.; Gorychev, A.; Raichlin, Y. Atomic and molecular emission of beryllium by LIBS. *Spectrochim. Acta Part B-At. Spectrosc.* **2021**, *182*, 106233. [CrossRef]
52. Nagli, L.; Gaft, M.; Raichlin, Y. LIBS-MLIBS-MLIF methods: Beryllium determination. *Spectrochim. Acta Part B-At. Spectrosc.* **2023**, *202*, 106631. [CrossRef]
53. Ashley, K.; Agrawal, A.; Cronin, J.; Tonazzi, J.; McCleskey, T.M.; Burrell, A.K.; Ehler, D.S. Ultra-trace determination of beryllium in occupational hygiene samples by ammonium bifluoride extraction and fluorescence detection using hydroxybenzoquinoline sulfonate. *Anal. Chim. Acta* **2007**, *584*, 281–286. [CrossRef]
54. Agrawal, A.; Cronin, J.; Tonazzi, J.; McCleskey, T.M.; Ehler, D.S.; Minogue, E.M.; Whitney, G.; Brink, C.; Burrell, A.K.; Warner, B.; et al. Validation of a standardized portable fluorescence method for determining trace beryllium in workplace air and wipe samples. *J. Environ. Monit.* **2006**, *8*, 619–624. [CrossRef] [PubMed]
55. Agrawal, A.; Lopez Tonazzi, J.C.; Cronin, J. High Sensitivity, Low-Cost Fluorescence Detection System for Beryllium Particulates. Available online: https://www.osti.gov/servlets/purl/902176-2kRhl1/ (accessed on 20 March 2025).
56. Ji, X.L.; Shi, W.Y.; Zhang, S.T.; Wei, M.; Evans, D.G.; Duan, X. A ratiometric fluorescence sensor for Be^{2+} based on Beryllon II/layered double hydroxide ultrathin films. *Anal. Chim. Acta* **2012**, *728*, 77–85. [CrossRef] [PubMed]
57. Amelin, V.G.; Aleshin, N.S.; Abramenkova, O.I.; Nikolaev, Y.N.; Lomonosov, I.A. Solid-phase fluorometric determination of Al(III), Be(II), and Ga(III) using dynamic preconcentration on reagent cellulose matrix. *J. Anal. Chem.* **2011**, *66*, 709–713. [CrossRef]
58. Fletcher, M.H. Fluorometric study of beryllium-morin system. *Anal. Chem.* **1965**, *37*, 550–557. [CrossRef]
59. Afkhami, A.; Zarei, A.R. Simultaneous kinetic determination of beryllium and aluminium by spectrophotometric H-point standard addition method. *Anal. Sci.* **2004**, *20*, 1711–1715. [CrossRef]
60. Afkhami, A.; Madrakian, T.; Bozorgzadeh, E.; Bahram, M. Spectrophotometric determination of beryllium in water samples after micelle-mediated extraction preconcentration. *Talanta* **2007**, *71*, 1103–1109. [CrossRef] [PubMed]
61. Bahram, M.; Madrakian, T.; Bozorgzadeh, E.; Afkhami, A. Micelle-mediated extraction for simultaneous spectrophotometric determination of aluminum and beryllium using mean centering of ratio spectra. *Talanta* **2007**, *72*, 408–414. [CrossRef]
62. Khan, N.; Kazi, T.G.; Tuzen, M.; Soylak, M. A multivariate study of solid phase extraction of beryllium(II) using human hair as adsorbent prior to its spectrophotometric detection. *Desalination Water Treat.* **2015**, *55*, 1088–1095. [CrossRef]
63. Fouad, H.K.; Atrees, M.S.; Badawy, W.I. Development of spectrophotometric determination of beryllium in beryl minerals using chrome azurol S. *Arab. J. Chem.* **2016**, *9*, S235–S239. [CrossRef]
64. Beiraghi, A.; Babaee, S. Spectrophotometric determination of trace amounts of beryllium using 1,8-dihydroxyanthrone as a new chromogenic reagent. *J. Iran. Chem. Soc.* **2007**, *4*, 459–466. [CrossRef]
65. Dayananda, B.P.; Revanasiddappa, H.D.; Kumar, T.N.K. Micellanized spectrophotometric method for the determination of beryllium using haematoxylin. *Spectrochim. Acta Part A-Mol. Biomol. Spectrosc.* **2007**, *67*, 1333–1338. [CrossRef] [PubMed]
66. Bysouth, S.R.; Tyson, J. Current Calibration Practices for Flame Atomic Absorption Spectrometry, Part 1. Initial Results from a Survey. Available online: https://scholarworks.umass.edu/server/api/core/bitstreams/4c39a6e8-eb68-4a86-a7dc-7c3961b7d1b1/content (accessed on 22 March 2025).

67. Husáková, L.; Urbanová, I.; Šafránková, M.; Šídová, T. Slurry sampling high-resolution continuum source electrothermal atomic absorption spectrometry for direct beryllium determination in soil and sediment samples after elimination of SiO interference by least-squares background correction. *Talanta* **2017**, *175*, 93–100. [CrossRef]
68. Li, C.C.; Kuo, M.S. Application of the acetylacetone chelation solid-phase extraction method to measurements of trace amounts of beryllium in human hair by GFAAS. *Anal. Sci.* **2002**, *18*, 607–609. [CrossRef]
69. Hsu, M.T.; Chen, M.H.; Yang, S.R.; Kuo, M.S. Application of acetylacetone chelation solid-phase extraction to GFAAS measurements of trace amounts of beryllium in marine organisms. *Anal. Sci.* **2004**, *20*, 1697–1700. [CrossRef]
70. Riss, P.E. ICP-MS Analysis of Low-Level Beryllium in Urine. *Spectroscopy* **2013**, *28*, 26.
71. AnalytikJena. Analysis of Low Level Beryllium in Urine Using the PlasmaQuant® M. Available online: https://www.analytik-jena.fr/fileadmin/content/pdf_analytical_instrumentation/ICP/ICP-MS/SpecialApp_ICP_MS_Be_urine_en.pdf (accessed on 19 March 2025).
72. Sun, Z.Y.; Jollands, M.; Palke, A.C. Chemical analysis in the gemological laboratory: XRF and LA-ICP-MS. *Gems Gemol.* **2024**, *60*, 536–559. [CrossRef]
73. Jin, W.K.; Che, X.D.; Wang, R.C.; Hu, H.; Rao, C.; Li, X.F. Accurate and precise in situ determination of beryllium contents in beryllium minerals using ablation spot size of 13 μm by LA-ICP-MS. *J. Geochem. Explor.* **2024**, *263*, 107512. [CrossRef]
74. Fernández-Peña, L.; Gutiérrez-Muro, S.; Guzmán, E.; Lucia, A.; Ortega, F.; Rubio, R.G. Oil-In-Water Microemulsions for Thymol Solubilization. *Colloids Interfaces* **2019**, *3*, 64. [CrossRef]
75. Sauer, M.; Hofkens, J.; Euderlein, J. *Handbook of Fluorescence Spectroscopy and Imaging: From Single Molecules to Ensembles*; Wiley-VCH Verlag GmbH & Co. KGaA: Weinheim, Germany, 2011.
76. Tesa, M. What Is Fluorescence Spectroscopy? What Can Fluorescence Spectroscopy Tell Us About Samples That Conventional Spectroscopy Cannot? Available online: https://www.azom.com/article.aspx?ArticleID=13958 (accessed on 20 March 2025).
77. Geisler, J. Choosing the Best Detection Method: Absorbance vs. Fluorescence. Available online: https://www.biocompare.com/Bench-Tips/173963-Choosing-the-Best-Detection-Method-Absorbance-vs-Fluorescence/ (accessed on 18 March 2025).
78. Peterson, W. The Measurement of Sensitivity in Fluorescence Spectroscopy. Available online: https://www.photonicsonline.com/doc/the-measurement-of-sensitivity-in-fluorescenc-0002 (accessed on 20 March 2025).
79. Ellis, J. Assessing Spectroscopy: Absorbance, Fluorescence, or Both? Available online: https://www.biocompare.com/Editorial-Articles/357719-Assessing-Spectroscopy-Absorbance-Fluorescence-or-Both/ (accessed on 10 March 2025).
80. Öztürk, B.; Ankan, A.; Özdemir, D. *Olive Oil Adulteration with Sunflower and Corn Oil Using Molecular Fluorescence Spectroscopy*; Academic Press: New York, NY, USA, 2010; pp. 451–461.
81. Minogue, E.M.; Ehler, E.D.; Burrell, A.K.; McCleskey, T.M.; Taylor, T.P. Development of a New Fluorescence Method for the Detection of Beryllium on Surfaces. Available online: https://doi.org/10.1520/JAI13168 (accessed on 18 March 2025).
82. Abate, C.; Giuffrè, O.; Amadeo, A.; Saija, F.; Cassone, G.; Foti, C. Experimental and computational study on morin and its complexes with Mg^{2+}, Mn^{2+}, Zn^{2+}, and Al^{3+}: Coordination and antioxidant properties. *J. Inorg. Biochem.* **2024**, *258*, 112635. [CrossRef]
83. Be. Beryllon II. Available online: https://www.benchchem.com/fr/product/b1200248 (accessed on 19 March 2025).
84. Taylor, T.P.; Sauer, N.N. Beryllium colorimetric detection for high speed monitoring of laboratory environments. *J. Hazard. Mater.* **2002**, *93*, 271–283. [CrossRef]
85. XRF. What Elements Cannot Be Detected by XRF? Key Limitations You Need to Know. Available online: https://kindle-tech.com/faqs/what-elements-cannot-be-detected-by-xrf/ (accessed on 21 March 2025).
86. LIBS. Expert-Approved LIBS Analyzers for Beryllium in Copper from Metal Analysis Group. Available online: https://metalanalysisgroup.com/mag-xrf-libs-alloy-beryllium-in-copper (accessed on 20 March 2025).
87. Hughes, R.W. LIBS—A New Beryllium Testing Method. Available online: https://www.palagems.com/beryllium-libs-testing (accessed on 22 March 2025).
88. Bolan, S.; Wijesekara, H.; Tanveer, M.; Boschi, V.; Padhye, L.P.; Wijesooriya, M.; Wang, L.; Jasemizad, T.; Wang, C.S.; Zhang, T.; et al. Beryllium contamination and its risk management in terrestrial and aquatic environmental settings. *Environ. Pollut.* **2023**, *320*, 121077. [CrossRef] [PubMed]
89. Thorat, D.D.; Mahadevan, T.N.; Ghosh, D.K.; Narayan, S. Beryllium concentrations in ambient air and its source identification. *Environ. Monit. Assess.* **2001**, *69*, 49–61. [CrossRef]
90. Anthemidis, A.N.; Ioannou, K.I.G. Recent developments in homogeneous and dispersive liquid-liquid extraction for inorganic elements determination. A review. *Talanta* **2009**, *80*, 413–421. [CrossRef] [PubMed]
91. Campillo, N.; Gavazov, K.; Viñas, P.; Hagarová, I.; Andruch, V. Liquid-phase microextraction: Update May 2016 to December 2018. *Appl. Spectrosc. Rev.* **2020**, *55*, 307–326. [CrossRef]

92. Bhattacharyya, S.S.; Das, A.K. Determination of beryllium in coal fly-ash by electrothermal atomic-absorption spectrometry. *J. Anal. At. Spectrom.* **1992**, *7*, 417–420. [CrossRef]
93. Meeravali, N.N.; Madhavi, K.; Kumar, S.J. A new ion pair-based surfactant-assisted dispersive liquid-liquid microextraction of ultratrace levels of beryllium from natural and effluent samples followed by ETAAS determination. *At. Spectrosc.* **2016**, *37*, 202–209. [CrossRef]
94. Krishna, D.S.; Madhavi, K.; Meeravali, N.N.; Sahayam, A.C. A sensitive vesicle mediated dispersive liquid-liquid microextraction of parts per quadrillion levels of beryllium from seawater samples prior to graphite furnace atomic absorption spectrometry determination. *Anal. Chim. Acta* **2022**, *1191*, 339313. [CrossRef]
95. Hagarová, I.; Nemček, L. Reliable quantification of ultratrace selenium in food, beverages, and water samples by cloud point extraction and spectrometric analysis. *Nutrients* **2022**, *14*, 3530. [CrossRef]
96. Hagarová, I.; Urík, M. Cloud point extraction in beverage analysis: Innovations and applications for trace elements. *Beverages* **2024**, *10*, 67. [CrossRef]
97. Hagarová, I.; Nemček, L. Recent advances in speciation analysis of trace antimony in environmental and biological samples based on cloud point extraction and spectrometric methods. In *Sustainable Agriculture Reviews*; Lichtfouse, E., Ed.; Springer Nature: Cham, Switzerland, 2021; pp. 49–77.
98. Krishna, D.S.; Meeravali, N.N.; Sahayam, A.C. A novel non-ionic nanoaggregate sensitized salt induced cloud point extraction of anionic beryllium-chrome azurol S for spectrophotometric determination of beryllium in environmental waters. *Microchem. J.* **2021**, *160*, 105651. [CrossRef]
99. Dundar, M.S.; Gucunlu, H.; Caner, C.; Altundag, H.; Gulec, Ö.; Arslan, M. Determination of lead and beryllium in boron samples using 4-sulfamoylphenyl dithiocarbamate salt by ICP-OES. *J. Chem. Metrol.* **2024**, *18*, 71–82. [CrossRef]
100. Beiraghi, A.; Zarei, A.R.; Babaee, S. Cloud-point formation based on mixed micelles for the extraction, preconcentration and spectrophotometric determination of trace amounts of beryllium in water samples. *Anal. Sci.* **2007**, *23*, 527–531. [CrossRef]
101. Beiraghi, A.; Babaee, S. Separation and preconcentration of ultra trace amounts of beryllium in water samples using mixed micelle-mediated extraction and determination by inductively coupled plasma-atomic emission spectrometry. *Anal. Chim. Acta* **2008**, *607*, 183–190. [CrossRef]
102. Hagarová, I.; Nemček, L. Analytical application of layered double hydroxides as high-capacity sorbents in dispersive solid phase extraction for the separation and preconcentration of (ultra)trace heavy metals. *Crit. Rev. Anal. Chem.* **2024**, *54*, 3114–3127. [CrossRef] [PubMed]
103. Peng, H.W.; Kuo, M.S. Determination of trace amounts of beryllium(II) in drinking water and of beryllium vapor in air by graphite-furnace atomic absorption spectrophotometry using acetylacetone as a chelating agent. *Anal. Sci.* **2000**, *16*, 157–161. [CrossRef]
104. Nukatsuka, I.; Sakai, K.; Kudo, R.; Ohzeki, K. Studies on the adsorption of trace amounts of beryllium(II) on the surface of silica fibres from an aqueous phase for the development of a novel enrichment technique for electrothermal atomic absorption spectrometry. *Analyst* **1995**, *120*, 2819–2822. [CrossRef]
105. Yamini, Y.; Hassan, J.; Mohandesi, R.; Bahramifar, N. Preconcentration of trace amounts of beryllium in water samples on octadecyl silica cartridges modified by quinalizarine and its determination with atomic absorption spectrometry. *Talanta* **2002**, *56*, 375–381. [CrossRef]
106. Hasegawa, S.I.; Yamaguchi, H.; Yamada, K.; Kobayashi, T. Determination of trace elements in high-purity molybdenum by solid-phase extraction/ICP-MS. *Mater. Trans.* **2004**, *45*, 925–929. [CrossRef]
107. Hasegawa, S.I. Determination of trace elements in high purity tungsten by solid-phase extraction/ICP-MS. *Mater. Trans.* **2008**, *49*, 2054–2057. [CrossRef]
108. Wen, Y.Y.; Chen, L.; Li, J.H.; Liu, D.Y.; Chen, L.X. Recent advances in solid-phase sorbents for sample preparation prior to chromatographic analysis. *Trac-Trends Anal. Chem.* **2014**, *59*, 26–41. [CrossRef]
109. Hashemi, B.; Rezania, S. Carbon-based sorbents and their nanocomposites for the enrichment of heavy metal ions: A review. *Microchim. Acta* **2019**, *186*, 578. [CrossRef] [PubMed]
110. Yaman, M.; Avci, H. Determination of beryllium in solid samples by flame atomic absorption spectrometry after preconcentration on activated carbon. *Anal. Sci.* **2006**, *22*, 721–725. [CrossRef] [PubMed]
111. Avci, H.; Yaman, M. Flame AAS determination of beryllium in water samples after preconcentration on activated carbon. *At. Spectrosc.* **2006**, *27*, 117–122.
112. Pena-Pereira, F.; Romero, V.; de la Calle, I.; Lavilla, I.; Bendicho, C. Graphene-based nanocomposites in analytical extraction processes. *Trac-Trends Anal. Chem.* **2021**, *142*, 116303. [CrossRef]

113. Devulapally, S.; Meeravali, N.N.; Sahayam, A.C. Interference free ultratrace beryllium determination in alkaline effluents of beryllium processing plants by graphite furnace atomic absorption spectrometry after a novel graphene oxide-assisted dispersive micro solid phase extraction without using a chelating agent. *J. Anal. At. Spectrom.* **2024**, *39*, 1322–1331. [CrossRef]
114. Taheri, Z.; Afkhami, A.; Madrakian, T.; Kamalabadi, M. Application of magnetic ion imprinted polymers for simultaneous quantification of $Al^{3+}$and Be^{2+} ions using the mean centering of ratio spectra method. *Talanta* **2021**, *225*, 122003. [CrossRef]
115. Liu, P.Y.; Chen, M.H.; Tsai, Y.Y.; Kuo, M.S. Application of acetylacetone chelation solid-phase extraction to GFAAS measurements of trace amounts of beryllium in livers and muscles of poultry and livestock. *Food Chem.* **2011**, *126*, 1460–1464. [CrossRef]
116. Kubová, J.; Nevoral, V.; Streško, V. Determination of beryllium trace concentrations in mineral waters after preconcentration on a chelating ion-exchanger. *Fresenius J. Anal. Chem.* **1994**, *348*, 287–290. [CrossRef]
117. Afkhami, A.; Madrakian, T.; Assl, A.A.; Sehhat, A.A. Solid phase extraction flame atomic absorption spectrometric determination of ultra-trace beryllium. *Anal. Chim. Acta* **2001**, *437*, 17–22. [CrossRef]

toxics

MDPI

Review

Uncovering the Potential Link Between Polychlorinated Biphenyls and Cardiovascular Diseases: A Comprehensive Analysis

Jingyu Liu [1,†], Qiuli Shan [1,*,†], Yang Yang [2] and Wenxing He [1,*]

[1] College of Biological Science and Technology, University of Jinan, Jinan 250022, China; jy18739485166@163.com
[2] College of Marine Life Science, Ocean University of China, Qingdao 266003, China; 21240613013@stu.ouc.edu.cn
* Correspondence: bio_shanql@ujn.edu.cn (Q.S.); chm_hewx@ujn.edu.cn (W.H.)
† These authors contributed equally to this work.

Abstract: Background: A family of persistent organic pollutants, known as polychlorinated biphenyls (PCBs), are extensively found in the environment and may be harmful to the cardiovascular system. Systematic reviews and meta-analyses are required to thoroughly evaluate the association between PCB exposure and cardiovascular disease (CVDs), despite the fact that studies on the subject have produced inconsistent results. Objective: The purpose of this study was to investigate the relationship between PCBs exposure and cardiovascular disease risk in order to provide more conclusive data to promote public health actions. Methods: The studies that met the inclusion criteria were screened out using the databases PubMed, Web of Science, ScienceDirect, and Cochrane Library. The comprehensive effect size (OR) was calculated using the random-effects model; the study's heterogeneity was analyzed using I^2 statistics; the major reasons of heterogeneity were identified using subgroup analysis; and publication bias graphically was measured using the Egger's test. Results: A meta-analysis of 11 studies revealed that total PCBs (OR = 1.56, 95% CI: 1.20–1.75), non-dioxin-like PCBs (NDL-PCBs) (OR = 1.33, 95% CI: 1.15–1.53), and dioxin-like PCBs (DL-PCBs) (OR = 1.31, 95% CI: 1.10–1.57) were all found to be positively associated with the risk of cardiovascular disease. Subgroup analysis revealed that study type, biomaterials, and literature quality were the most significant drivers of variation. Furthermore, certain PCB homologues, such as non-dioxin-like (NDL)-PCB153 and dioxin-like (DL)-PCB118, are highly related with cardiovascular disease. Conclusions: According to this meta-analysis, exposure to PCBs may increase the risk of cardiovascular disease. Notwithstanding major drawbacks, our results emphasize the significance of lowering exposure to PCBs and offering a solid theoretical basis for public health initiatives.

Keywords: PCBs; CVDs; meta-analysis; systematic review; public health

1. Introduction

Cardiovascular diseases (CVDs) are disorders that affect the heart and blood vessels, including coronary heart disease, myocardial infarction, stroke, and arteriosclerosis [1]. These situations interrupt normal blood circulation and oxygen flow, which may cause organ damage [2]. CVDs pose a significant global health threat and are among the main causes of death [3]. They can lead to serious complications such as myocardial infarction and thrombosis, significantly impairing patients' quality of life and posing potentially life-threatening risks [4]. Obesity, hypertension, diabetes, high cholesterol and triglyceride levels, chronic psychological stress, genetic susceptibility, and bad lifestyle choices have all been identified as risk factors for CVDs [5,6]. Persistent organic pollutants (POPs) have received more attention lately. Studies show that POP exposure in the environment plays a major role in the development and progression of CVDs [7].

POPs are natural or manmade organic contaminants that remain in environmental media such as air, water, soil, and living organisms for long periods, posing major hazards to the environment and human health [8]. PCBs are a common class of POPs. According to studies, PCBs are persistent, bioaccumulative, semi-volatile, and highly poisonous [9]. These compounds possess the potential to induce permanent damage to the neurological, endocrine, and reproductive systems. As lipophilic substances, they can disrupt intracellular lipid metabolism, thereby affecting metabolic and endocrine functions. There is a strong link between PCBs and chronic metabolic disorders, such as diabetes, obesity, CVDs, and other chronic diseases, according to recent epidemiological research [10,11]. PCBs have been linked to metabolic syndrome (MetS), which is linked to the type and homologue of PCBs, according to a meta-analysis [12]. The findings of another meta-analysis indicate that PCBs, particularly DL-PCBs, constitute a significant risk factor for the development of hypertension [13].

The number of articles and reports discussing the link between PCBs and CVDs has significantly increased in recent years, raising public awareness of PCBs. Individual studies produced inconsistent or contradictory results, and there has been some research on the association between PCBs and CVDs, but it has not been systematically integrated as of late. A 2016 cohort study of men who were Swedish citizens in 1997 discovered a link between dietary PCB exposure and an increased risk of myocardial infarction [14]. On the other hand, a cross-sectional examination in 2020 revealed a common association between coronary artery calcification and PCB exposure not seen in the diet [15]. A 2021 study linked six serum PCB homologues to CVD prevalence [16]. In contrast, Laura Deen et al. found no such association [17]. Therefore, more research is required to validate the link between PCBs and CVDs.

The objectives we set in doing this meta-analysis were to better understand the variations in PCBs levels across individuals with and without CVDs and to assess the correlation between PCBs and CVDs. Additionally, we performed a subgroup analysis of research design, PCB type, and article quality, three possible impacting factors.

2. Materials and Methods

2.1. Methods

This study was conducted in accordance with the PRISMA 2020 (Preferred Reporting Items for Systematic Reviews and Meta-Analyses) [18] statement and the MOOSE (Meta-analyses of Observational Studies in Epidemiology) guidelines [19]. This study has been registered as PROSPERO, Registration number CRD42024563475. The following is the Population, Exposure, Comparator, and Outcome (PECO) [20] for this topic: Population (P): General population, including those exposed to PCBs. Exposure (E): Exposure to or increased exposure to PCBs as indicated by the results of human blood, serum, or adipose tissue tests. Comparator (C): Unexposed or less exposed to PCBs (if applicable) or lowest PCB exposure group. Outcome (O): Occurrence of CVDs.

2.2. Exposure and Outcome Measures

Assessments were conducted individually for PCBs, dioxin-like (DL) PCBs, non-dioxin-like (NDL) PCBs, and selected individual congeners. The primary outcome was incidence or prevalence of CVDs.

2.3. Literature Sources and Search Methodologies

Our research team looked through PubMed, ScienceDirect, Web of Science, and the Cochrane Library for pertinent literature. Database retrieval period began on 1 March 2024. Due to variations in search methods across different websites, the keywords used for searches may differ. Please refer to Supplementary Materials for specific search strategies.

2.4. Criteria for Study Selection

Studies that fulfilled the following criteria were considered epidemiological: (1) any demographic or subject group; (2) case-control, cross-sectional, and queuing study designs (the literature that is included needs to address the connection between cardiovascular illnesses and homologues of polychlorinated biphenyls); (3) biological samples (blood, serum, or adipose tissue) for the purpose of measuring PCBs directly or indirectly through consumption of PCB-estimating foods; (4) the incidence or prevalence of cardiovascular disease, together with the related 95% confidence intervals (CI) for the hazard ratio (HR), relative risk ratio (RR), and odds ratio (OR); (5) English should be the language used for the included books; (6) original research should be the genre of the incorporated literature.

2.5. Criteria for Study Exclusion

Our exclusion criteria were: (1) Studies that are not research-focused on PCBs and CVDs; (2) literature encompassing both animal and in vitro experiments; (3) the language of literature is not English; (4) topics for literature include reviews, analyses, abstracts, and so on; (5) studies lacking valid data in their findings.

2.6. Quality Evaluation

For the cohort and case-control studies included in the literature, the Newcastle–Ottawa Quality-Assessment Scale (NOS) was used for evaluation [21]; for cross-sectional studies, a modified NOS scale [22] was applied.

2.7. Data Extraction

We will extract the following information from all included studies: authors, publication year, design of the study, location, study population, study period, sample size, gender ratio, age distribution, biological substances, types of PCBs, methods of PCBs measurement, outcomes, and main findings.

2.8. Result Analysis

The effect sizes and confidence intervals between PCBs and CVDs will be calculated using the raw data from the literature. The relationship between PCBs and CVDs will be investigated through the synthesis of effect sizes. The heterogeneity of the combined effect was examined using the Q test. A significant level of heterogeneity is indicated by an effect size of the Q test (I^2) larger than 50%, at which point the random-effects model ought to be applied. A fixed-effect model should be used when the heterogeneity is deemed low [23] and the I^2 value is less than 50%.

Subgroup analysis will be used to investigate the sources of heterogeneity when they are high. Utilizing the funnel plot and Egger test method, the publication bias of the included literature was quantified. To determine how each study affected the total effect size, we conducted sensitivity analyses. After removing one study per round, we ran the meta-analysis. Using stratified analyses, potential causes of heterogeneity related to the quality of the literature, research design, or PCB type were evaluated. The amount of possible confounding (unmeasured, unknown, OR residual) was estimated using the total PCBs measured with OR as the effect, and the e values were provided.

A smaller e value indicates that less unmeasurable confounding is needed to explain the impact estimate, whereas a greater e value indicates the necessity for substantial unmeasurable confounding. Stata MP14 (521.14.0.366) and Review Manager 5.3 (5.3.5.0) were used for the statistical analysis.

3. Result

3.1. Screening Process

The Cochrane Library, Web of Science, ScienceDirect, and PubMed were the sources of 749 papers that we retrieved. Following a literature search, two researchers (Jingyu Liu and Yang Yang) separately chose the literature. For any objections, the third reviewer (Qiuli Shan) provides additional feedback.

Six hundred forty articles were initially removed based on our inclusion and exclusion criteria after reviewing the titles and abstracts. Following the completion of the literature extraction, the articles that did not meet the requirements and those for which the complete text could not be retrieved were rejected individually by two researchers. After reviewing the full text of the remaining publications using the inclusion and exclusion criteria, a total of 11 papers were included in this analysis, with no articles eliminated due to a lack of complete text (Figure 1).

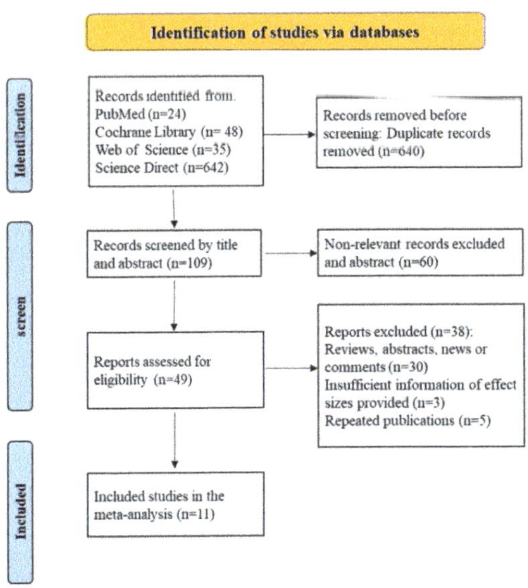

Figure 1. A literature screening flow chart identified a total of 11 articles.

3.2. Research Characteristics

The characteristics of the included studies are presented in Table 1. This systematic review comprised seven cohort studies, three case-control studies, and one cross-sectional research. Five investigations were undertaken in Sweden, two in Spain, and one each in

Denmark, Italy, China, and the Republic of Korea. Considering five studies including more than 300 participants and six studies involving more than 1300 participants, the study population was generally big. Eight of the studies included high-exposure subgroups, and three examined the overall population. The majority of research calculates exposure by adding up all of the PCB homologues. Nine studies measured PCB concentrations in serum or plasma, one study measured PCB concentrations in adipose tissue, and one study tested PCB concentrations in lipids. These findings provide insight into the methodologies used to estimate PCB exposure. Nine of the nine studies that assessed PCBs in blood or serum did so as a ratio of total lipids to PCB serum levels (standardized). Almost all studies controlled for age ($n = 10$), smoking habits ($n = 10$), education ($n = 9$), and body mass index ($n = 9$), and most also adjusted for alcohol consumption ($n = 8$), physical activity ($n = 7$), sex ($n = 7$), and sex ($n = 7$). Some studies also adjusted for triglycerides or cholesterol ($n = 8$), family history of genetic disease ($n = 5$), and diabetes ($n = 4$) (Supplemental Materials Table S1).

Table 1. Main features of the included literature.

Reference	Location	Study Design	Study Population	Time-Period	Sample Size	Age (Year)	Ratio of Sex	Biomaterials	PCBs Type	Method of Measurement	Results [a]	Main Finding
Charlotte Bergkvist et al. (2016) [14]	Swedish	Cohort study	Lived in Central Sweden and did not have cardiovascular disease.	1998–2009	36,759	45–79	All male	Serum	6 PCB congeners	Unclear	ΣPCBs OR 1.97 95% CI [1.42–2.75)] [b]	Exposure to PCBs via diet was associated with increased risk of myocardial infarction in men.
Carolina Donat-Vargas et al. (2020) [15]	Aragon	Cross-sectional	Men without cardiovascular disease enrolled in the Aragon Workers' Health Study	2011–2014	1844	40–60	All male	Serum	4 PCB Congeners	Computerized tomography	ΣPCBs OR 2.03, 95% CI [1.21–3.40]	PCB exposure seems to increase the risk of coronary disease in men from the very early stages.
Francisco Miguel P ´erez-Carrascosa et al. (2021) [16]	Spanish	Cohort study	Participants were recruited in two hospitals in Granada province, Southern Spain.	15-year follow-up study	387	Unclear	Unclear	Adipose tissue	3 PCB congeners	Gas chromatography coupled to mass spectrometry in tandem mode	Main PCB138 OR 1.75, 95% CI [1.18–2.60]	Long-term PCB exposure might represent a modifiable risk factor for CVD.
Laura Deen et al. (2023) [17]	Danish	Cohort study	The HESPAIR cohort includes all residents of two residential areas in the Greater Copenhagen area	21-year follow-up study	51,249	Children and adults	Unclear	Plasma	7 PCB congeners	Unclear	ΣPCBs HR 1.02, 95% CI [0.94–1.10]	Cumulative residential exposure to airborne PCB was not associated with a higher overall risk for CVD.
Duk-Hee Lee et al. (2012) [24]	Swedish	Cohort study	Study subjects at baseline were 1016 subjects who were 70 years old and residents of Uppsala	5-year follow-up study	898	70	Unclear	Plasma	16 PCB congeners	HRGC/HRMS	ΣPCBs OR 5.5 95% CI [1.7–18.1]	Background exposure to POPs may play an important role in development or progression of stroke in the elderly.
Charlotte Bergkvist et al. (2014) [25]	Swedish	Cohort study	Women residing in central Sweden	12-year follow-up study	34,591	Unclear	All women	Serum	6 PCBs	Unclear	ΣPCBs OR 1.65; 95% CI [1.27–2.15]	Dietary exposure to PCBs was associated with an increased stroke risk in women, especially haemorrhagic stroke.
Jung-eun Lim et al. (2018) [26]	Korean	Case-control study	Participants in routine health assessment at 11 health promotion centers in Seoul and Gyeonggi Province	2004–2013	637	>20	Unclear	Serum	32 PCBs	GC/HRMS	ΣPCBs OR 1.66; 95% CI [0.8–3.45] ΣDL-PCBs OR: 3.17; 95% CI [1.29–7.77] ΣNDL-PCBs OR: 1.76; 95% CI [0.88–3.5]	Elevated serum POPs levels were associated with an increased risk of stroke, especially ischemic stroke.
Elena Raffetti et al. (2018) [27]	North Italy	Cohort study	Urban residents near chemical plants that produce PCBs	2001–2013	1331	Mean age 50.6 years	45.7% males and 54.3% women	Serum	24 PCBs	Hewlett–Packard 6890 N gas chromatograph coupled with an MSD HP 5973.	ΣPCBs RR 2.07, 95% CI [1.18–3.63]	These results suggest that PCBs might play a role in the development of possibly cardiovascular disease, though alternative explanations are to be considered, too.
PingLi et al. (2020) [28]	China	Case-control study	Stroke Patients and Healthy Population Recruited at Tianjin Hospital, China	2017–2019	482	>20	56% males and 44% women	Serum	17 PCBs	GC/MS	ΣPCBs OR 1.704; 95% CI [1.073–2.506] ΣDL-PCBs OR: 1.846; 95% CI [1.156–2.949]	The results suggest detrimental roles of PCBs, mainly dioxin-like PCBs, in stroke risk, irrespective of stroke subtypes.

Table 1. *Cont.*

Reference	Location	Study Design	Study Population	Time-Period	Sample Size	Age (Year)	Ratio of Sex	Biomaterials	PCBs Type	Method of Measurement	Results [a]	Main Finding
Carolina Donat-Vargas et al. (2023) [29]	Swedish	Cohort study	The SMC included women born from 1914 to 1948 residing in central Sweden	Mean age 61: 15-year follow-up study Mean age	1528	Mean age 61	33% males and 67% women	Blood lipids	12 PCBs	Gas chromatography–triple quadrupole mass spectrometry	ΣPCBs OR 1.28; 95% CI, [0.92–1.79]	Dioxin-like PCBs and non-dioxin-like PCBs were significantly associated with cardiovascular disease.
Tessa Schillemans et al. (2024) [30]	Swedish	Nested case-control design	The study used data from the SMC-C, which is part of the Swedish Infrastructure for Medical Population-Based Life-Course and Environmental Research	2003–2009	657	<85	All Women	Plasma	13 PCB con-geners	GC-MS/MS	ΣPCBs OR 1.55; 95% CI [1.16–2.09]	PCBs correlated positively with omics associated with increased MI and stroke risk.

[a] The estimation is presented for the highest category compared with the lowest for the most adjusted model.
[b] Estimated full intake.

3.3. Comprehensive Analysis

We carefully read the 11 included articles [14–17,24–30], extracted the effect indicators of PCBs and CVDs, combined them for meta-analysis, and the results were represented by forest maps, as shown in Figure 2. Through data extraction and analysis, a summary of PCBs and CVDs was produced from the article. When the data were merged, they showed a strong correlation between PCB exposure and the risk of cardiovascular disease (OR = 1.56, 95% CI: 1.28, 1.90, $p < 0.001$). The next section will address the reasons for the significant heterogeneity in this analysis ($I^2 = 81.3\%$), as indicated by the meta-analysis.

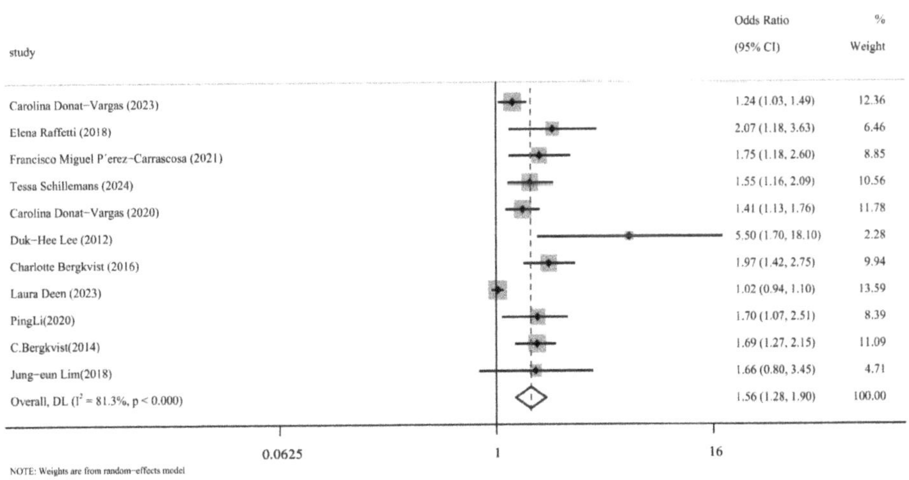

Figure 2. Forest plot of overall analysis of PCBs and CVDs [14–17,24–30].

First, we tested for publication bias using the collected literature. The findings were plotted as a funnel plot in Figure 3, suggesting that the meta-analysis may have some publication bias. To investigate the possibility of publication bias, we used the Egger test on the compiled literature. The test results are displayed in Supplemental Materials Table S2. There is publication bias in the included literature, as indicated by the p-value of 0.001. Subsequently, sensitivity analysis was performed on the included studies, and the results are displayed in Figure 4, which demonstrates the robustness of the findings. Consequently, in order to investigate the reasons for heterogeneity, we performed a subgroup analysis.

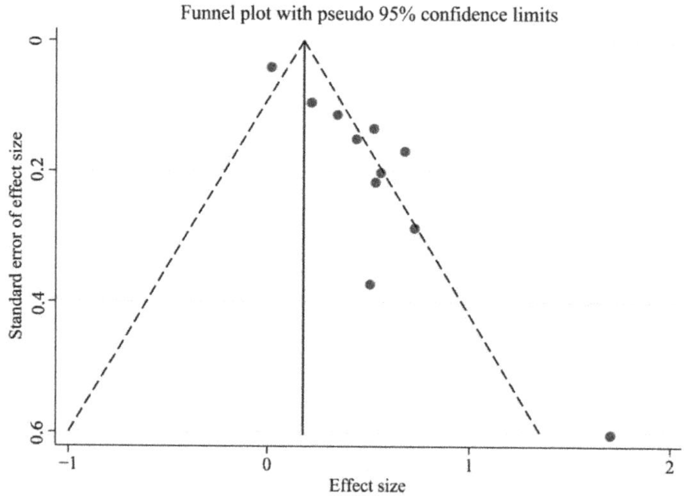

Figure 3. Funnel plot of total PCBs and CVDs overall analysis.

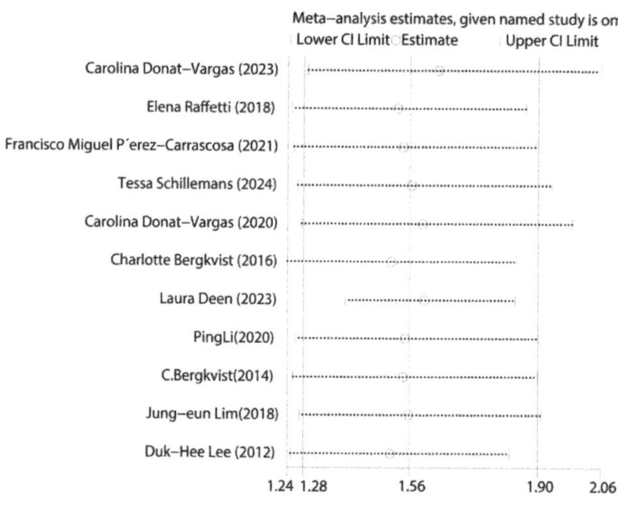

Figure 4. Graph of sensitivity analysis results for the overall analysis of total PCBs and CVDs [14–17,24–30].

3.3.1. Subgroup Analysis of Literature Quality

The case-control, cohort, and cross-sectional studies were assessed separately, and the quality of the 11 included publications was assessed using the NOS scoring technique (Figure 5). It can be seen from the figure that there are three kinds of literature of high quality [14,15,17] and eight kinds of literature of medium quality [16,24–30]. The analysis results are shown in Figure 6, including the group of high quality (OR = 1.38, 95% CI: 0.95, 1.99, $p < 0.001$, $I^2 = 90.1\%$) and the medium-quality group (OR = 1.61, 95% CI: 1.35, 1.92, $p = 0.107$, $I^2 = 40.8\%$). The results demonstrate that, whereas the medium-quality group has minimal variability, the high-quality group has significant heterogeneity. According to this analysis, one of the factors contributing to the high consistency of comprehensive results is the high caliber of the literature.

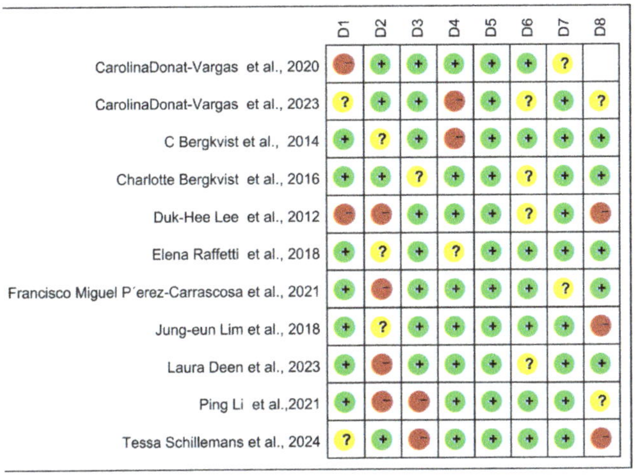

Figure 5. Newcastle–Ottawa Scale (NOS)—Quality assessment. The quality of the studies was evaluated using the NOS. D1–D8 represent NOS items for case-control and cohort studies, while D1–D7 represent adapted NOS items for cross-sectional studies. + for low risk, − for high risk, ? Unclear representation [14–17,24–30].

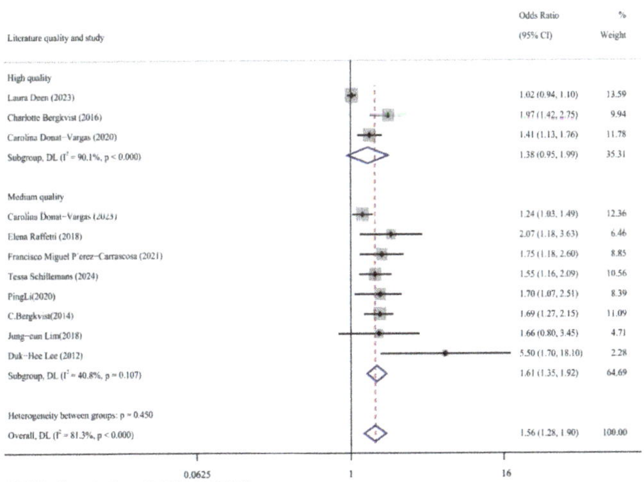

Figure 6. Forest plots with literature quality as subgroup [14–17,24–30].

3.3.2. Subgroup Analysis Based on the Kind of Biomaterials Was Conducted

The types of biomaterials included in the literature were subgroups analyzed by serum and plasma. The results of the subgroup analysis are shown in Figure 7. The results in the serum group were as follows: (OR = 1.64, 95% CI: 1.43, 1.88, $p = 0.592$, $I^2 = 0\%$). The results of plasma group were as follows: (OR = 1.51, 95% CI: 0.91, 2.52, $p < 0.001$, $I^2 = 86.4\%$). According to the data, the plasma group had a significant degree of heterogeneity compared to the serum group's low level. It is possible to argue that one of the causes of the significant heterogeneity of the overall results was the type of biomaterial called plasma.

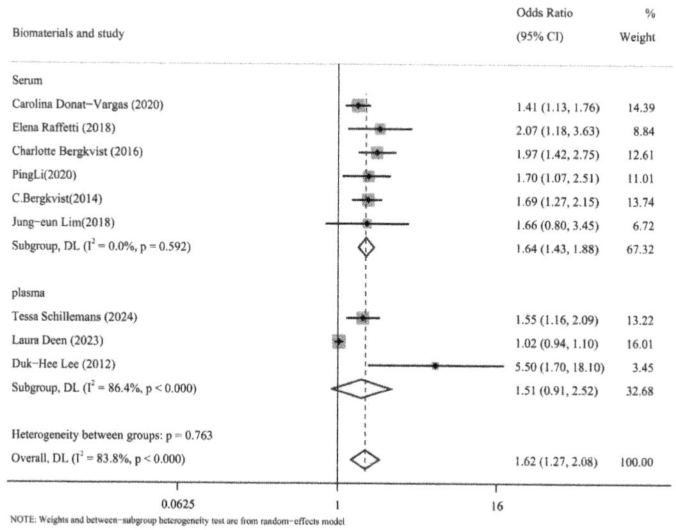

Figure 7. Forest plots of PCBs and CVDs with biomaterial as a subgroup [14,15,17,24–28,30].

3.3.3. Subgroup Analysis Took out Based on the Type of Study

Subgroup analysis was conducted in accordance with the study's design. Figure 8 displays the findings of the analysis. The following are the cohort study's findings: (OR = 1.59, 95% CI: 1.22, 2.09, $p < 0.001$, $I^2 = 86.1\%$); The case-control analysis yielded the following results: (OR = 1.60, 95% CI: 1.28, 2.02, $p = 0.933$, $I^2 = 0\%$). As can be observed, the cohort study group has a high level of heterogeneity compared to the case-control study group, which has a low level. The significant degree of variation in the comprehensive results is thought to be caused, in part, by the type of study that was included in the literature.

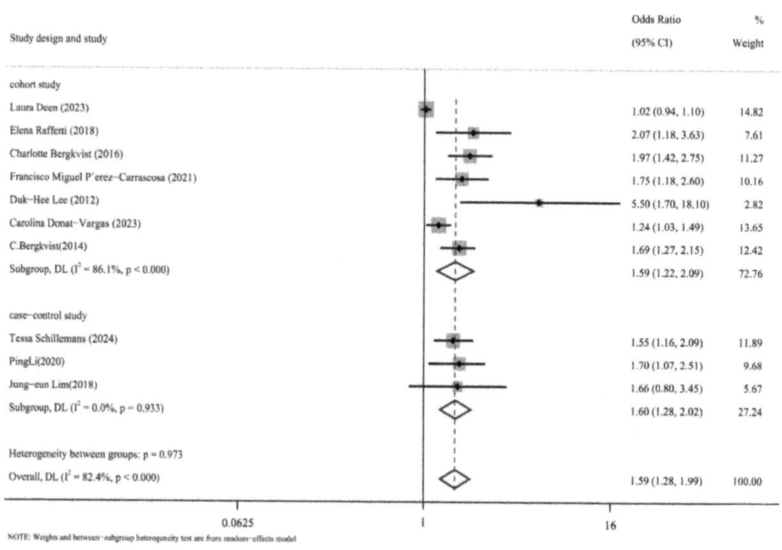

Figure 8. Forest map with research method as subgroup [14,16,17,24–30].

3.3.4. Subpopulation Analysis Based on PCB Type Was Conducted

According to the types of PCBs, the literature was divided into the DL-PCB group [16,24,26,29] and the NDL-PCB group [24,26,28,29]. Figure 9 displays the outcomes of the subgroup analysis. The following were the NDL-PCB group's findings: DL-PCB group results were as follows (OR = 1.31, 95% CI: 1.10, 1.57, p = 0.199, I^2 = 31.6%; OR = 1.33, 95% CI: 1.15, 1.53, p = 0.347, I^2 = 9.3%). The substantial heterogeneity of the comprehensive results cannot be attributed to the type of PCBs, as the heterogeneity of the DL-PCB group and the NDL-PCB group is both low and not significant. The findings suggested that there was a higher risk of cardiovascular illness associated with both DL-PCBs and NDL-PCBs.

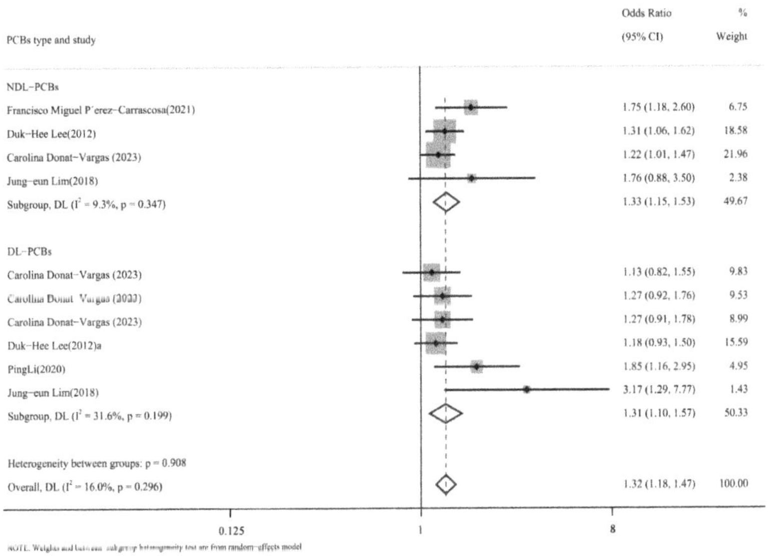

Figure 9. Forest map with PCB types as subgroup [24,26–29].

In addition, we conducted a subpopulation analysis of different homologues of PCB types. As for the effects of different PCBs on cardiovascular diseases, four articles [16,24,27,29] reported PCB153, PCB138, and PCB180 for NDL-PCBs. Supplementary Figure S1 displays the findings for PCB153 (OR = 1.32, 95% CI: 1.19, 1.45, p = 0.411, I^2 = 0%); PCB138 (OR = 1.19, 95% CI: 0.93, 1.54, p = 0.021, I^2 = 69.2%); and PCB180 (OR = 1.09, 95% CI: 0.99, 1.19, p = 0.705, I^2 = 0%). A strong conclusion was reached by using the fixed-effect model, which demonstrated a positive correlation between PCB153 and the incidence of cardiovascular illnesses without any heterogeneity.

This was followed by DL-PCBs, with three articles [24,26,29] reporting PCB118 and PCB156. Supplemental Materials Figure S2 displays the findings for PCB118 (OR = 1.26, 95% CI: 1.04, 1.52, p = 0.408, I^2 = 1.2%) and PCB156 (OR = 1.18, 95% CI: 0.83, 1.67, p = 0.060, I^2 = 52.8%). PCB118 was shown to have a significant increase in the risk of cardiovascular disease among them. The conclusion was supported by the low level of heterogeneity.

4. Discussion

We conducted a meta-analysis and systematic review to examine the link between cardiovascular disease and PCB exposure. We draw the conclusion that, due to its great heterogeneity, PCB exposure is a risk factor for cardiovascular disease based on a selection of 11 epidemiological studies conducted up until March 2024 among six nations. As a result, we performed subgroup analysis based on the biological material, research type, article quality, and PCB type. We discovered that these factors could be the cause of the article's high heterogeneity.

The results of the subgroup analysis of PCB types for NDL-PCBs (OR = 1.33, 95% CI: 1.15, 1.53) and DL-PCBs (OR = 1.31, 95% CI: 1.10, 1.57) all indicated a low degree of heterogeneity in the positive association between PCBs and the risk of cardiovascular disease. NDL-PCB-153 (OR = 1.32, 95% CI: 1.19, 1.45) and DL-PCB-118 (OR = 1.26, 95% CI: 1.04, 1.52) were found to be risk variables for cardiovascular disease in homologous subgroup analysis. The E value of the PCB effect on cardiovascular disease was calculated in this study, and the result was 2.259, indicating a high degree of confidence and relative robustness. As a result, we think that our analysis's findings are more precise and compelling.

The molecular pathways that could link PCBs to cardiovascular disease have been examined in earlier research. PCBs are well-known endocrine disruptors that mimic or obstruct the body's hormonal functions, particularly those of the thyroid and sex hormones [31]. The changes in the metabolic rate induced by this disruption may affect the functioning of the cardiovascular system. For example, an imbalance in thyroid hormones can lead to abnormal blood pressure, altered cholesterol levels, and irregular heart rhythms, each of which is a known risk factor for cardiovascular disease [32]. Research has indicated that estrogen functions as a cardiac protective agent, regulating cardiovascular health and lowering blood pressure, vasoconstriction, vascular resistance, and heart hypertrophy [33]. These effects provide protection against cardiovascular disease, and an excess of estrogen may actually exacerbate the condition [33].

Chronic inflammation is closely linked to the onset of cardiovascular disease, particularly when atherosclerosis is forming. The growth and accumulation of plaque may be aided by the activation and deposition of inflammatory cells in the blood vessel wall [34]. The accumulation and activation of inflammatory cells in the vascular wall can promote the formation and progression of plaques. Dioxin-like PCBs (DL-PCBs) can initiate intracellular signaling by binding to the aryl hydrocarbon receptor (AHR), thereby activating inflammatory pathways in the body. For example, PCB126 induces inflammation by increasing the production of the inflammatory cytokine tumor necrosis factor-α (TNF-α) [35]. Studies have demonstrated that non-dioxin-like PCBs (NDL-PCBs) can stimulate the production of reactive oxygen species (ROS), leading to oxidative stress [36]. The oxidative stress induced by PCB118 may contribute to endothelial dysfunction, increased lipid peroxidation, and the degradation of nitric oxide in the endothelium, thereby impairing vascular relaxation and exacerbating hypertension and arteriosclerosis [36]. Furthermore, exposure to PCB153, a dioxin-like PCB (DL-PCB), may lead to the downregulation of lipoprotein lipase (LPL) activity, thereby affecting the hydrolysis and absorption of lipids. This, in turn, results in elevated levels of low-density lipoprotein (LDL) in the blood, thereby increasing the risk of cardiovascular disease [37].

The shortcomings of this meta-analysis are numerous. With only 11 studies included, it has a small sample size and low representativeness, which increases the risk of bias. Significant variability between the studies was also discovered in the analysis, with differing levels of research quality, measurement errors in exposure levels, and inadequate management of confounding variables. Generally speaking, a significant cause of heterogeneity is the variable quality of the included research. According to this research, high-quality studies could contain selection biases that impede their findings from accurately representing the target population's real circumstances. Moreover, variations in sample size, follow-up duration, and data-processing techniques between the studies could impact the consistency and dependability of the findings. A dearth of high-caliber studies may also affect the results. The main focus of this investigation was on biological materials containing serum and plasma. Due to their high lipophilicity, PCBs usually attach to blood proteins. The changes in serum and plasma composition, especially the presence of coagulation factors, may have an impact on PCB binding status [38,39].

The action of coagulation factors may cause changes in plasma during storage, which could have an impact on PCB stability and measurement outcomes. Serum, on the other hand, remains reasonably stable following separation, which could lead to more accurate measurement results [40]. Cross-sectional, case-control, and cohort studies are the study types that are considered; an additional source of heterogeneity is the variations in these study designs. Subgroup analysis on case-control and cohort studies is the main focus of this research. Recall and selection bias are common problems in case-control research. On the other hand, longitudinal cohort studies, which frequently necessitate lengthy follow-up periods and substantial resources, are better able to evaluate the temporal association between exposure and disease. Moreover, a number of confounding variables, including nutrition, physical activity, education level, socioeconomic position, smoking, drinking alcohol, and exposure to other environmental contaminants, can affect the association between PCB exposure and cardiovascular disease. Variations in the degree to which these characteristics are adjusted in different studies may lead to biased findings. Furthermore, while examining the connection between PCBs and cardiovascular illness, it is important to consider the level of exposure, the length of exposure, and the relevant lifetime periods of sensitivity.

5. Conclusions

The connection between PCB exposure and the risk of CVDs was thoroughly assessed in this meta-analysis, which found that exposure to PCBs considerably raises the risk of CVDs. This discovery offers crucial scientific support for our comprehension of how environmental contaminants affect human health. Despite certain methodological limitations, the study's findings generally show a favorable association between exposure to PCBs and cardiovascular diseases. The current findings provide preliminary evidence for a potential association between PCBs and cardiovascular disease. However, this field still requires more detailed studies to further elucidate the underlying mechanisms and the diversity of effects. In conclusion, this study emphasizes the significance of lowering exposure to PCBs and offers a solid scientific foundation for therapeutic and public health actions. It highlights the need for individuals and society to take measures to reduce PCB exposure in order to lower the risk of CVDs.

Supplementary Materials: The following supporting information can be downloaded at: https://www.mdpi.com/article/10.3390/toxics13020071/s1, Search term; Table S1: Control for confounding; Table S2: Egger's test of total PCBs and CVDs; Figure S1: Forest map with NDL-PCB homolog as a grouping; Figure S2: Forest map featuring DL-PCB homolog as a distinct subgroup.

Author Contributions: Conceptualization, J.L., methodology, data curation, software, formal analysis, writing—original draft; Q.S., data curation, writing—original draft, writing—review and editing; Y.Y., methodology, software; W.H., funding acquisition, resources, supervision, writing—review and editing. This work is original research that has not been published previously and is not under publication consideration elsewhere. All authors have read and agreed to the published version of the manuscript.

Funding: This research was funded by The National Natural Science Foundation of China (NSFC), grant numbers 21507040 and 31872415.

Institutional Review Board Statement: Not applicable.

Informed Consent Statement: Not applicable.

Data Availability Statement: The data that support the findings of this study are available from the corresponding author upon reasonable request.

Conflicts of Interest: There is no potential conflict of interest to disclose.

References

1. Piepoli, M.F. 2016 European Guidelines on cardiovascular disease prevention in clinical practice: The Sixth Joint Task Force of the European Society of Cardiology and Other Societies on Cardiovascular Disease Prevention in Clinical Practice (constituted by representatives of 10 societies and by invited experts). *Int. J. Behav. Med.* **2017**, *24*, 321–419. [CrossRef]
2. Teshale, A.B.; Htun, H.L.; Hu, J.; Dalli, L.L.; Lim, M.H.; Neves, B.B.; Baker, J.; Phyo, A.Z.Z.; Reid, C.M.; Ryan, J.; et al. The relationship between social isolation, social support, and loneliness with cardiovascular disease and shared risk factors: A narrative review. *Arch. Gerontol. Geriatr.* **2023**, *111*, 105008. [CrossRef] [PubMed]
3. Fang, N.; Jiang, M.; Fan, Y. Ideal cardiovascular health metrics and risk of cardiovascular disease or mortality: A meta-analysis. *Int. J. Cardiol.* **2016**, *214*, 280–284. [CrossRef] [PubMed]
4. Machaalani, M.; Fakhry, B.; Zwaihed, M.; Mendelek, K.; Mahmoud, N.; Hammoud, T.; Chahine, M.N. Knowledge, Attitude, and Practice Toward Cardiovascular Diseases in the Lebanese Population. *Glob. Heart* **2022**, *17*, 47. [CrossRef] [PubMed]
5. Arrebola, J.P.; Fernández, M.F.; Martin-Olmedo, P.; Bonde, J.P.; Martín-Rodriguez, J.L.; Expósito, J.; Rubio-Domínguez, A.; Olea, N. Historical exposure to persistent organic pollutants and risk of incident hypertension. *Environ. Res.* **2015**, *138*, 217–223. [CrossRef]
6. Ge, L.; Guyatt, G.; Tian, J.; Pan, B.; Chang, Y.; Chen, Y.; Li, H.; Zhang, J.; Li, Y.; Ling, J.; et al. Insomnia and risk of mortality from all-cause, cardiovascular disease, and cancer: Systematic review and meta-analysis of prospective cohort studies. *Sleep Med. Rev.* **2019**, *48*, 101215. [CrossRef]
7. Peng, F.-J.; Lin, C.-A.; Wada, R.; Bodinier, B.; Iglesias-González, A.; Palazzi, P.; Streel, S.; Guillaume, M.; Vuckovic, D.; Chadeau-Hyam, M.; et al. Association of hair polychlorinated biphenyls and multiclass pesticides with obesity, diabetes, hypertension and dyslipidemia in NESCAV study. *J. Hazard. Mater.* **2024**, *461*, 132637. [CrossRef]
8. Hoyeck, M.P.; Matteo, G.; MacFarlane, E.M.; Perera, I.; Bruin, J.E. Persistent organic pollutants and β-cell toxicity: A comprehensive review. *Am. J. Physiol.-Endocrinol. Metab.* **2022**, *322*, E383–E413. [CrossRef]
9. Alharbi, O.M.; Basheer, A.A.; Khattab, R.A.; Ali, I. Health and environmental effects of persistent organic pollutants. *J. Mol. Liq.* **2018**, *263*, 442–453. [CrossRef]
10. Dzierlenga, M.; Yoon, M.; Wania, F.; Ward, P.; Armitage, J.; Wood, S.; Clewell, H.; Longnecker, M. Quantitative bias analysis of the association of type 2 diabetes mellitus with 2,2′,4,4′,5,5′-hexachlorobiphenyl (PCB-153). *Environ. Int.* **2019**, *125*, 291–299. [CrossRef]
11. Yang, B.; Qin, Q.; Xu, L.; Lv, X.; Liu, Z.; Song, E.; Song, Y. Polychlorinated Biphenyl Quinone Promotes Atherosclerosis through Lipid Accumulation and Endoplasmic Reticulum Stress via CD36. *Chem. Res. Toxicol.* **2020**, *33*, 1497–1507. [CrossRef] [PubMed]
12. Gao, X.; Yan, D.; Li, G.; Wei, Y.; He, H.; Zhai, J. Polychlorinated biphenyls and risk of metabolic syndrome and comparison with the risk of diabetes: A systematic review and meta-analysis. *Sci. Total Environ.* **2023**, *900*, 165773. [CrossRef] [PubMed]
13. Raffetti, E.; Donat-Vargas, C.; Mentasti, S.; Chinotti, A.; Donato, F. Association between exposure to polychlorinated biphenyls and risk of hypertension: A systematic review and meta-analysis. *Chemosphere* **2020**, *255*, 126984. [CrossRef] [PubMed]
14. Bergkvist, C.; Berglund, M.; Glynn, A.; Julin, B.; Wolk, A.; Åkesson, A. Dietary exposure to polychlorinated biphenyls and risk of myocardial infarction in men—A population-based prospective cohort study. *Environ. Int.* **2016**, *88*, 9–14. [CrossRef]
15. Donat-Vargas, C.; Moreno-Franco, B.; Laclaustra, M.; Sandoval-Insausti, H.; Jarauta, E.; Guallar-Castillon, P. Exposure to dietary polychlorinated biphenyls and dioxins, and its relationship with subclinical coronary atherosclerosis: The Aragon Workers' Health Study. *Environ. Int.* **2020**, *136*, 105433. [CrossRef]
16. Pérez-Carrascosa, F.M.; Gómez-Peña, C.; Echeverría, R.; Moleón, J.J.J.; Melchor, J.M.; García-Ruiz, A.; Navarro-Espigares, J.L.; Cabeza-Barrera, J.; Martin-Olmedo, P.; Ortigosa-García, J.C.; et al. Historical exposure to persistent organic pollutants and cardiovascular disease: A 15-year longitudinal analysis focused on pharmaceutical consumption in primary care. *Environ. Int.* **2021**, *156*, 106734. [CrossRef]
17. Deen, L.; Clark, A.; Hougaard, K.S.; Meyer, H.W.; Frederiksen, M.; Pedersen, E.B.; Petersen, K.U.; Flachs, E.M.; Bonde, J.P.E.; Tøttenborg, S.S. Risk of cardiovascular diseases following residential exposure to airborne polychlorinated biphenyls: A register-based cohort study. *Environ. Res.* **2023**, *222*, 115354. [CrossRef]

18. Page, M.J.; McKenzie, J.E.; Bossuyt, P.M.; Boutron, I.; Hoffmann, T.C.; Mulrow, C.D.; Shamseer, L.; Tetzlaff, J.M.; Akl, E.A.; Brennan, S.E.; et al. The PRISMA 2020 statement: An updated guideline for reporting systematic reviews. *J. Clin. Epidemiol.* **2021**, *134*, 178–189. [CrossRef]
19. Stroup, D.F.; Berlin, J.A.; Morton, S.C.; Olkin, I.; Williamson, G.D.; Rennie, D.; Moher, D.; Becker, B.J.; Sipe, T.A.; Thacker, S.B. Meta-analysis of observational studies in epidemiology: A proposal for reporting. Meta-analysis of Observational Studies in Epidemiology (MOOSE) group. *JAMA* **2000**, *283*, 2008–2012. [CrossRef]
20. Morgan, R.L.; Whaley, P.; Thayer, K.A.; Schünemann, H.J. Identifying the PECO: A framework for formulating good questions to explore the association of environmental and other exposures with health outcomes. *Environ. Int.* **2018**, *121*, 1027–1031. [CrossRef]
21. Masuda, Y. Toxic effects of PCB/PCDF to human observed in Yusho and other poisonings. *Fukuoka Igaku Zasshi = Hukuoka Acta Medica* **2009**, *100*, 141–155. [PubMed]
22. Tang, X.; Tang, S.; Ren, Z.; Wong, D.F.K. Psychological risk and protective factors associated with depressive symptoms among adolescents in secondary schools in China: A systematic review and meta-analysis. *Child. Youth Serv. Rev.* **2020**, *108*, 104680. [CrossRef]
23. Lee, Y.H. An overview of meta-analysis for clinicians. *Korean J. Intern. Med.* **2018**, *33*, 277–283. [CrossRef] [PubMed]
24. Lee, D.-H.; Lind, P.M.; Jacobs, D.R.; Salihovic, S.; van Bavel, B.; Lind, L. Background exposure to persistent organic pollutants predicts stroke in the elderly. *Environ. Int.* **2012**, *47*, 115–120. [CrossRef]
25. Bergkvist, C.; Kippler, M.; Larsson, S.C.; Berglund, M.; Glynn, A.; Wolk, A.; Åkesson, A. Dietary exposure to polychlorinated biphenyls is associated with increased risk of stroke in women. *J. Intern. Med.* **2014**, *276*, 248–259. [CrossRef]
26. Lim, J.-E.; Lee, S.; Lee, S.; Jee, S.H. Serum persistent organic pollutants levels and stroke risk. *Environ. Pollut.* **2018**, *233*, 855–861. [CrossRef]
27. Raffetti, E.; Donato, F.; Speziani, F.; Scarcella, C.; Gaia, A.; Magoni, M. Polychlorinated biphenyls (PCBs) exposure and cardiovascular, endocrine and metabolic diseases: A population-based cohort study in a North Italian highly polluted area. *Environ. Int.* **2018**, *120*, 215–222. [CrossRef]
28. Li, P.; Dan, Y.; Li, S.; Zhang, Q.; Su, Y.; Lu, M. Serum levels of polychlorinated biphenyls and stroke risk among Chinese: A hospital-based case-control study. *Acta Neurol. Belg.* **2020**, *121*, 1217–1224. [CrossRef]
29. Donat-Vargas, C.; Schillemans, T.; Kiviranta, H.; Rantakokko, P.; de Faire, U.; Arrebola, J.P.; Wolk, A.; Leander, K.; Åkesson, A. Blood Levels of Organochlorine Contaminants Mixtures and Cardiovascular Disease. *JAMA Netw. Open* **2023**, *6*, e2333347. [CrossRef]
30. Schillemans, T.; Yan, Y.; Ribbenstedt, A.; Donat-Vargas, C.; Lindh, C.H.; Kiviranta, H.; Rantakokko, P.; Wolk, A.; Landberg, R.; Åkesson, A.; et al. OMICs Signatures Linking Persistent Organic Pollutants to Cardiovascular Disease in the Swedish Mammography Cohort. *Environ. Sci. Technol.* **2024**, *58*, 1036–1047. [CrossRef]
31. Brouwer, A.; Longnecker, M.P.; Birnbaum, L.S.; Cogliano, J.; Kostyniak, P.; Moore, J.; Schantz, S.; Winneke, G. Characterization of potential endocrine-related health effects at low-dose levels of exposure to PCBs. *Environ. Health Perspect.* **1999**, *107* (Suppl. S4), 639–649. [CrossRef] [PubMed]
32. Ma, R.; Sassoon, D.A. PCBs exert an estrogenic effect through repression of the Wnt7a signaling pathway in the female reproductive tract. *Environ. Health Perspect.* **2006**, *114*, 898–904. [CrossRef] [PubMed]
33. Murphy, M.O.; Petriello, M.C.; Han, S.G.; Sunkara, M.; Morris, A.J.; Esser, K.; Hennig, B. Exercise protects against PCB-induced inflammation and associated cardiovascular risk factors. *Environ. Sci. Pollut. Res.* **2015**, *23*, 2201–2211. [CrossRef] [PubMed]
34. Jabbar, A.; Pingitore, A.; Pearce, S.H.S.; Zaman, A.; Iervasi, G.; Razvi, S. Thyroid hormones and cardiovascular disease. *Nat. Rev. Cardiol.* **2016**, *14*, 39–55. [CrossRef] [PubMed]
35. El Amine, Z.; Mauger, J.-F.; Imbeault, P. CYP1A1, VEGFA and Adipokine Responses of Human Adipocytes Co-Exposed to PCB126 and Hypoxia. *Cells* **2022**, *11*, 2282. [CrossRef]
36. Long, Y.; Liu, X.; Tan, X.-Z.; Jiang, C.-X.; Chen, S.-W.; Liang, G.-N.; He, X.-M.; Wu, J.; Chen, T.; Xu, Y. ROS-induced NLRP3 inflammasome priming and activation mediate PCB 118-induced pyroptosis in endothelial cells. *Ecotox. Environ. Saf.* **2020**, *189*, 109937. [CrossRef]
37. Mesnier, A.; Champion, S.; Louis, L.; Sauzet, C.; May, P.; Portugal, H.; Benbrahim, K.; Abraldes, J.; Alessi, M.-C.; Amiot-Carlin, M.-J.; et al. The Transcriptional Effects of PCB118 and PCB153 on the Liver, Adipose Tissue, Muscle and Colon of Mice: Highlighting of Glut4 and Lipin1 as Main Target Genes for PCB Induced Metabolic Disorders. *PLoS ONE* **2015**, *10*, e0128847. [CrossRef]
38. Li, Z.; Sandau, C.D.; Romanoff, L.C.; Caudill, S.P.; Sjodin, A.; Needham, L.L.; Patterson, D.G. Concentration and profile of 22 urinary polycyclic aromatic hydrocarbon metabolites in the US population. *Environ. Res.* **2008**, *107*, 320–331. [CrossRef]
39. Hansen, L.G. Stepping backward to improve assessment of PCB congener toxicities. *Environ. Health Perspect.* **1998**, *106* (Suppl. S1), 171–189. [CrossRef]

40. Patterson, D.G.; Todd, G.D.; E Turner, W.; Maggio, V.; Alexander, L.R.; Needham, L.L. Levels of non-ortho-substituted (coplanar), mono- and di-ortho-substituted polychlorinated biphenyls, dibenzo-p-dioxins, and dibenzofurans in human serum and adipose tissue. *Environ. Health Perspect.* **1994**, *102* (Suppl. S1), 195–204. [CrossRef]

toxics

MDPI

Review

Reproductive Toxicity and Multi/Transgenerational Effects of Emerging Pollutants on *C. elegans*

Zhiling Wu [1,†], Lingqiao Wang [1,†], Weihua Chen [2], Yiqi Wang [1], Ke Cui [1], Weiyan Chen [1], Jijun Liu [3], Huidong Jin [1] and Ziyuan Zhou [1,*]

1 Department of Environmental Health, College of Preventive Medicine, Army Medical University (Third Military Medical University), Chongqing 400038, China; wzl2023@tmmu.edu.cn (Z.W.); mamababa520qq@163.com (L.W.); wangyiqi@tmmu.edu.cn (Y.W.); cuike777777@163.com (K.C.); weiyanchen@tmmu.edu.cn (W.C.); 17640061992@163.com (H.J.)

2 Central & Southern China Municipal Engineering Design and Research Institute Co., Ltd., Wuhan 430010, China; cwh361028@126.com

3 Chongqing Center for Disease Control and Prevention, Chongqing 400707, China; cqliujijun2007@163.com

* Correspondence: ziyuanzhou@tmmu.edu.cn

† These authors contributed equally to this work.

Abstract: Emerging pollutants (EPs) are receiving increasing attention due to the threats they pose to the environment and human health. As EPs continue to emerge, risk assessment requires many model animals. *Caenorhabditis elegans* (*C. elegans*) has been an outstanding toxicological model organism due to its growth and development characteristics. Particularly, in studying the transgenerational influences of EPs, *C. elegans* has advantages in saving time and cost due to its short generation cycle. As infertility has become a major problem in human reproductive health, reproductive toxicities of EPs on contemporary nematodes and across generations of *C. elegans* were introduced in this review. Moreover, the underlying mechanisms involved in germ cell apoptosis, spermatogenesis, and epigenetic alteration were discussed. Future research opportunities and challenges are also discussed to expand our understanding of the reproductive influences of EPs.

Keywords: emerging pollutant; reproductive toxicity; parental exposure; successive exposure; *C. elegans*

1. Introduction

Infertility has become a global health issue [1]. There are many factors contributing to infertility, such as age, lifestyle, and environmental factors [2,3]. One of the major causes of increasing infertility is high exposure to environmental pollutants, which are pervasive and ensue via numerous routes [4]. Unlike conventional pollutants, emerging pollutants (EPs) refer to newly discovered or concerned pollutants that pose risks to the ecological environment or human health, with characteristics such as biological toxicity, environmental persistence, and bioaccumulation [5]. EPs include many chemicals used in daily life [6]. In China, the dominant types include perfluorinated compounds (PFCs), endocrine disruptors, microplastics (MPs), and antibiotics [7]. EPs can widely exist in water, soil, dust, air, and living organisms. As a result of their entry into the human body, they can cause adverse health effects, including organ injury, neurological damage, reproductive disorder, developmental disturbance, etc. To understand the EP-related reproductive disorders and fertility threat, a lot of research has been conducted [1,8]. Human exposure to EPs can have adverse effects on reproduction. For example, a study of a Chinese adult male population suggests that exposure to high doses of perfluoroalkyl and polyfluoroalkyl substances (PFAS) may be harmful to men's reproductive health. Compared to serum PFAS, semen PFAS might serve as a more accurate indicator for men's reproductive system [9]. Another Canadian population study showed a negative correlation between hair 2,2′,4,4′-tetrabromodiphenyl ether (BDE-47) concentration and sperm motility [10]. However, due to the limitations of research in humans, elucidating the molecular and biochemical mechanisms of human reproduction is challenging [11]. To gain a deeper view of the molecular and biochemical mechanisms of human reproduction, suitable animal models like rats and mice were selected for in vivo studies [12]. Prenatal exposure to Di-(2-ethylhexyl) phthalate (DEHP) had a significant effect on reproduction of male mice [13]. After exposure to perfluorooctanoic acid (PFOA) during pregnancy, fewer mice survived, their testicles were damaged, and their reproductive hormones were disrupted [14].

Although, mammalian models remain the gold standard for toxicology experiments, considering that many new pollutants in the environment are constantly detected, millions of individuals would be sacrificed in animal experiments. In addition to animal ethics, lots of labor, time, and materials would be consumed. A small, nonparasitic nematode, *Caenorhabditis elegans* (*C. elegans*) has been applied for studying many human diseases and has been one of the optimal animal models ever used. Based on these advantages, it is an extremely fascinating experimental model [15,16]: small size, short life span, high reproductive rate, and self-fertilize ability, which make it easy to obtain a mass of experimental worms. As the worm is transparent and easy to grow, reporter gene fusions, protein expression, and cell morphology can be observed in vivo. Moreover, it is the first multicellular organism in the world to complete full gene sequencing [17], which makes it possible to study toxicological mechanisms from a genetic angle. From nematodes to humans, many of the critical genetic pathways that regulate reproductive function are conserved.

This paper summarizes the recent progress of the reproductive effects of EPs using the model organism *C. elegans*. As shown in Figure 1, this article will mainly conduct a systematic discussion and put forward a prospect focusing on the reproductive toxicity induced by EPs, as represented by PFCs, endocrine disruptors, microplastics, and antibiotics.

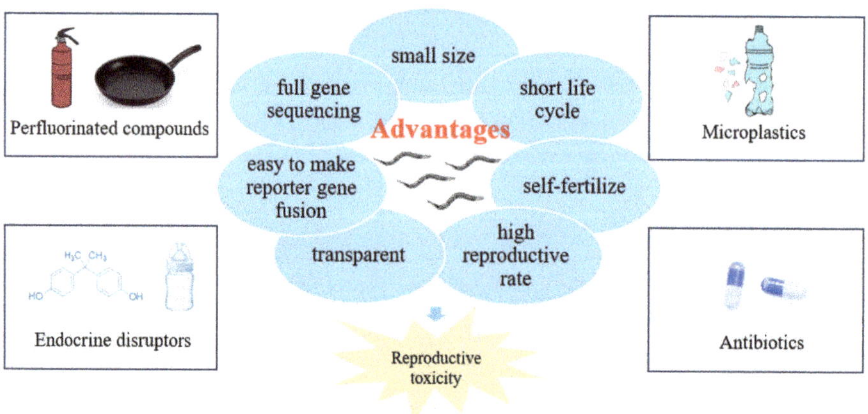

Figure 1. Advantages of the nematode model and the types of EPs discussed in this review.

2. Methods

This review searched for articles related to the reproductive toxicity of EPs in *C. elegans* since 2018. Three major databases including Web of Science, Embase, and PubMed were searched with combinations of these search terms: "*Caenorhabditis elegans*", "*C. elegans*", "reproduction", "reproductive", "transgenerational", "multigenerational", "cross-generation", "offspring", "progeny", "exposure".

3. Reproductive Toxicity of EPs on Contemporary *C. elegans*

The reproductive toxicity of EPs on the worms was generally assessed from fertility, development of reproductive organs, and visible cellular biomarkers, which is shown in Figure 2. Table 1 summarizes the reproductive influence of the selected EPs. Visualized endpoints of reproductive toxicity were listed. As is shown, the brood size was selected as the endpoint in nearly all research listed to evaluate reproductive capacity. In addition to brood size, the number of oocytes, egg hatching, embryonic lethality, spermatid-related parameters, and generation time can also be used to evaluate fertility. Development of reproductive organs is another classification of endpoints, including the length of germline arm, gonadal area, and morphology of vulva. For the transparent body of *C. elegans*, germline apoptosis becomes visible cellular biomarkers to assess reproductive toxicity. Based on the findings, exposure to selected EPs caused reproductive damage.

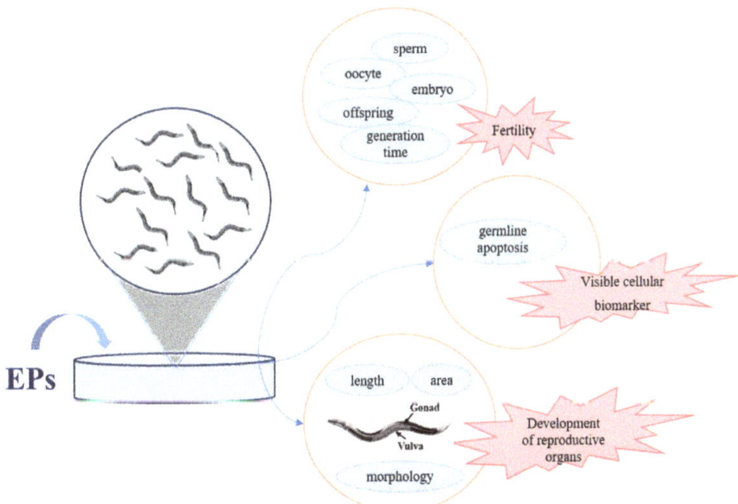

Figure 2. Assessment indicators of reproductive toxicity of *C. elegans*.

3.1. PFCs

PFCs are synthetic alkane organic compounds, which have been widely used in many fields including food packaging materials, nonstick cookware, detergents, oil-proof treatment agents, and foam fire extinguishing agents [18].

Of the thousands of PFCs, PFOA and perfluorooctane sulfonate (PFOS) are the most studied. There were decreases in the number of germ cells, brood size, the size and motility of spermatid, and a rise in the rate of spermatid malformation observed following the exposure to PFOS and PFOA [19]. Reproductive toxicity effects were observed following perfluorobutane sulfonate (PFBS) and PFOS treatment in another study including significant reductions in brood number and egg production, and an increase in apoptosis in the gonads. By comparison, PFOS exhibits a greater capacity for bioaccumulation, while PFBS necessitates higher concentrations of exposure to induce reproductive toxicity [20]. However, the reproductive influences of additional PFCs have been less explored, including perfluorooctane sulfonamide (PFOSA), 6:2 chlorinated polyfluorinated ether sulfonate (F-53B), and perfluorohexanesulfonate (PFHxS).

3.2. Endocrine Disrupting Chemicals (EDCs)

EDCs, also known as environmental hormones or environmental estrogens, generally refer to exogenous chemicals to influence the endocrine system of organisms. There are a lot of EDCs and common examples including phenols, flame retardants, plastic additives, and pesticides. Previous studies have confirmed that EDCs could induce significant reproductive effects on *C. elegans*.

For instance, the brood size decrease was discovered under both nonylphenol (NP) and 4-nitrophenol (4-NP) exposure [21,22]. Abnormal reproductive systems, particularly irregular vulvas characterized by swelling, absence, and asymmetry, were also noted following exposure to NP. The overall count of germ cells was utilized to evaluate the impact on gonadal development toxicity under 4-NP exposure. Three studies researched the reproductive influences of di-(2-ethylhexyl) phthalate (DEHP) using identical concentrations [23–25]. These investigations revealed that DEHP has the potential to diminish reproductive capacity. One research focused on brood sizes, generation time, oocyte numbers, and apoptotic cells [23]. Alongside aspects of reproductive capacity like brood size, the quantity of fertilized eggs, the ratio of egg laying, and the hatchability of eggs, another study also focused on the advancement of the reproductive system, including the relative area of the gonadal arm [24]. Zongur's study only focused on the number of eggs [25]. Fosthiazate and fenitrothion (FNT) are organophosphorus insecticides, and both of them can induce brood size reduction [26,27]. Atrazine (ATR) ($\geq$0.04 mg/L) and carbendazim (10 μg/L) significantly decreased the worm's reproduction with reduction rates of 17.06–35.41% and 43.71% in brood size [28,29]. Another experimental research exhibited that compared with 2,4-dichlorophenoxyacetic acid (2,4-D), cypermethrin (CYP), chlorpyrifos (CPF), and mancozeb (MCZ), ATR was the pesticide that had the greatest impact on brood size with a decrease rate of nearly 30% at the highest concentrations [30]. Tri-n-butyl phosphate (TnBP) and triphenyl phosphate (TPHP) are organophosphate flame retardants, while tetrabromobisphenol A (TBBPA) and BDE-47 are brominated flame retardants. All of them could impair the fertility of *C. elegans*. For example, following exposure to TnBP, significant effects on the reproductive ability and gonadal development of *C. elegans* were noted, along with a marked rise in germline apoptosis [31]. Treatment with BDE-47 may lead to a notable reduction in offspring numbers and promote germ cell apoptosis [32].

3.3. MPs

Global plastic production has grown exponentially since the invention of plastics in the early 19th century. Plastic fragments smaller than 5 mm in diameter are often considered MPs. There are a lot of types of MPs, including polypropylene (PP), polyamide (PA), polyvinyl chloride (PVC), polyethylene (PE), and polystyrene (PS) [33]. As a synthetic organic polymer, MPs possess traits such as small particle size, lightweight, extensive specific surface area, strong hydrophobicity, variable density, etc., allowing them to remain stable in the environment for an extended period. Because of the ubiquity and persistence of MPs, their toxic effects on organisms are of increasing concern.

PS is among the plastics that are frequently identified in the environment. Nano-sized PS soil exposure resulted in a decrease in eggs' quantity presented in utero and the percentage of hatching, with reduction rates of 7–33% and 2.6–4.4%, and increase rates of 12–55% in the incidence of apoptotic germ cells within the gonads [34]. Media and particle size can affect reproductive toxicity. Research indicated that *C. elegans* responded more sensitively to the number of progeny in soil medium than in liquid medium. Additionally, in soil environments, *C. elegans* demonstrated increased sensitivity towards larger particles [35]. Chemical modifications to the surface can alter the physicochemical characteristics of MPs/nanoplastics (NPs) and influence their toxicity. Studies have indicated that amino modification groups may increase the toxicity of nanopolystyrene (NPS) on reproductive abilities and gonadal development [36]. Microplastics existing in the environment are susceptible to environmental factors (such as temperature, light, and mechanical stress), and undergo aging processes, which could lead to significant changes in the physicochemical properties and ecotoxicity of microplastics. Aged MPs were obtained by UV irradiation in two studies [37,38]. The reproductive effects of aged MPs were more severe compared to those of pristine MPs. MPs can absorb a large number of environmental pollutants due to their extensive surface area, so they can become transport carriers of environmental pollutants such as organic pollutants. Therefore, combinational effects between MPs and other contaminants were conducted. Research [39] demonstrated that NPS could significantly increase the toxicity of Microcystins-LR (MC-LR), leading to a decrease in brood size. However, the effect was affected by the concentration of NPS.

3.4. Antibiotics

Antibiotics have been used to treat disease and promote the growth of livestock. Antibiotics in the environment mainly come from the livestock and poultry industry, the aquaculture industry, and pharmaceutical wastewater. Antibiotics can directly influence the diversity of microbial communities, the growth and development of animals and plants, and human health. Recently, there have been limited studies relating to the effect of antibiotics on the reproductive toxicity of *C. elegans*. Huang et al. [40] surveyed exposing nematodes to Fluoroquinolone antibiotics (FQs), including enrofloxacin (ENR), ciprofloxacin (CIP), norfloxacin (NOR), ofloxacin (OFL), fleroxacin (FLE), lomefloxacin hydrochloride (LOM), and sarafloxacin hydrochloride (SAR). The result showed that all the FQ exposures could cause reproductive toxicity of *C. elegans*, resulting in a reduced brood size and lower egg hatchability. ENR exhibited the strongest inhibitory effect on reproduction among the seven FQs [40]. In addition, early-life long-term exposure to sulfamethoxazole (SMX) could also result in significant reproductive impairment [41].

Table 1. Summary of reproductive toxicity of EPs on *C. elegans*.

EPs		Exposure Condition	Visualized Endpoints of Reproductive Toxicity	Reference
PFCs	PFOS PFBS	0.1 μM (50.0 μg/L) 500, 1000, 1500 μM (150.0, 300.1, 450.15 mg/L)	egg production, brood size, apoptosis	[20]
	PFOS PFOA	0.001, 0.01, 0.1 mmol/L (0.5, 5.0, 50.0 mg/L) 0.001, 0.01, 0.1 mmol/L (0.4, 4.1, 41.4 mg/L)	brood size, spermatid (size, morphology, and activation), number of germ cells	[19]
EDCs	DEHP	0.1, 1, 10 mg/L	brood size, generation time, oocyte numbers, gonadal structure, apoptosis	[23]
	BDE-47	1, 3, 10, 30 μg/mL	offspring number, average time of egg-laying, apoptosis	[32]
	BPA	100, 500 μM (22.8, 114.1 mg/L)	egg number, brood size, embryonic lethality, apoptosis	[42]
	NP	1, 10, 200, 400 μg/L	brood size, gonad system	[22]
	Carbendazim	0.01, 0.1, 10, 100 μg/L	brood size	[29]
	ATR	0.0004, 0.004, 0.04, 0.4, 4, 40 mg/L	brood size, generation time	[28]
	TnBP	0.1, 1, 10, 100, 1000 μg/L	brood size, numbers of germline cells and fertilized eggs, area of gonad arm, apoptosis	[31]
	DEHP	0.1, 1, 10 mg/L	brood size, egg-laying rate, eggs in the uterus, gonadal area, germline cell numbers	[24]
	TCBPA	0.01, 0.1, 1, 10, 100 μg/L	brood size, apoptosis	[43]
	Fosthiazate	0.01, 0.1, 1, 10 mg/L	brood size	[26]
	ATR/2,4-D CPF/CYP/MCZ	1, 10, 100, 1000 μg/L 0.1, 1, 10, 100 μg/L	brood size, percentage of gravid nematodes	[30]
	FNT	0.4, 4, 40, 400 μg/L	brood size, germ cell numbers, generation time, gonadal development	[27]
	TPHP	1, 10, 100, 500 μg/L	germline apoptotic cells, number of embryos, total progeny per worm	[44]
	DEHP	0.625, 1.25, 2.5, 5, 10 mM (0.2, 0.5, 1.0, 2.0, 3.9 g/L)	number of eggs	[25]
	4-NP	8 ng/L, 8 μg/L	brood size, oosperm numbers, ovulation rate, total number of germ cells	[21]
MPs/NPs	Pristine/NPS-NH_2	1, 10, 100, 1000 μg/L	brood size, number of fertilized eggs, length of gonad arm, relative area of gonad arm, germline apoptosis	[36]
	MC-LR NPS	0.1, 1, 10 μg/L 0.1, 1 μg/L	brood size	[39]
	PS	0.01, 0.1, 1, 10, 100 mg/L 0.01, 0.1, 1, 10, 100 mg/kg	number of offspring	[35]
	NPS	1, 10, 100, 1000 mg/kg	number of eggs in utero and hatched eggs, apoptosis	[34]
	Pristine/UV-PS	0.1, 1, 10, 100 μg/L	brood size, number of egg ejections, apoptosis	[37]
	Pristine/aged PLA-MPs	0.1, 1, 10, 100 μg/L	brood size, number of hatched eggs and fertilized eggs in the uterus, number of total germline cells, area and length of gonad arm, apoptosis	[38]
Antibiotics	ENR/CIP/NOR/OFL/FLE/LOM/SAR	5.56, 13.9, 27.8, 55.6, 139, 209, 278, 556 μmol/kg	brood size, egg hatchability, morphology of eggs in the uterus, apoptosis	[40]
	SMX	0.001, 1, 10, 100 mg/L	cumulative offspring	[41]

Abbreviations: PFOS: Perfluorooctane sulfonate; PFBS: Perfluorobutane sulfonate; PFOA: Perfluorooctanoic acid; DEHP: Di-(2-ethylhexyl) phthalate; BDE-47: 2,2′,4,4′-tetrabromodiphenyl ether; BPA: Bisphenol A; NP: Nonylphenol; ATR: Atrazine; TnBP: Tri-n-butyl phosphate; TCBPA: Tetrachlorobisphenol A; 2,4-D: 2,4-dichlorophenoxyacetic acid; CPF: Chlorpyrifos; CYP: Cypermethrin; MCZ: Mancozeb; FNT: Fenitrothion; TPHP: Triphenyl phosphate; 4-NP: 4-nitrophenol; NPS: Nanopolystyrene; NPS-NH_2: Amino modified NPS; MC-LR: Microcystins-LR; PS: Polystyrene; UV-PS: UV-photodegraded PS; PLA-MPs: Polylactic acid MPs; ENR: Enrofloxacin; CIP: Ciprofloxacin; NOR: Norfloxacin; OFL: Ofloxacin; FLE: Fleroxacin; LOM: Lomefloxacin hydrochloride; SAR: Sarafloxacin hydrochloride; SMX: Sulfamethoxazole.

4. Multi/Trans-Generational Reproductive Toxicity of EPs on *C. elegans*

The generation time of *C. elegans* is 3–4 days, while the sexual maturity time of zebrafish and mice is approximately 3–4 months and 6–8 weeks, respectively [45–47]. Moreover, cultivating nematodes is both simple and inexpensive, allowing for the rapid collection of numerous samples [48,49]. Therefore, *C. elegans* have the advantage as model organisms to study multi/trans-generational toxicity. To confirm whether the toxic influences of EPs on the parent organisms would be passed on to their offspring, studies on the multi/trans-generational reproductive toxicity of EPs were carried out and are presented in Table 2. There are two categories of exposure in the assessment system for multi/trans-generational toxicity: parental exposure and successive exposure (Figure 3). Parental exposure refers to the scenario where only the parent generation (F0) is subjected to exposure, whereas successive exposure involves conducting exposure experiments on both the F0 nematodes and their subsequent offspring [50,51].

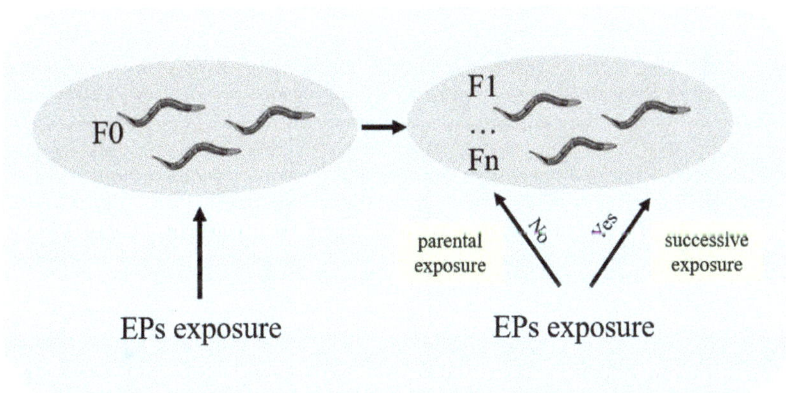

Figure 3. Diagram showing two types of exposure (F0, parent generation; Fn, the nth generation).

4.1. PFCs

Both parent and successive PFOS exposure were conducted in Chowdhury's research. After PFOS parental exposure (0.01, 0.1, 1 μM), in all the P0 generations, significant reductions in brood size were found compared to the control, and in the later generations (F1–F5), the defects of brood size were recovered completely. Under conditions of exposure to PFOS over successive generations (0.001 μM), there was no notable variation in the overall number of offspring from P0 to F5 when compared to the control [52]. This may be associated with the low levels of PFOS; future studies could focus on higher concentrations of PFOS to examine the impact of ongoing exposure on reproductive toxicity in offspring.

4.2. EDCs

Prolonged exposure of parents to 200 nM of hexabromocyclododecane (HBCD) could greatly diminish the brood size of the F0 generation, but the brood size of the F1 generation did not change significantly, indicating that exposure of the F0 generation to HBCD would not have adverse reproductive effects on F1 generation [53]. However, under DEHP, tebuconazole (TEB), and tetrabromobisphenol A (TBBPA) exposure, reproductive toxicities could be caused in the parental generation, and these detrimental influences might also be detected in the offspring even in the absence of toxicant. Take DEHP as an example, after prolonged parental exposure, the total brood size among the F0–F4 generations significantly decreased when a light recovery was detected in the F5 generation [54]. The findings indicated that DEHP has the potential to influence the reproductive capabilities of the initial generations, yet the nematodes appeared to regain their functionality after experiencing multigenerational impacts. This recovery may be linked to the restoration of certain biological processes, including patterns of methylation. The results of parentally TEB exposure were similar to DEHP exposure when the reproduction defects gradually recovered starting from F3 [55]. Under exposure to TBBPA, reproductive toxicities were observed in both the G1 and G2 generations [56]. The brood size of G1 nematodes decreased significantly under TBBPA treatment of 10–1000 mg/L, while in G2 nematodes, the brood size decreased only in the highest treatment group, indicating that the reproductive toxicity of offspring recovered. Similar to PFOS exposure [52], bisphenol S (BPS) successive exposure (0.001 μM) had no significant influence on the brood size of G1 to G4 generations [57]. However, when the concentration increased (0.01 to 100 μM), the brood size across the four generations reduced significantly compared to the control. Both successive and parental exposure were conducted to identify the multi/transgenerational reproductive influence of Atrazine (ATR) [58]. Continuous exposure to ATR significantly increased the reproductive toxicity of the subsequent generations, and the damage to the F2 generation was most significant under parental ATR exposure.

4.3. MPs

Research showed that exposure to MPs/NPs could cause transgenerational reproductive toxicity, and the influences were affected by the plastic concentration, particle size, and the modification of the particles. For instance, exposure to PS-NPs at concentrations ranging from 1 to 100 μg/L during the P0 generation inhibited brood size, and reproduction defects were additionally noted in the offspring. However, the reproduction defects recovered starting from the F3, F4, and F5 generations, respectively [59]. PLA-MPs could also cause transgenerational reproduction inhibition [60]. To explore whether PS-NPs induced transgenerational reproductive toxicity was size-dependent, toxicity experiments exposure to 20 and 100 nm PS-NPs were conducted. The findings indicated that exposure to 20 nm particles led to more pronounced transgenerational toxicity compared to larger particles. The 20 nm PS-NPs exhibited reproductive toxicity in F1–F6 generations, whereas the 100 nm PS-NPs demonstrated toxic effects solely in the F1–F3 generations at identical concentrations [61]. As mentioned above, microplastic modification was another important factor affecting transgenerational toxicity. Pristine NPS was modified with amino groups, which were defined as NPS-NH_2, and NPS-NH_2 showed severe transgenerational reproductive toxicity [62]. In addition, compared with carboxyl-modified PS (PS-COOH), PS-NH_2 still exhibited more severe transgenerational reproductive toxicity [63].

4.4. Antibiotics

Zhang's group previously investigated the multi/trans-generational reproductive toxicity of several antibiotics [64–66]. For instance, sulfamethoxazole (SMZ) and erythromycin (ERY) were selected as the contaminants in Yu's research. Both ERY and SMZ could inhibit reproduction across all generations, although the level of inhibition decreased over successive generations with ongoing exposure to ERY. In the case of SMZ, reduced inhibition was only noted in the F4 generation. Furthermore, even after complete cessation of exposure, ERY and SMZ continued to affect reproduction [66].

Until now, there have been relatively limited studies focusing on multi/transgenerational reproductive toxicity in *C. elegans*, and more attention should be focused on this aspect in the future.

Table 2. Summary of multi/trans-generational reproductive toxicity of EPs on *C. elegans*.

EPs		Exposure Condition	Exposure Method	Number of Generations	Visualized Endpoints	Reference
PFCs	PFOS	0.01, 0.1, 1 μM (5.0, 50.0, 500.13 μg/L) 0.001 μM (0.5 μg/L)	parental exposure successive exposure	six (P0–F5)	brood size	[52]
EDCs	DEHP	20 mg/L	parental exposure	six (F0–F5)	brood size	[54]
	HBCD	0.2, 2, 20, 200 nM (0.13, 1.3, 12.8, 128.3 μg/L)	parental exposure	two (F0–F1)	brood size	[53]
	BPS	0.001, 0.01, 0.1, 1, 10, 100 μM (0.3, 2.5, 25.0, 250.3, 2502.7, 25,027 μg/L)	successive exposure	four (G1–G4)	brood size	[57]
	TEB	0.01, 0.1, 1, 10 μg/L	parental exposure	five (P0–F4)	brood size, reproductive system abnormality, embryo hatchability	[55]
	TBBPA	0.1, 1, 10, 100, 1000 μg/L	parental exposure	two (G1–G2)	brood size	[56]
	Glufosinate	0.1, 1, 10, 100 μg/L	successive exposure	three (F0–F2)	brood size, number of pregnant eggs	[67]
	ATR	0.0004, 0.004, 0.04, 0.4, 4, 40 mg/L	successive and parental exposure	six (P0–F5)	brood size, fertilized eggs, oocytes, ovulation rate, bag of worms, germ cell numbers, relative area of gonad arm	[58]
MPs/NPs	PS-NPs	1, 10, 50, 100 mg/L/ 100 mg/L	successive exposure parental exposure	five (F0–F4)	brood size, germline apoptosis	[68]
	NPS/NPS-NH_2	1, 10, 100 μg/L	parental exposure	five (P0–F4)	brood size, number of fertilized eggs and germline cells, length and area of gonad arm, apoptosis	[62]
	NPS	0.1, 1, 10, 100 μg/L	parental exposure	eight (P0–F7)	brood size	[61]
	NPS	1, 10, 100 μg/L	parental exposure	six (P0–F5)	brood size	[59]
	NPS-S	1, 10, 100 μg/L	parental exposure	five (P0–F4)	brood size, number of fertilized eggs	[69]
	PLA-MPs	1, 10, 100 μg/L	parental exposure	four (P0–F3)	brood size, number of fertilized eggs, gonad development, germline apoptosis	[60]
	PS/PS-NH_2/PS-COOH	100 μg/L	parental exposure	five (P0–F4)	brood size, fertilized eggs, egg ejection rate, cell corpses per gonad	[63]
	NPS-NH_2	0.1, 1, 10 μg/L	parental exposure	five (P0–F4)	brood size, number of fertilized eggs	[70]
Antibiotics	OFL NOR	2.6 ng/L 6.5 ng/L	successive and parental exposure	nine (F1–F9)	number of offspring	[64]
	ENR	229 ng/L	successive exposure	nine (F1–F9)	number of offspring	[65]
	ERY SMZ	0.022, 22.0 mg/L 0.036, 36.0 mg/L	successive and parental exposure	four (F1–F4)	number of offspring	[66]

Abbreviations: PFOS: Perfluorooctane sulfonate; DEHP: Di-(2-ethylhexyl) phthalate; HBCD: Hexabromocyclododecane; BPS: Bisphenol S; TEB: Tebuconazole; TBBPA: Tetrabromobisphenol A; ATR: Atrazine; PS: Polystyrene; PS-NPs: Polystyrene nanoplastics; NPS: Nanopolystyrene; NPS-NH_2: Amino modified NPS; NPS-S: Sulfonate-modified NPS; PLA-MPs: Polylactic acid MPs; PS-NH_2: Amino modified PS; PS-COOH: Carboxyl modified PS; OFL: Ofloxacin; NOR: Norfloxacin; ENR: Enrofloxacin; ERY: Erythromycin; SMZ: Sulfamethoxazole.

5. Underlying Mechanisms of Reproductive Toxicity Induced by EPs

Numerous mechanisms may function in the reproductive toxic influences of EPs on *C. elegans*. Potential mechanisms and associated genes are detailed in Tables 3 and 4. As illustrated, the primary mechanisms are predominantly related to germ cell apoptosis, spermatogenesis, and epigenetic modifications.

5.1. Apoptosis in Germ Cell

The mechanism related to apoptosis is the most studied. Apoptosis represents a biologically conserved mechanism that is vital for the development and maintenance of homeostasis in the majority of multicellular organisms. Apoptosis usually occurs in the germ line of hermaphrodite nematodes and accounts for about 50% of developing oocytes [71]. As listed above, germ cell apoptosis is a sensitive endpoint for evaluating reproductive toxicity. In *C. elegans*, critical elements that contributed to the process of apoptosis comprise Apaf-1, along with Bcl-2 homologs CED-4 and CED-9, the BH3-only domain protein EGL-1, and the caspase CED-3 [72]. CED-4 dimers are sequestered through their contact with a single CED-9 molecule in living cells. EGL-1 associates with CED-9, prompting conformational alterations in CED-9 that ultimately disrupt the binding between CED-4 dimers and CED-9 in cells that are programmed for apoptosis. CED-4 dimers aggregate to form tetramers that subsequently engage with CED-3, facilitating its intrinsic activation upon dissociation from CED-9 [71]. Studies revealed that EPs could modulate the expression of genes related to apoptosis. Following exposure to TnBP, a reduction in the expression levels of the *ced-9* gene was observed, whereas the levels of the *ced-3* and *ced-4* genes exhibited an increase. This suggested that TnBP exposure had a significant impact on the CED-9-CED-4-CED-3 signaling pathway associated with apoptosis [31]. The signaling cascade could persist in the subsequent generations under the exposure of NPs [68]. Likewise, DEHP exposure upregulated *ced-3* and *ced-4* expressions and downregulated *ced-9* gene expression [23].

DNA damage can trigger germline apoptosis, and the mechanisms that trigger apoptosis are particularly complex. One of the most prominent examples is the worm protein CEP-1, which can enhance germline apoptosis caused by DNA damage through the modulation of EGL-1 activity [73–75]. DNA damage elevates the expression of *egl-1* (the proapoptotic gene), and the response relies on the involvement of *hus-1* and *cep-1* [73]. In nematodes, HUS-1, which is the ortholog of Hus1, functions as a checkpoint protein for DNA damage [73–75]. The *hus-1* gene regulates the expression of the *cep-1* gene [37]. To sum up, the HUS-1-CEP-1-EGL-1 signaling cascade is the upstream of the core apoptosis pathway to regulate the germline apoptosis. One research showed that apoptosis induced by TCBPA may be induced by DNA damage. The potential molecular mechanism appeared to be involved in DNA damage facilitated by *hus-1*, resulting in apoptosis through a *cep-1* dependent pathway [43].

The damage induced by oxidative stress is also significant in the reproductive toxicity of nematodes exposed to EPs [24]. Reactive oxygen species (ROS) are typically characterized as small, short-lived, and highly reactive molecules. Within cellular environments, the production of ROS is balanced by a diverse array of antioxidant defenses. These defenses encompass both enzymatic scavengers and non-enzymatic scavenging mechanisms [76,77]. When the antioxidant defense mechanisms are compromised, cells may suffer damage due to an overabundance of ROS, subsequently leading to the occurrence of apoptosis [77]. High concentrations of carbendazim exposure could cause severe oxidative stress, thus disrupting cell homeostasis and promoting cell apoptosis [29]. Another study further illustrated that germline apoptosis, triggered by oxidative stress, was a crucial factor in the reproductive toxicity caused by ENR [40]. BDE-47 has the potential to trigger oxidative stress, leading to germline apoptosis through a MAPK-mediated pathway that operates independently of p53 [32].

Table 3. Underlying mechanisms for reproductive toxicity of EPs on *C. elegans*.

EPs	Possible Mechanisms Involved	Genes Involved	References
PFOS/PFBS	ROS, germ cell apoptosis	*sod-3, ctl-2, gst-4, ced-13, egl-1*	[20]
DEHP	oxidative stress, DNA damage, oocyte apoptosis	*cep-1, ced-4, ced-3, ced-9, egl-1, mev-1, gas-1*	[23]
BDE-47	oxidative stress, oocyte apoptosis (p53-independent MAPK pathway)	*cep-1, sek-1, abl-1, mek-1, hus-1, egl-1*	[32]
BPA	StAR-mediated mitochondrial cholesterol transport	*strl-1, tspo-1*	[42]
TnBP	DNA damage, oxidative stress, germ cell apoptosis	*ced-4, ced-3, ced-9, hus-1, egl-1, clk-2, mev-1, gas-1, cep-1*	[31]
DEHP	autophagy, ROS	*unc-86, atg-7, atg-18, lgg-1, bec-1, unc-51*	[24]
PFOS/PFOA	spermatogenesis	*spe-4, spe-6, spe-10, spe-15, spe-17, fer-1, wee-1.3, swm-1, puf-8, try-5*	[19]
TCBPA	germ cell apoptosis, DNA damage	*cep-1, ced-4, ced-3, ced-9, hus-1, egl-1, efl-2, egl-38, lin-35, dpl-1, sir-2.1, pax-2*	[43]
Fosthiazate	oxidative stress, spermatogenesis	*puf-8, fer-1, swm-1, try-5, spe-5, wee-1.3, sod-3, sod-1, isp-1, sod-2, sod-5, gst-4, mlt-1, mlt-2*	[26]
Pristine/NPS-NH_2	germline apoptosis, DNA damage	*cep-1, ced-4, ced-3, ced-9, hus-1, egl-1, clk-2*	[43]
Pristine/UV-PS	DNA damage, germline apoptosis	*ced-4, ced-3, ced-9, hus-1, egl-1, clk-2, cep-1,*	[37]
FNT	germ cell meiosis and sperm formation (androgen receptor signaling)	*nhr-69, gld-2, gld-3, fbf-1, fbf-2, fog-1, fog-3*	[27]
TPHP	JNK signaling pathway	*mkk-4, dlk-1, egl-15, jnk-1, vhp-1, kgb-2, kgb-1,*	[44]
ENR/CIP/NOR/OFL/FLE/LOM/SAR	oxidative stress, germ cell apoptosis	*gst-1, gst-4, mev-1, sod-2, gst-5, gpx-2, ctl-1, ctl-2, gst-3, gst-8, sod-1, gpx-3, egl-5, egl-38, pax2-b, dpl-1, ced-11, egl-13, pax3, ced-7, egl-3*	[40]
Pristine/aged PLA-MPs	DNA damage, germline apoptosis	*cep-1, hus-1, egl-1, clk-2, mrt-2, ced-4, ced-3, ced-9*	[38]

Abbreviations: PFOS: Perfluorooctane sulfonate; PFBS: Perfluorobutane sulfonate; DEHP: Di-(2-ethylhexyl) phthalate; BDE-47: 2,2′,4,4′-tetrabromodiphenyl ether; BPA: Bisphenol A; TnBP: Tri-n-butyl phosphate; PFOA: Perfluorooctanoic acid; TCBPA: Tetrachlorobisphenol A; NPS: Nanopolystyrene; NPS-NH_2: Amino modified NPS; UV-PS: UV-photodegraded PS; FNT: Fenitrothion; TPHP: Triphenyl phosphate; ENR: Enrofloxacin; CIP: Ciprofloxacin; NOR: Norfloxacin; OFL: Ofloxacin; FLE: Fleroxacin; LOM: Lomefloxacin hydrochloride; SAR: Sarafloxacin hydrochloride; PLA-MPs: Polylactic acid MPs.

Table 4. Underlying mechanisms for multi/trans-generational reproductive toxicity of EPs on *C. elegans*.

EPs	Possible Mechanisms Involved	Genes Involved	References
DEHP	production of inadequate vitellogenin, malfunction of H3Kme2 demethylase	*vit-2, spr-5, vit-6*	[54]
HBCD	oxidative stress, cell apoptosis	*hsp-16.2, hsp-16.48, sod-1, sod-3, cep-1*	[53]
PS-NPs	epigenetic regulation	*ced-4, ced-3, ced-9, met-2, spr-5, set-2*	[68]
NPS/NPS-NH_2	germ cell apoptosis	*ced-4, ced-3, ced-9*	[62]
NPS	oxidative stress	*daf-2, sod-3, mev-1*	[59]
NPS-S	germline Notch signal	*lag-2, glp-1, glb-10, ins-3, daf-28, ins-39, daf-7, dbl-1*	[69]
ATR	epigenetic modification (methylation of DNA and histones)	*damt-1, nmad-1, set-2, set-25, met-2, mes-4, utx-1, pat-12, wrt-3, flwr-1, lnp-1, fbxa-108, ZC317.7, atfs-1, hsp-6, hsp-60*	[58]
PS/PS-NH_2/PS-COOH	histone methylation	*set-30, met-2*	[63]
PLA-MPs	histone methylation, secreted ligands	*ced-4, ced-3, ced-9, egl-1, cep-1, mrt-2, clk-2, hus-1, ins-39, wrt-3, met-2, set-6, mes-2, set-24, set-31, set-2, set-16*	[60]

Abbreviations: DEHP: Di-(2-ethylhexyl) phthalate; HBCD: Hexabromocyclododecane; PS: Polystyrene; PS-NPs: Polystyrene nanoplastics; NPS: Nanopolystyrene; NPS-NH_2: Amino modified NPS; NPS-S: Sulfonate-modified NPS; ATR: Atrazine; PS-NH_2: Amino modified PS; PS-COOH: Carboxyl modified PS; PLA-MPs: Polylactic acid MPs.

5.2. Spermatogenesis

Hermaphrodites and male nematodes both undergo spermatogenesis, which creates functional sperm from an undifferentiated germ cell. Spermatogenesis involves a sequence of critical events, encompassing mitotic and meiotic divisions, the transport of fibrous body-membranous organelles (FB-MO), and the activation of spermatozoa [19]. Research showed that some environmental pollutants may interfere with the expression of spermatogenesis-related genes so reproductive ability was affected [19,26]. Another study revealed that fenitrothion could impact the expression of androgen receptors via the modulation of cortisol and melatonin levels, thereby influencing androgen receptor signaling pathways that are critical for germ cell meiosis and sperm formation [27].

From current studies, mechanisms involved in spermatogenesis are still lacking and require further investigation.

5.3. Epigenetic Alteration

A single parental (F0) exposure to EPs can lead to alterations in reproductive toxicity, which are subsequently passed on to future generations. However, understanding of the transfer mechanism to subsequent generations is limited. Epigenetic inheritance is a potential mechanism for trans-generational effects. Epigenetics refers to heritable changes in gene function without changes to the DNA sequence [78]. Among the epigenetic modifications, DNA methylation is the most extensively researched and understood, followed by histone modifications and non-coding RNAs [79,80].

Under ATR exposure, transgenerational toxicity may arise from mitochondrial stress in the P0 generation, which was influenced by transcriptional 6 mA modifiers. Furthermore, these epigenetic marks could also be established in the offspring [58]. Reproductive toxic memory may be transmitted to subsequent generations via alterations in epigenetic modifications, such as 6-methyladenine (6mdA), which possess the potential for inheritance. MET-2 and SPR-5 collaboratively controlled histone methylation in the germline, and their deletion could cause transgenerational inheritance of H3K4me2, leading to offspring sterility [81,82]. Findings [68] also suggested that MET-2, SPR-5, and SET-2 were involved in NPs-induced transgenerational effects. Except for H3K4me2, H3K9me3 may also play an important role in regulating transgenerational toxicity [63].

6. Conclusions and Perspectives

In summary, this paper reviews the reproductive toxicity of EPs on *C. elegans* and discusses whether this toxicity can be transmitted to the next generation or subsequent generations. The potential mechanisms were also discussed. Studies based on nematodes as model organisms can provide references for investigating the detrimental impacts of EPs on other organisms or humans. However, to further understand the reproductive toxicity of EPs, many problems remain to be addressed. For example, (1) most of the studies are under single pollutant exposure, while there are relatively few studies on co-exposure. Combined exposure can better reflect the influences of environmental pollution on the reproductive toxicity of *C. elegans*; therefore, more attention needs to be paid in the future. (2) Parent exposure obtained more attention than successive exposure. For EPs to persist in the environment, successive exposure deserves future study. (3) For mechanisms, although many potential mechanisms have been proposed, most of them are not thorough enough, only detect changes in relevant genes and speculate on possible mechanisms based on the literature. In addition, these mechanisms may not cover all aspects, as exposure to pollutants can trigger a variety of cellular responses in *C. elegans*. Therefore, more in-depth and comprehensive potential mechanisms need to be explored and presented in the future. (4) As a model organism, *C. elegans* poses several limitations which should not be omitted. *C. elegans* lacks any specific organs. When studying complex conditions, the evolutionary distance from humans might pose a significant constraint. In the future, the impact of EPs on reproduction should be comprehensively conducted in combination with *C. elegans* and other animal models. Concurrently, it is essential to emphasize the thorough assessment and mechanistic investigation of various chemical compounds to enhance our comprehension of their impacts on the physiological and genetic characteristics of living organisms. Furthermore, the development of environmental protection policies holds significant importance. Policies that are informed by scientific evidence can substantially decrease the release of environmental pollutants and mitigate harm to the ecological system.

Author Contributions: Z.W. and L.W.: Conception and design, literature collecting, writing draft, editing. Z.Z.: Conception and design, editing, funding acquisition, validation. W.C. (Weihua Chen), Y.W. and K.C.: Literature collecting, visualization. W.C. (Weiyan Chen), J.L. and H.J.: Editing. All authors have read and agreed to the published version of the manuscript.

Funding: This research was funded by the National Natural Science Foundation of China (Key Program U23A20494) and the Natural Science Foundation of Chongqing, China (CSTB2024NSCQ-LZX0142).

Institutional Review Board Statement: Not applicable.

Informed Consent Statement: Not applicable.

Data Availability Statement: Not applicable.

Conflicts of Interest: Author Weihua Chen was employed by the company Central & Southern China Municipal Engineering Design and Research Institute Co., Ltd. The remaining authors declare that the research was conducted in the absence of any commercial or financial relationships that could be construed as a potential conflict of interest.

References

1. Ma, Y.; He, X.; Qi, K.; Wang, T.; Qi, Y.; Cui, L.; Wang, F.; Song, M. Effects of environmental contaminants on fertility and reproductive health. *J. Environ. Sci.* **2019**, *77*, 210–217. [CrossRef]
2. Carson, S.A.; Kallen, A.N. Diagnosis and Management of Infertility. *JAMA* **2021**, *326*, 65–76. [CrossRef]
3. Pedro, J.; Brandão, T.; Schmidt, L.; Costa, M.E.; Martins, M.V. What do people know about fertility? A systematic review on fertility awareness and its associated factors. *Upsala J. Med. Sci.* **2018**, *123*, 71–81. [CrossRef]
4. Dutta, S.; Gorain, B.; Choudhury, H.; Roychoudhury, S.; Sengupta, P. Environmental and occupational exposure of metals and female reproductive health. *Environ. Sci. Pollut. Res.* **2022**, *29*, 62067–62092. [CrossRef] [PubMed]
5. Chia, X.K.; Hadibarata, T.; Jusoh, M.N.H.; Sutiknowati, L.I.; Tan, I.S.; Foo, H.C.Y. Role of Extremophiles in Biodegradation of Emerging Pollutants. *Top. Catal.* **2024**, 1–18. [CrossRef]
6. Matei, E.; Covaliu-Mierla, C.I.; Ţurcanu, A.A.; Râpă, M.; Predescu, A.M.; Predescu, C. Multifunctional Membranes-A Versatile Approach for Emerging Pollutants Removal. *Membranes* **2022**, *12*, 67. [CrossRef] [PubMed]
7. Niu, H.; Xu, M.; Tu, P.; Xu, Y.; Li, X.; Xing, M.; Chen, Z.; Wang, X.; Lou, X.; Wu, L.; et al. Emerging Contaminants: An Emerging Risk Factor for Diabetes Mellitus. *Toxics* **2024**, *12*, 47. [CrossRef] [PubMed]
8. Khasin, L.G.; Della Rosa, J.; Petersen, N.; Moeller, J.; Kriegsfeld, L.J.; Lishko, P.V. The Impact of Di-2-Ethylhexyl Phthalate on Sperm Fertility. *Front. Cell Dev. Biol.* **2020**, *8*, 426. [CrossRef]
9. Cui, Q.; Pan, Y.; Wang, J.; Liu, H.; Yao, B.; Dai, J. Exposure to per- and polyfluoroalkyl substances (PFASs) in serum versus semen and their association with male reproductive hormones. *Environ. Pollut.* **2020**, *266*, 115330. [CrossRef]
10. Albert, O.; Huang, J.Y.; Aleksa, K.; Hales, B.F.; Goodyer, C.G.; Robaire, B.; Chevrier, J.; Chan, P. Exposure to polybrominated diphenyl ethers and phthalates in healthy men living in the greater Montreal area: A study of hormonal balance and semen quality. *Environ. Int.* **2018**, *116*, 165–175. [CrossRef]
11. Kim, Y.; Park, Y.; Hwang, J.; Kwack, K. Comparative genomic analysis of the human and nematode *Caenorhabditis elegans* uncovers potential reproductive genes and disease associations in humans. *Physiol. Genom.* **2018**, *50*, 1002–1014. [CrossRef] [PubMed]
12. Habas, K.; Demir, E.; Guo, C.; Brinkworth, M.H.; Anderson, D. Toxicity mechanisms of nanoparticles in the male reproductive system. *Drug Metab. Rev.* **2021**, *53*, 604–617. [CrossRef]
13. Barakat, R.; Lin, P.P.; Rattan, S.; Brehm, E.; Canisso, I.F.; Abosalum, M.E.; Flaws, J.A.; Hess, R.; Ko, C. Prenatal Exposure to DEHP Induces Premature Reproductive Senescence in Male Mice. *Toxicol. Sci.* **2017**, *156*, 96–108. [CrossRef]
14. Song, P.; Li, D.; Wang, X.; Zhong, X. Effects of perfluorooctanoic acid exposure during pregnancy on the reproduction and development of male offspring mice. *Andrologia* **2018**, *50*, e13059. [CrossRef]
15. Ruszkiewicz, J.A.; Pinkas, A.; Miah, M.R.; Weitz, R.L.; Lawes, M.J.A.; Akinyemi, A.J.; Ijomone, O.M.; Aschner, M.C. *C. Elegans* as a model in developmental neurotoxicology. *Toxicol. Appl. Pharmacol.* **2018**, *354*, 126–135. [CrossRef] [PubMed]
16. Yao, Y.; Zhang, T.; Tang, M. A critical review of advances in reproductive toxicity of common nanomaterials to *Caenorhabditis elegans* and influencing factors. *Environ. Pollut.* **2022**, *306*, 119270. [CrossRef] [PubMed]
17. *C. elegans* Sequencing Consortium. Genome sequence of the nematode *C. elegans*: A platform for investigating biology. *Science* **1998**, *282*, 2012–2018. [CrossRef]

18. Zitouni, F.; Kumar, M.; Uday, V.; Srivastava, P.; Deka, B.J.; Zitouni, F.; Mahlknecht, J. EI/IOT of PFCs: Environmental impacts/interactions, occurrences, and toxicities of perfluorochemicals. *Environ. Res.* **2023**, *218*, 114707.
19. Yin, J.; Jian, Z.; Zhu, G.; Yu, X.; Pu, Y.; Yin, L.; Wang, D.; Bu, Y.; Liu, R. Male reproductive toxicity involved in spermatogenesis induced by perfluorooctane sulfonate and perfluorooctanoic acid in *Caenorhabditis elegans*. *Environ. Sci. Pollut. Res.* **2021**, *28*, 1443–1453. [CrossRef]
20. Chen, F.; Wei, C.; Chen, Q.; Zhang, J.; Wang, L.; Zhou, Z.; Chen, M.; Liang, Y. Internal concentrations of perfluorobutane sulfonate (PFBS) comparable to those of perfluorooctane sulfonate (PFOS) induce reproductive toxicity in *Caenorhabditis elegans*. *Ecotoxicol. Environ. Saf.* **2018**, *158*, 223–229. [CrossRef]
21. Wang, J.; Yin, J.; Peng, D.; Zhang, X.; Shi, Z.; Li, W.; Shi, Y.; Sun, M.; Jiang, N.; Cheng, B.; et al. 4-Nitrophenol at environmentally relevant concentrations mediates reproductive toxicity in *Caenorhabditis elegans* via metabolic disorders-induced estrogen signaling pathway. *J. Environ. Sci.* **2025**, *147*, 244–258. [CrossRef] [PubMed]
22. Cao, X.; Yan, C.; Wu, X.; Zhou, L.; Xiu, G. Nonylphenol induced individual and population fluctuation of *Caenorhabditis elegans*: Disturbances on developmental and reproductive system. *Environ. Res.* **2020**, *186*, 109486. [CrossRef] [PubMed]
23. Yin, J.; Liu, R.; Jian, Z.; Yang, D.; Pu, Y.; Yin, L.; Wang, D. Di (2-ethylhexyl) phthalate-induced reproductive toxicity involved in DNA damage-dependent oocyte apoptosis and oxidative stress in *Caenorhabditis elegans*. *Ecotoxicol. Environ. Saf.* **2018**, *163*, 298–306. [CrossRef]
24. Li, J.; Qu, M.; Wang, M.; Yue, Y.; Chen, Z.; Liu, R.; Bu, Y.; Li, Y. Reproductive toxicity and underlying mechanisms of di(2-ethylhexyl) phthalate in nematode *Caenorhabditis elegans*. *J. Environ. Sci.* **2021**, *105*, 1–10. [CrossRef] [PubMed]
25. Zongur, A. Evaluation of the Effects of Di-(2-ethylhexyl) phthalate (DEHP) on *Caenorhabditis elegans* Survival and Fertility. *Appl. Biochem. Biotecnolh.* **2024**, 1–12.
26. Liu, S.; Wu, Q.; Zhong, Y.; He, Z.; Wang, Z.; Li, R.; Wang, M. Fosthiazate exposure induces oxidative stress, nerve damage, and reproductive disorders in nontarget nematodes. *Environ. Sci. Pollut. Res.* **2022**, *30*, 12522–12531. [CrossRef]
27. Li, W.; Ma, L.; Shi, Y.; Wang, J.; Yin, J.; Wang, D.; Luo, K.; Liu, R. Meiosis-mediated reproductive toxicity by fenitrothion in *Caenorhabditis elegans* from metabolomic perspective. *Ecotoxicol. Environ. Saf.* **2023**, *253*, 114680.
28. Yin, J.; Hong, X.; Ma, L.; Liu, R.; Bu, Y. Non-targeted metabolomic profiling of atrazine in *Caenorhabditis elegans* using UHPLC-QE Orbitrap/MS. *Ecotoxicol. Environ. Saf.* **2020**, *206*, 111170. [CrossRef]
29. Li, J.; Zhou, X.; Zhang, C.; Zhao, Y.; Zhu, Y.; Zhang, J.; Bai, J.; Xiao, X. The Effects of Carbendazim on Acute Toxicity, Development, and Reproduction in *Caenorhabditis elegans*. *J. Food Qual.* **2020**, *2020*, 8853537. [CrossRef]
30. Moya, A.; Tejedor, D.; Manetti, M.; Clavijo, A.; Pagano, E.; Munarriz, E.; Kronberg, M.F. Reproductive toxicity by exposure to low concentrations of pesticides in *Caenorhabditis elegans*. *Toxicology* **2022**, *475*, 153229. [CrossRef]
31. Zhang, H.; Liu, T.; Song, X.; Zhou, Q.; Tang, J.; Sun, Q.; Pu, Y.; Yin, L.; Zhang, J. Study on the reproductive toxicity and mechanism of tri-n-butyl phosphate (TnBP) in *Caenorhabditis elegans*. *Ecotoxicol. Environ. Saf.* **2021**, *227*, 112896. [CrossRef] [PubMed]
32. You, X.; Xi, J.; Liu, W.; Cao, Y.; Tang, W.; Zhang, X.; Yu, Y.; Luan, Y. 2,2′,4,4′-tetrabromodiphenyl ether induces germ cell apoptosis through oxidative stress by a MAPK-mediated p53-independent pathway. *Environ. Pollut.* **2018**, *242*, 887–893. [CrossRef] [PubMed]
33. Lei, L.; Wu, S.; Lu, S.; Liu, M.; Song, Y.; Fu, Z.; Shi, H.; Raley-Susman, K.M.; He, D. Microplastic particles cause intestinal damage and other adverse effects in zebrafish Danio rerio and nematode *Caenorhabditis elegans*. *Sci. Total Environ.* **2018**, *619–620*, 1–8. [CrossRef] [PubMed]
34. Huang, C.; Yen, P.; Kuo, Y.; Chang, C.; Liao, V.H. Nanoplastic exposure in soil compromises the energy budget of the soil nematode *C. elegans* and decreases reproductive fitness. *Environ. Pollut.* **2022**, *312*, 120071. [CrossRef] [PubMed]
35. Kim, S.W.; Kim, D.; Jeong, S.W.; An, Y.J. Size-dependent effects of polystyrene plastic particles on the nematode *Caenorhabditis elegans* as related to soil physicochemical properties. *Environ. Pollut.* **2020**, *258*, 113740. [CrossRef]
36. Qu, M.; Qiu, Y.; Kong, Y.; Wang, D. Amino modification enhances reproductive toxicity of nanopolystyrene on gonad development and reproductive capacity in nematode *Caenorhabditis elegans*. *Environ. Pollut.* **2019**, *254*, 112978. [CrossRef]
37. Chen, H.; Yang, Y.; Wang, C.; Hua, X.; Li, H.; Xie, D.; Xiang, M.; Yu, Y. Reproductive toxicity of UV-photodegraded polystyrene microplastics induced by DNA damage-dependent cell apoptosis in *Caenorhabditis elegans*. *Sci. Total Environ.* **2022**, *811*, 152350. [CrossRef]
38. Shao, Y.; Hua, X.; Li, Y.; Wang, D. Comparison of reproductive toxicity between pristine and aged polylactic acid microplastics in *Caenorhabditis elegans*. *J. Hazard. Mater.* **2024**, *466*, 133545. [CrossRef] [PubMed]
39. Qu, M.; Nida, A.; Kong, Y.; Du, H.; Xiao, G.; Wang, D. Nanopolystyrene at predicted environmental concentration enhances microcystin-LR toxicity by inducing intestinal damage in *Caenorhabditis elegans*. *Ecotoxicol. Environ. Saf.* **2019**, *183*, 109568. [CrossRef]
40. Huang, J.; Liao, L.; Wang, G.; Du, Z.; Wu, Z. Reproductive toxicity of enrofloxacin in *Caenorhabditis elegans* involves oxidative stress-induced cell apoptosis. *J. Environ. Sci.* **2023**, *127*, 726–737. [CrossRef]
41. Kuo, Y.; How, C.M.; Huang, C.; Yen, P.; Yu, C.; Chang, C.; Liao, V.H. Co-contaminants of ethinylestradiol and sulfamethoxazole in groundwater exacerbate ecotoxicity and ecological risk and compromise the energy budget of *C. elegans*. *Aquat. Toxicol.* **2023**, *257*, 106473. [CrossRef] [PubMed]
42. Chen, Y.; Panter, B.; Hussain, A.; Gibbs, K.; Ferreira, D.; Allard, P. BPA interferes with StAR-mediated mitochondrial cholesterol transport to induce germline dysfunctions. *Reprod. Toxicol.* **2019**, *90*, 24–32. [CrossRef] [PubMed]

43. Yu, Y.; Hua, X.; Chen, H.; Yang, Y.; Dang, Y.; Xiang, M. Tetrachlorobisphenol A mediates reproductive toxicity in *Caenorhabditis elegans* via DNA damage-induced apoptosis. *Chemosphere* **2022**, *300*, 134588. [CrossRef] [PubMed]
44. Shi, C.; Wang, C.; Zeng, L.; Peng, Y.; Li, Y.; Hao, H.; Zheng, Y.; Chen, C.; Chen, H.; Zhang, J.; et al. Triphenyl phosphate induced reproductive toxicity through the JNK signaling pathway in *Caenorhabditis elegans*. *J. Hazard. Mater.* **2023**, *446*, 130643. [CrossRef] [PubMed]
45. Hunt, P.R. The *C. elegans model in toxicity testing*. *J. Appl. Toxicol.* **2017**, *37*, 50–59.
46. Lohr, H.; Hammerschmidt, M. Zebrafish in endocrine systems: Recent advances and implications for human disease. *Annu. Rev. Physiol.* **2011**, *73*, 183–211. [CrossRef]
47. McNamara, M.P.; Singleton, J.M.; Cadney, M.D.; Ruegger, P.M.; Borneman, J.; Garland, T. Early-life effects of juvenile Western diet and exercise on adult gut microbiome composition in mice. *J. Exp. Biol.* **2021**, *224*, jeb239699. [CrossRef]
48. Long, N.P.; Kang, J.S.; Kim, H.M. *Caenorhabditis elegans*: A model organism in the toxicity assessment of environmental pollutants. *Environ. Sci. Pollut. Res. Int.* **2023**, *30*, 39273–39287. [CrossRef]
49. Scharf, A.; Pohl, F.; Egan, B.M.; Kocsisova, Z.; Kornfeld, K. Reproductive Aging in *Caenorhabditis elegans*: From Molecules to Ecology. *Front. Cell Dev. Biol.* **2021**, *9*, 718522. [CrossRef]
50. Li, H.; Zeng, L.; Wang, C.; Shi, C.; Li, Y.; Peng, Y.; Chen, H.; Zhang, J.; Cheng, B.; Chen, C.; et al. Review of the toxicity and potential molecular mechanisms of parental or successive exposure to environmental pollutants in the model organism *Caenorhabditis elegans*. *Environ. Pollut.* **2022**, *311*, 119927. [CrossRef]
51. Wamucho, A.; Unrine, J.; May, J.; Tsyusko, O. Global DNA Adenine Methylation in *Caenorhabditis elegans* after Multigenerational Exposure to Silver Nanoparticles and Silver Nitrate. *Int. J. Mol. Sci.* **2023**, *24*, 6168. [CrossRef] [PubMed]
52. Chowdhury, M.I.; Sana, T.; Panneerselvan, L.; Sivaram, A.K.; Megharaj, M. Perfluorooctane sulfonate (PFOS) induces several behavioral defects in *Caenorhabditis elegans* that can also be transferred to the next generations. *Chemosphere* **2022**, *291*, 132896. [CrossRef] [PubMed]
53. Chen, H.; Guo, S.; Li, H.; Zhou, D.; Cao, X.; Wang, C.; Liu, Y.; Xiang, M.; Li, L.; Yu, Y. Multi-generational effects and variations of stress response by hexabromocyclododecane (HBCD) exposure in the nematode *Caenorhabditis elegans*. *J. Environ. Manag.* **2019**, *245*, 216–222. [CrossRef] [PubMed]
54. Li, S.; How, C.M.; Liao, V.H. Prolonged exposure of di(2-ethylhexyl) phthalate induces multigenerational toxic effects in *Caenorhabditis elegans*. *Sci. Total Environ.* **2018**, *634*, 260–266. [CrossRef]
55. Lu, Q.; Bu, Y.; Ma, L.; Liu, R. Transgenerational reproductive and developmental toxicity of tebuconazole in *Caenorhabditis elegans*. *J. Appl. Toxicol.* **2020**, *40*, 578–591. [CrossRef]
56. Liu, F.; Luo, Q.; Zhang, Y.; Huang, K.; Cao, X.; Cui, C.; Lin, K.; Zhang, M. Trans-generational effect of neurotoxicity and related stress response in *Caenorhabditis elegans* exposed to tetrabromobisphenol A. *Sci. Total Environ.* **2020**, *703*, 134920. [CrossRef]
57. Xiao, X.; Zhang, X.; Zhang, C.; Li, J.; Zhao, Y.; Zhu, Y.; Zhang, J.; Zhou, X. Toxicity and multigenerational effects of bisphenol S exposure to *Caenorhabditis elegans* on developmental, biochemical, reproductive and oxidative stress. *Toxicol. Res.* **2019**, *8*, 630–640. [CrossRef]
58. Yin, J.; Hong, X.; Wang, J.; Li, W., Shi, Y.; Wang, D.; Liu, R. DNA methylation 6 mA and histone methylation involved in multi-/trans-generational reproductive effects in *Caenorhabditis elegans* induced by Atrazine. *Ecotoxicol. Environ. Saf.* **2023**, *249*, 114348. [CrossRef]
59. Zhang, L.; Wang, S.; Zhao, Y.; Nurdebek, B.; Bu, Y.; Wang, D. Long-term exposure to polystyrene nanoparticles causes transgenerational toxicity by affecting the function and expression of MEV-1 and DAF-2 signals in *Caenorhabditis elegans*. *Nanoimpact* **2022**, *26*, 100403. [CrossRef]
60. Shao, Y.; Li, Y.; Wang, D. Polylactic acid microplastics cause transgenerational reproductive toxicity associated with activation of insulin and hedgehog ligands in *C. elegans*. *Sci. Total Environ.* **2024**, *942*, 173746. [CrossRef]
61. Liu, H.; Tian, L.; Wang, S.; Wang, D. Size-dependent transgenerational toxicity induced by nanoplastics in nematode *Caenorhabditis elegans*. *Sci. Total Environ.* **2021**, *790*, 148217. [CrossRef] [PubMed]
62. Sun, L.; Liao, K.; Wang, D. Comparison of transgenerational reproductive toxicity induced by pristine and amino modified nanoplastics in *Caenorhabditis elegans*. *Sci. Total Environ.* **2021**, *768*, 144362. [CrossRef] [PubMed]
63. Chen, H.; Chen, X.; Gu, Y.; Jiang, Y.; Guo, H.; Chen, J.; Yu, J.; Wang, C.; Chen, C.; Li, H. Transgenerational reproductive toxicity induced by carboxyl and amino charged microplastics at environmental concentrations in *Caenorhabditis elegans*: Involvement of histone methylation. *Sci. Total Environ.* **2024**, *949*, 175132. [CrossRef] [PubMed]
64. Zhang, J.; Zheng, Y.; Yu, Z. Reproductive toxicities of ofloxacin and norfloxacin on *Caenorhabditis elegans* with multi-generational oscillatory effects and trans-generational residual influences. *Environ. Toxicol. Phar.* **2022**, *95*, 103962. [CrossRef] [PubMed]
65. Zheng, Y.; Yu, Z.; Zhang, J. Multi-generational effects of enrofloxacin on lifespan and reproduction of *Caenorhabditis elegans* with SKN-1-mediated antioxidant responses and lipid metabolism disturbances. *Sci. Total Environ.* **2022**, *804*, 150250. [CrossRef] [PubMed]
66. Yu, Z.; Wang, L.; Li, G.; Zhang, J. Reproductive Influences of Erythromycin and Sulfamethoxazole on *Caenorhabditis elegans* over Generations Mediated by Lipid Metabolism. *Chem. Res. Chin.* **2023**, *39*, 434–440. [CrossRef]
67. Zhao, X.; Fu, K.; Xiang, K.; Wang, L.; Zhang, Y.; Luo, Y. Comparison of the chronic and multigenerational toxicity of racemic glufosinate and -glufosinate to *Caenorhabditis elegans* at environmental concentrations. *Chemosphere* **2023**, *316*, 137863. [CrossRef]

68. Yu, C.; Luk, T.C.; Liao, V.H. Long-term nanoplastics exposure results in multi and trans-generational reproduction decline associated with germline toxicity and epigenetic regulation in *Caenorhabditis elegans*. *J. Hazard. Mater.* **2021**, *412*, 125173. [CrossRef]
69. He, W.; Gu, A.; Wang, D. Sulfonate-Modified Polystyrene Nanoparticle at Precited Environmental Concentrations Induces Transgenerational Toxicity Associated with Increase in Germline Notch Signal of *Caenorhabditis elegans*. *Toxics* **2023**, *11*, 511. [CrossRef]
70. Liu, H.; Tan, X.; Li, X.; Wu, Y.; Lei, S.; Wang, Z. Amino-modified nanoplastics at predicted environmental concentrations cause transgenerational toxicity through activating germline EGF signal in *Caenorhabditis elegans*. *Sci. Total Environ.* **2024**, *947*, 174766. [CrossRef]
71. Lettre, G.; Hengartner, M.O. Developmental apoptosis in *C. elegans*: A complex CEDnario. *Nat. Rev. Mol. Cell Biol.* **2006**, *7*, 97–108. [CrossRef] [PubMed]
72. Pourkarimi, E.; Greiss, S.; Gartner, A. Evidence that CED-9/Bcl2 and CED-4/Apaf-1 localization is not consistent with the current model for *C. elegans apoptosis induction*. *Cell. Death Differ.* **2012**, *19*, 406–415. [CrossRef] [PubMed]
73. Hofmann, E.R.; Milstein, S.; Boulton, S.J.; Ye, M.; Hofmann, J.J.; Stergiou, L.; Gartner, A.; Vidal, M.; Hengartner, M.O. *Caenorhabditis elegans* HUS-1 is a DNA damage checkpoint protein required for genome stability and EGL-1-mediated apoptosis. *Curr. Biol.* **2002**, *12*, 1908–1918. [CrossRef] [PubMed]
74. Zhao, Y.; Wu, Q.; Wang, D. An epigenetic signal encoded protection mechanism is activated by graphene oxide to inhibit its induced reproductive toxicity in *Caenorhabditis elegans*. *Biomaterials* **2016**, *79*, 15–24. [CrossRef] [PubMed]
75. Derry, W.B.; Putzke, A.P.; Rothman, J.H. *Caenorhabditis elegans* p53: Role in apoptosis, meiosis, and stress resistance. *Science* **2001**, *294*, 591–595. [CrossRef]
76. Halliwell, B. Free radicals and antioxidants—Quo vadis? *Trends Pharmacol. Sci.* **2011**, *32*, 125–130. [CrossRef]
77. Redza-Dutordoir, M.; Averill-Bates, D.A. Activation of apoptosis signaling pathways by reactive oxygen species. *Biochim. Biophys. Acta (BBA) Mol. Cell. Res.* **2016**, *1863*, 2977–2992. [CrossRef]
78. Kaliman, P. Epigenetics and meditation. *Curr. Opin. Psychol.* **2019**, *28*, 76–80. [CrossRef]
79. Ashapkin, V.; Suvorov, A.; Pilsner, J.R.; Krawetz, S.A.; Sergeyev, O. Age-associated epigenetic changes in mammalian sperm: Implications for offspring health and development. *Hum. Reprod.* **2023**, *29*, 24–44. [CrossRef]
80. Lee, G.S.; Conine, C.C. The Transmission of Intergenerational Epigenetic Information by Sperm microRNAs. *Epigenomes* **2022**, *6*, 12. [CrossRef]
81. Wei, C.; Yen, P.; Chaikritsadakarn, A.; Huang, C.; Chang, C.; Liao, V.H. Parental CuO nanoparticles exposure results in transgenerational toxicity in *Caenorhabditis elegans* associated with possible epigenetic regulation. *Ecotoxicol. Environ. Saf.* **2020**, *203*, 111001. [CrossRef] [PubMed]
82. Kerr, S.C.; Ruppersburg, C.C.; Francis, J.W.; Katz, D.J. SPR-5 and MET-2 function cooperatively to reestablish an epigenetic ground state during passage through the germ line. *Proc. Natl. Acad. Sci. USA* **2014**, *111*, 9509–9514. [CrossRef] [PubMed]

toxics

MDPI

Systematic Review

The Association Between Per- and Polyfluoroalkyl Substances Exposure and Thyroid Hormones in Men and Non-Pregnant Women: A Systematic Review and Meta-Analysis

Bin Zhang [1,†], Meizi Zhao [2,†], Xiangru Cong [1], Chunyu Liu [1], Chaofei Li [3], Yu Qiu [4], Sha Li [3], Yanying Chen [3], Xiaoxue Li [5,*,‡] and Penghui Li [1,*,‡]

1 School of Environmental Science and Safety Engineering, Tianjin University of Technology, Tianjin 300384, China; 15588245258@163.com (B.Z.); congxiangru719@163.com (X.C.); liuchunyu981002@163.com (C.L.)

2 Tianjin Eco-Environmental Monitoring Center, Tianjin 300191, China; zhaomz_2004@126.com

3 Zhonghuan (Fujian) Environmental Technology Co., Ltd., Fuzhou 350025, China; lichaofei1985@hotmail.com (C.L.); fzhkjc@163.com (S.L.); chenyanying_60@126.com (Y.C.)

4 Fujian Jinhuang Environmental Protection Technology Co., Ltd., Fuzhou 350025, China; qiuyu075@163.com

5 Disaster Medicine Research Center, Medical Innovation Research Division of the Chinese PLA General Hospital, Beijing 100853, China

* Correspondence: lixiaoxue@301hospital.com.cn (X.L.); lipenghui406@163.com (P.L.)

† These authors contributed equally to this work.

‡ Penghui Li is the 1st correspondence and Xiaoxue Li is 2nd correspondence.

Abstract: Studies have shown that per- and polyfluoroalkyl substances (PFAS) may impact thyroid function in human health. While the consistency between PFAS exposure and thyroid health effects in pregnant women has been validated, the effects on men and non-pregnant women remains inconclusive. To address this, a meta-analysis was carried out in this paper, with 14 eligible studies retrieved from Embase, PubMed, and Web of Science that were published up to 2 June 2024, focusing on the relationship between PFAS exposure and its effect on thyroid hormone levels in the human body. The thyroid function indexes analyzed included thyroid stimulating hormone (TSH), triiodothyronine (T3), thyroxine (T4), free T3 (FT3), and free T4 (FT4). The estimated value (β) and the corresponding confidence interval (95% CI) were extracted from the literature. A heterogeneity test was carried out, and the sensitivity analysis and publication bias of the studies were analyzed using Stata 18.0. The results revealed that in men and non-pregnant women, PFOA was positively correlated with FT3 ($\beta = 0.011$, 95% CI = 0.001, 0.02, $I^2 = 13.4$). However, no significant associations were found between exposure to other PFAS and thyroid hormones. A subgroup analysis further indicated that the correlations between PFAS exposure and thyroid hormone levels were more significant in adolescents, in both America and Europe.

Keywords: per- and polyfluoroalkyl substances; thyroid hormones; non-pregnant women; meta-analysis

1. Introduction

The normal synthesis and release of thyroid hormone are crucial for human growth and development. Research shows that the impaired signaling of thyroid hormone (TH) and thyroid hormone receptor beta (TRβ) in the liver can trigger hepatic steatosis [1]. Thyroid hormones are of great significance for the development of the brain (including the cerebellum) [2]. A deficiency of thyroid hormones can lead to abnormal cerebellar development, and the abnormalities caused by perinatal hypothyroidism are difficult to fully recover from [3]. At the same time, thyroid hormones and insulin jointly regulate glucose metabolism. A decrease in thyroid hormone sensitivity is associated with a decline in body mass index (BMI), total cholesterol (TC), high-density lipoprotein (HDL), and low-density lipoprotein (LDL) [4,5]. The growing evidence in humans and experimental animals shows that the perturbations of thyroid hormone are associated with specific environmental chemical exposure to heavy metals [6], polybrominated diphenylethers (PBDEs), hydroxylated metabolites (OH-PBDEs) [7], per- and polyfluoroalkyl substances (PFAS) [8], and polychlorinated biphenyls (PCBs) [9].

PFAS are persistent organic pollutants that widely exist in the environment. Due to their potential harm to the environment and health, they have become a research focus in public health [10]. This class of compounds has excellent hydrophobicity and oil-repellent properties [11]; since the 1950s, these compounds have been used in a wide range of industrial and consumer products, such as surfactants, fire protection, textiles, food packaging, lubricants, cosmetics, cleaning products, and many other types [12]. Meanwhile, due to their hydrophobic, oil-repellent properties, and other characteristics, PFAS have a long environmental retention time and are not easily decomposed, leading to more significant environmental damage [13,14]. PFAS that are widely used in the environment include perfluorooctanoate (PFOA), perfluorooctane sulfonate (PFOS), perfluorohexane sulfonate (PFHxS), perfluorononanoic acid (PFNA), perfluorodecanoic acid (PFDA), perfluorododecane sulfonate (PFDoDS), and perfluorodecane sulfonic acid (PFDS). PFAS with long chains, such as PFOA, PFNA, PFDA, PFOS, and PFHxS, were more toxic when compared to ultrashort-chain PFAS (TFA) [15]. Research has revealed that the half-life of PFAS in humans varies depending on the length of the carbon chain, and the half-lives of PFOA, PFNA, PFDA, PFOS, and PFHxS are 3–12 years [16,17].

PFAS have been widely detected in various environmental media, locally and globally, such as aquatic systems, terrestrial sediments, and ecological communities [18]. Extensive human exposure to PFAS has also been confirmed by testing of human blood in multiple countries [19–21]. Some studies have pointed out that PFAS will continue to bioaccumulate with the amplification of trophic levels in the food chain. Compared with aquatic food chains, the bioaccumulation process of terrestrial food chains is more complex and more harmful. This bioaccumulation enables PFAS to accumulate to biologically relevant concentrations in the human body, potentially activate the proliferator-activated receptor-alpha (PPARα) signaling pathway, trigger oxidative stress, and induce endocrine disruption [22–24]. Notably, PFAS exhibit a pronounced interference with thyroid hormone, which are essential for the growth and development of the body [25–27].

A meta-analysis of maternal exposures to PFAS on thyroid hormones showed a positive association between thyroid stimulating hormone (TSH) and PFAS [28]. Pregnant women and their fetuses are susceptible to external factors owing to the special physiological changes during pregnancy [29,30]. This might be due to a higher probability of pregnant women ingesting certain foods (such as seafood and meat, which are rich in specific nutrients) that contain elevated levels of PFAS [31]. For men and non-pregnant women, the association between PFAS and thyroid hormone is inconsistent and controversial. A previous study indicated a negative relation between PFAS exposure and triiodothyronine (T3) and thyroxine (T4) in adults [32]. The exposure of adolescents to PFAS was negatively associated with free T4 (FT4) levels [33]. Other epidemiological studies found a positive correlation between PFAS exposure and T4 [34,35], while another study indicated that the lack of conclusive evidence substantiated a specific association between thyroid hormone levels and PFAS [36]. As a result, a meta-analysis of the potential association between PFAS exposure and thyroid hormone levels in men and non-pregnant women (removing pregnant women from the study population) needs to be conducted. Thus, we systematically retrieved relevant studies and performed a quantitative analysis using a meta-analysis model to assess the relationship between PFAS exposure and changes in thyroid levels in men and non-pregnant women. This study carefully screened high-quality research to ensure that the data were reliable and scientific. Rigorous statistical methods were used to accurately reveal the potential association pattern between them.

2. Methods

The study was conducted using the methods proposed in the Preferred Reporting Items for Systematic Review and Meta-analysis Protocol (PRISMA-P) statement [37]. It has been registered with PROSPERO (ID 1001533).

2.1. Keywords Search

Perfluoroalkyl acids (PFAA) are the most widely studied category of PFAS. In the scientific literature, PFAA is generally divided into two categories: one of these is long-chain compounds containing seven or more carbon–fluorine bonds; the other category is short-chain compounds with fewer than seven carbon–fluorine bonds [38,39]. Meanwhile, long-chain perfluoroalkyl carboxylic acids (PFCAs, $C_nF_{2n+1}COOH$, $n \geq 7$) and long-chain perfluoroalkyl sulfonic acids ($PFSA_S$, $C_nF_{2n+1}SO_3H$, $n \geq 6$) are the focus of international due to their environmental persistence and bioaccumulation [40,41]. Thus, we chose PFOA, PFNA, PFDA, PFOS, and PFHxS, which belong to the long-chain PFAA, to explore the correlation between PFAS with thyroid hormone (thyroid stimulating hormone (TSH), triiodothyronine (T3), thyroxine (T4), free T3 (FT3), and free T4 (FT4)).

All relevant articles were retrieved from the Embase, PubMed, and Web of Science databases by setting specific keywords and the latest publication date as 2 June 2024. The following keywords were included:

1. PFAS exposure: "fluorocarbons" or "perfluorinated" or "polyfluorinated" or "polyfluoroalkyl" or "perfluoroalkyl" or "perfluorochemicals" or "PFAs" or "per-and polyfluoroalkyl substances" or "Perfluorohexane sulfonic acid" or "PFHxS" or "perfluorobutane sulfonic acid" or "Perfluorononanoic acid" or "PFNA" or "perfluorooctanoic acid" or "PFOA" or "perfluorooctane sulfonate acid" or "PFOs" or "Perfluorodecaoic acid" or "PFDA".
2. Five thyroid hormones: "thyroid hormone levels" or "T3" or "T4" or "TSH" or "thyroid dysfunction" or "hypothyroidism" or "hyperthyroidism" or "FT3" or "FT4".
3. The keywords should contain "1" and "2".

To minimize the risk of information omission, all relevant references to this topic were meticulously reviewed by two authors (B.Z. and M.Z.) individually. In the event of discrepancies between their assessments, a third party (P.L.) with expertise in the field was consulted to assist in making the final selection decision. Subsequently, during the data collation and in-depth analysis phases, a rigorous double-check system was adhered to, ensuring the accuracy of the data and the reliability of the analysis outcomes.

2.2. Inclusion and Exclusion Criteria

Inclusion criteria:

- The study was conducted with men and non-pregnant women;
- The study design was a cohort or cross-sectional study;
- The study included an association between PFAS exposure (at least one pollutant) and thyroid health effects (at least one metric);
- The study included basic statistical data such as the estimated value beta and the 95% CI;
- English-language articles were used.

Exclusion criteria:

- Duplicate studies;
- Off-topic studies;
- Studies reporting only PFAS exposure or thyroid hormone levels with no association between the two;
- Literature reviews, conference reports, case reports, letters, in vivo studies, in vitro studies;
- Studies with incomplete or unaccountable data.

2.3. Data Extraction and Quality Assessment

According to the established search strategy, we selected articles from the database and imported them into the EndNote 21.0 software, automatically eliminating duplicate entries. Subsequently, the titles and abstracts were filtered according to the predefined inclusion and exclusion criteria. After a comprehensive and detailed reading of the retained articles, relevant data were extracted from the eligible articles to construct a feature table. The extracted data covered the following aspects: author name, publication year, study area, study period duration, study population (including their age range), sample number type of PFAS, effect indicator, and adjustment variable information. We independently assessed the quality of each study using the Joanna Briggs Institute (JBI) criteria. The JBI evaluation criteria have a total of eight items, and each item is evaluated as "yes", "no", "unclear", and "not applicable" (Table S1).

2.4. Statistical Methods

The data were processed and analyzed using Stata 18 and Endnote X9 software. Relevant data were meticulously extracted from the included literature to construct a database and subsequently analyzed using the meta-analysis module of the Stata plug-in. We used beta (β) values to represent the combined association between human exposure to PFAs and thyroid hormone levels. The specific statistical methods were as follows: (1) The exposure levels of PFAS were evaluated by means of median (interquartile range (IQR)), while the thyroid function was presented in terms of serum thyroid hormone levels. If the original article presented the percentage change (%ch) along with their 95% confidence intervals (CIs) in thyroid hormones associated with a 2-fold increase in the exposure variable, the formula ln [%ch or upper confidence interval (UCI) or lower confidence interval (LCI)) ÷ 100 + 1] ÷ 2 was employed to calculate the β value and its corresponding 95% CIs. If the original article presented the % difference along with their 95% CIs in thyroid hormones associated with an elevated IQR in the PFAS concentration, the formula ln [(% difference or UCI or LCI) ÷ 100 + 1] was used to calculate the β-value and its 95% CI. We uniformly carried out the conversion to β (95% CI) in strict accordance with the above formula prior to the data summarization process [28]. (2) Heterogeneity test (q-test): When no heterogeneity was found in the included literature ($I^2 < 50\%$ and $p > 0.1$), we used the fixed-effects model; otherwise, we used the random-effects model. The forest plots showed the study's pooled effect sizes. (3) Subgroup analysis: The original literature was analyzed based on the characteristics, stratified according to the possible confounding factors during the research process, and both the effect sizes and 95% CIs for each subgroup were calculated, respectively. (4) Sensitivity analysis: The included articles were removed successively to obtain the new effect values. The stability of the results and the influencing factors were evaluated. (5) Test and correction for publication bias: The funnel plot was used to observe the size of publication bias. The Begg's funnel plot and Egger's linear regression test method were combined to undertake testing (Figures S1–S3). In the test, publication bias was considered if the p value < 0.05. Publication bias was considered to be absent if the p-value ≥ 0.05 [42].

3. Results

3.1. Selected Study Results

A total of 774 records were retrieved from three databases (Web of Science—276; Pub Med—246; Embase—252). After 442 duplicate records were removed, 332 study records remained. By screening the titles and abstracts, 234 records were excluded. A total of 46 records were excluded for unrelated population and 42 articles were assessed for full text eligibility, of which 28 were excluded for various reasons. Ultimately, 14 studies were included in the meta-analysis [26,32–35,43–51]. The screening process is shown in Figure 1.

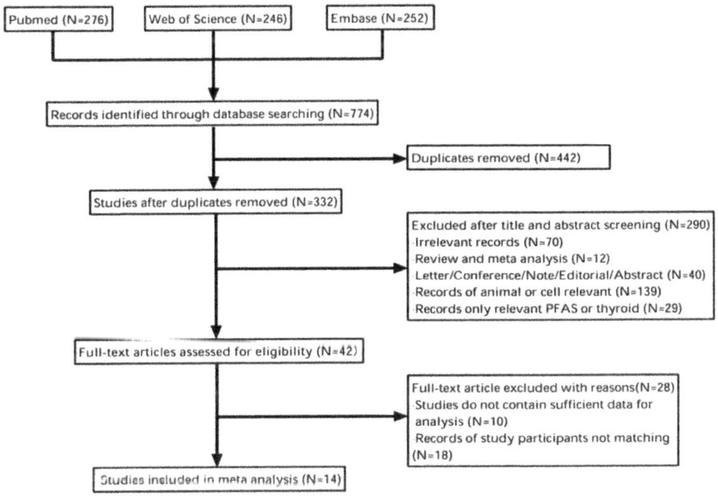

Figure 1. Flowchart of the screening process for meta-analysis.

3.2. Characteristics of the Study Included

The fourteen cross-sectional studies published between 2010 and 2024 included 38,956 participants [26,32–35,43–51]. Six of the fourteen studies were published in the last five years (2019–2024) [26,32,45–48]. Four of the fourteen studies were implemented in Europe [26,46,47, 49], six in North America [35,43–45,50,51], and four in Asia [32–34,48]. All the participants of the fourteen studies were over 12 years of age. Additionally, we collected the sample period, exposures, effect indicator, sample detection type (sample detected), and adjustment factors from 14 studies (Tables 1 and 2).

Table 1. Characteristics of studies included in the meta-analysis.

Author (Year)	Region	Period	Sample Size	Age	Design
Carmen Freire (2023)	Spain	2017–2019	129	15–17	cross-section
Elisa Gallo (2022)	Veneto	2017–2019	21,424	14–39	cross-section
Yanan Xing (2024)	China	2017–2018	10,853	≥18	cross-section
Kai Tan (2024)	China	May 2023–June 2023	746	>60	cross-section
Andrea Rodríguez-Carrillo (2023)	Belgium, Slovakia, Spain	2014–2020	733	12–19	cross-section
Élyse Caron-Beaudoin (2019)	Quebec	May 2015–October 2015	186	3–19	cross-section
Srishti Shrestha (2015)	New York	2005	84	55–74	cross-section
Samuel C. Byrne (2018)	Alaska	2013–2014	85	18–45	cross-section
Hélène Tillaut (2022)	France	2014–2018	476	12	cross-section

Table 1. *Cont.*

Author (Year)	Region	Period	Sample Size	Age	Design
Michael S. Bloom (2010)	New York	2006	31	31–45	cross-section
Kyunghee Ji (2012)	Korea	July 2008–August 2008	633	12–75	cross-section
Lili Wen (2013)	USA	2007–2010	1181	≥20	cross-section
Glenys M. Webster (2016)	USA	2007–2008	1525	≥18	cross-section
Linna Xie (2024)	China	2018	836	11–15	cross-section

Table 2. Exposure, effect indicator, and adjustment factors.

Author (Year)	Sample Detected	Exposures	Effect Indicator	Adjustment Factors
Carmen Freire (2023)	serum	PFOA, PFNA, PFDA, PFOS, PFHxS	T3, FT4, TSH	Child passive smoking, alcohol intake, total fish intake, iodine intake, physician-diagnosed thyroid disease history, maternal schooling, and the use of current or recent medication
Elisa Gallo (2022)	serum	PFOA, PFNA, PFOS, PFHxS	TSH	BMI, time lag between the enrolment and the beginning of the study, gender, physical activity, smoking habits, food consumption, country of birth, alcohol consumption, education level, and laboratory in charge of the TSH analyses
Yanan Xing (2024)	serum	PFOA, PFNA, PFDA, PFOS, PFHxS	T4, T3	Age, BMI, sex, nationality, education level, residence, marital status, annual family income, current smoking, current alcohol consumption, and multivitamin supplementation
Kai Tan (2024)	serum	PFOA, PFNA, PFDA, PFOS, PFHxS	TSH, T3, T4, FT3, FT4	Sex, age, BMI, smoking, and alcohol
Andrea Rodríguez-Carrillo (2023)	serum	PFOA, PFNA, PFOS	TSH, FT3, FT4	Random effect, age, sex, z-BMI, household education, and urinary creatinine concentration
Élyse Caron-Beaudoin (2019)	serum	PFOA, PFNA, PFOS, PFHxS	TSH, FT4	Age, sex, studied nation, urinary iodine, urinary cotinine, parent's education, and BMI z-score
Srishti Shrestha (2015)	serum	PFOA, PFOS	TSH, T3, T4, FT4	Age, sex, years of education, and serum ∑ PCBs
Samuel C. Byrne (2018)	serum	PFOA, PFNA, PFOS	TSH, T3, T4	Using total T3, fT3, total T4, fT4 or TSH as the dependent variables, adjusted for age, sex, and smoking habits
Hélène Tillaut (2022)	serum	PFOA, PFNA, PFDA, PFOS, PFHxS	TSH, FT3, FT4	Namely parental history of thyroid hormonal disorders, season, and time of day for the blood draw
Michael S. Bloom (2010)	serum	PFOA, PFNA, PFDA, PFOS, PFHxS	TSH, FT4	Age, gender, BMI, cigarette smoking, history of physician-diagnosed goiter or thyroid condition, race/ethnicity, the use of medication, and the consumption situation of sportfish from self-report
Kyunghee Ji (2012)	serum	PFOA, PFNA, PFDA, PFOS, PFHxS	TSH, T4	Age, sex, and BMI
Lili Wen (2013)	serum	PFOA, PFNA, PFOS, PFHxS	TSH, T3, T4, FT3, FT4	Age, gender, race, alcohol consumption, smoking status, and urinary iodine
Glenys M. Webster (2016)	serum	PFOA, PFNA, PFOS, PFHxS	TSH, T3, T4, FT3, FT4	Rage, race, log serum cotinine, sex, parity, pregnancy, and menopause status
Linna Xie (2024)	serum	PFOA, PFNA, PFDA, PFOS, PFHxS	TSH, FT3, FT4	Sex, age, BMI, and household income levels

3.3. Association Between PFAs and Thyroid Hormones

In this meta-analysis, the relationship between exposure to five per- and polyfluoroalkyl substances (PFOA, PFNA, PFDA, PFOS, and PFHxS) and five thyroid hormones (TSH, T3, T4, FT3, and FT4) was analyzed. The number of documents included is shown in Figure 2. The pooled analysis showed a significant effect between PFOA exposure and FT3 ($\beta = 0.011$, 95% CI = 0.003, 0.019, $I^2 = 0$), but no significant association was found in other PFAS.

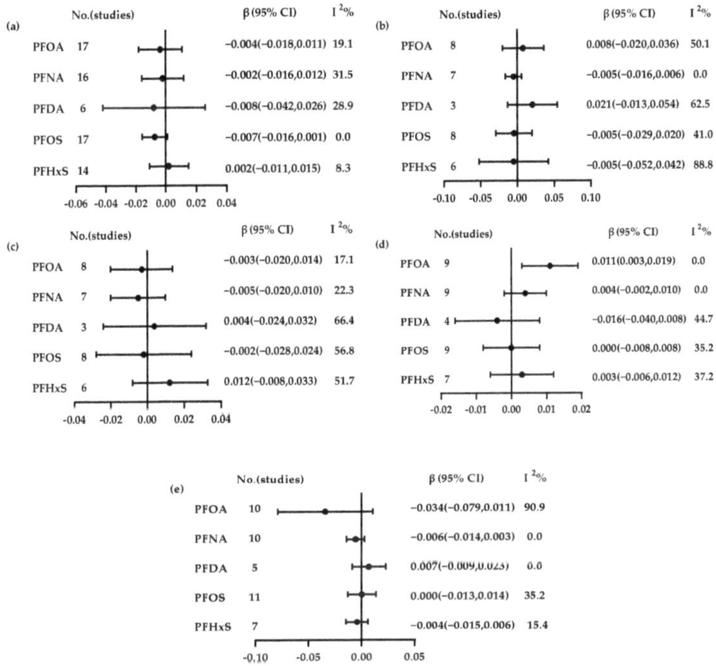

Figure 2. Forest plots showing the associations between PFAS exposure and thyroid hormones: (**a**) PFASs and TSH; (**b**) PFASs and T3; (**c**) PFASs and T4; (**d**) PFASs and FT3; (**e**) PFASs and FT4.

3.4. Subgroup Analysis

In the comprehensive assessment of the overall effect of PFAS exposure on thyroid hormone levels, potential interference factors were considered. To better understand the effects of PFAS exposure on thyroid hormones under different conditions and to explore potential sources of heterogeneity, a subgroup analysis was carried out with different subgroup sample sizes (>500 and <500), regions (North America, Asia, and Europe), sexes, ages (≥19 and <19), and under the consideration of whether the model was adjusted for BMI.

3.4.1. PFOA

In the subgroup of the sample size > 500, we discovered that PFOA exposure was positively associated with FT3 levels ($\beta = 0.011$, 95% CI = 0.001, 0.02, $I^2 = 13.4$). However, in the subgroup of the sample size ≤ 500, no significant correlation was found between PFOA exposure and FT3 ($\beta = -0.014$, 95% CI = −0.107, 0.079, $I^2 = 0$). No significant connection was found between PFOA and other thyroid hormones in the subgroup of the sample size. In the subgroup of North America, PFOA exposure was found to be positively associated with FT3 levels ($\beta = 0.014$, 95% CI = 0.005, 0.02, $I^2 = 0$), while no association was found in Asia ($\beta = -0.037$, 95% CI = −0.124, 0.049, $I^2 = 41.90$) and Europe ($\beta = 0.01$, 95% CI = −0.012,

0.032, $I^2 = 0$). In the subgroup of Europe, we discovered PFOA exposure with a positive effect on T4 levels ($\beta = 0.72$, 95% CI = 0.06, 1.38). PFOA exposure was positively associated with FT3 levels ($\beta = 0.014$, 95% CI = 0.003, 0.026, $I^2 = 0$) in the group without BMI adjustment. In <19 years subgroup, a significant positive association between PFOA exposure and FT3 level ($\beta = 0.014$, 95% CI = 0.003, 0.026, $I^2 = 0$) was observed, whereas no significant effect was found in the older than 19 years subgroup ($\beta = -0.001$, 95 % CI = −0.027, 0.025, $I^2 = 41.5$) (Table 3 and Table S2).

Table 3. Subgroup associations of PFOA exposure with thyroid health effects.

Subgroup		FT3			FT4		
		No	β (95% CI)	I^2	No	β (95% CI)	I^2
Sample size	<500	3	−0.014 (−0.107, 0.079)	0.0	4	0.006 (−0.028, 0.049)	0.0
	>500	6	**0.011 (0.001, 0.020)**	13.4	6	−0.057 (−0.118, 0.005)	94.7
Region	Asia	2	−0.037 (−0.124, 0.049)	41.9	2	−0.760 (−2.250, 0.730)	98.2
	North America	4	**0.014 (0.005, 0.022)**	0.0	6	−0.001 (−0.017, 0.014)	0.0
	Europe	3	0.010 (−0.012, 0.032)	0.0	2	−0.045 (−0.146, 0.056)	92.1
Adjusted for BMI	yes	2	−0.037 (−0.124, 0.0491)	41.9	3	−0.445 (−0.896, 0.006)	96.4
	no	7	**0.013 (0.005, 0.021)**	0.0	7	−0.017 (−0.055, 0.020)	85.9
Sex	male	9	0.001 (−0.006, 0.007)	38.0	9	−0.003 (−0.020, 0.014)	84.3
	female	9	0.002 (−0.003, 0.006)	32.8	10	0.000 (−0.007, 0.007)	64.0
Age	<19	5	**0.014 (0.003, 0.026)**	0.0	4	−0.152 (−0.289, −0.015)	96.2
	≥19	4	−0.001 (−0.027, 0.025)	41.5	7	−0.004 (−0.017, 0.010)	0.0

Bold font: used to highlight associated results.

3.4.2. PFNA

No significant association was found between PFNA exposure and thyroid hormone levels, which may be due to the small number of relevant studies. A significant positive association between PFNA exposure and T4 levels was observed in the <19 years subgroup ($\beta = 0.278$, 95% CI = 0.065, 0.491, $I^2 = 0$); no significant effects were found in ≥19 years subgroup ($\beta = -0.005$, 95% CI = −0.019, 0.009, $I^2 = 0$) (Table 4 and Table S3).

Table 4. Subgroup associations of PFNA exposure with thyroid health effects.

Subgroup		TSH			T3			T4		
		No	β (95% CI)	I^2	No	β(95% CI)	I^2	No	β (95% CI)	I^2
Age	<19	7	0.005 (−0.012, 0.021)	0.0	1	0.020 (−0.030, 0.080)	--	2	**0.278 (0.065, 0.491)**	0.0
	≥19	5	−0.000 (−0.061, 0.060)	53.4	5	−0.005 (−0.017, 0.008)	0.0	5	−0.005 (−0.019, 0.009)	0.0

Bold font: used to highlight associated results; (--): no value.

3.4.3. PFDA

In the subgroup of sample size ≤ 500, PFDA exposure was negatively correlated with FT3 levels ($\beta = -0.032$, 95% CI = −0.056, −0.007, $I^2 = 0$). In the subgroup of the sample size > 500, no significant correlation was found between PFDA and FT3 ($\beta = 0.023$, 95% CI = −0.068, 0.114, $I^2 = 0$). In the subgroup of Europe, PFDA exposure was found to be negatively correlated with FT3 levels ($\beta = -0.032$, 95% CI = −0.056, −0.007, $I^2 = 0$). However, no association was found in Asia ($\beta = 0.023$, 95% CI = −0.068, 0.114, $I^2 = 57.5$) and the data of North America were unable to be found. In the group without BMI adjustment, PFDA exposure was negatively associated with FT3 levels ($\beta = -0.032$, 95% CI = −0.056, −0.007, $I^2 = 0$), whereas no significant correlation was observed in the group with BMI adjustment ($\beta = 0.023$, 95% CI = −0.068, 0.114, $I^2 = 57.5$). In the <19 years subgroup ($\beta = -0.018$, 95% CI = −0.093, 0.058, $I^2 = 46.5$) and ≥19 years subgroup ($\beta = -0.007$, 95% CI = −0.026, 0.011), no significant effects were found (Table 5 and Table S4).

Table 5. Subgroup associations of PFDA exposure with thyroid health effects.

Subgroup		No	TSH β (95% CI)	I^2	No	T3 β(95% CI)	I^2	No	T4 β (95% CI)	I^2
Age	<19	3	−0.018 (−0.093, 0.058)	35.3	1	0.040 (−0.040, 0.120)	--	1	−0.080 (−0.660, 0.500)	--
	≥19	2	**−0.022 (−0.041, −0.003)**	0.0	1	−0.001 (−0.022, 0.019)	--	1	−0.007 (−0.027, 0.130)	--

Subgroup		No	FT3 β(95%CI)	I^2	No	FT4 β(95%CI)	I^2
Sample size	<500	2	**−0.032 (−0.056, −0.007)**	0.0	3	0.014 (−0.012, 0.041)	0.0
	>500	2	0.023 (−0.068, 0.114)	57.5	2	0.003 (−0.016, 0.023)	0.0
Region	Asia	2	0.023 (−0.068, 0.114)	57.5	2	0.003 (−0.016, 0.023)	0.0
	North America	0	--	--	1	0.090 (−0.020, 0.210)	--
	Europe	2	**−0.032 (−0.056, −0.007)**	0.0	2	0.010 (−0.017, 0.037)	0.0
Adjusted for BMI	yes	2	0.023 (−0.068, 0.114)	57.5	3	0.011 (−0.024, 0.046)	7.6
	no	2	**−0.032 (−0.056, −0.007)**	0.0	2	0.010 (−0.017, 0.037)	0.0

Bold font: used to highlight associated results; (--): no value.

3.4.4. PFOS

No significant association between PFOS exposure and thyroid level was found in subgroup analysis. Still, further studies are needed to determine other potential factors (Table S5).

3.4.5. PFHxS

In the non-adjustment of the BMI group, PFHxS exposure was negatively associated with FT3 levels (β = −0.011, 95% CI = −0.021, −0.001, I^2 = 0), while no significant association was found in the adjustment of the BMI group (β = −0.001, 95% CI = −0.006, 0.003, I^2 = 58.2) (Table 6 and Table S6).

Table 6. Subgroup associations of PFHxS exposure with thyroid health effects.

Subgroup		No	FT3 β (95%CI)	I^2	No	FT4 β (95%CI)	I^2
Adjusted for BMI	yes	4	0.015 (−0.015, 0.044)	67.0	5	−0.001 (−0.014, 0.030)	0.0
	no	5	0.005 (−0.001, 0.011)	0.0	3	**−0.011 (−0.021, −0.001)**	**0.0**

Bold font: used to highlight associated results.

3.5. *Sensitivity Analysis and Publication Bias*

A sensitivity analysis was carried out to ensure the reliability of the results. In recalculating effect sizes after removing studies individually, no significant change was found in the result (Figure S1), indicating that the results are relatively robust. Meanwhile, the publication bias of the studies was examined by the Begg's test (Table 7) and Egger's test (Figures S2 and S3). The Begg's test results between PFDA and T3 showed publication bias, and the Egger test results between PFHxS and T3 and FT4 showed publication bias ($p < 0.05$). No publication bias was detected in other studies ($p > 0.05$).

Table 7. Begg's test for the associations of PFASs exposure and thyroid hormones.

	TSH Z-Value	TSH *p*	T3 Z-Value	T3 *p*	T4 Z-Value	T4 *p*	FT3 Z-Value	FT3 *p*	FT4 Z-Value	FT4 *p*
PFOA	0.04	0.967	0.62	0.536	1.08	0.279	1.77	0.076	0.81	0.419
PFNA	1.22	0.224	0.24	0.806	0.52	0.602	0.00	1.000	1.62	0.105
PFDA	0.00	1.000	0.00	1.000	0.34	0.734	0.34	0.734	0.73	0.462
PFOS	0.87	0.386	0.12	0.902	0.89	0.371	0.00	1.000	0.86	0.390
PFHxS	0.05	0.956	0.96	0.339	0.75	0.454	0.46	0.649	2.10	0.035

4. Discussion

This study aims to comprehensively evaluate the association between PFAS exposure and thyroid health risks in men and non-pregnant women. Without considering confounding factors, we discovered that the variation of FT3 levels in men and non-pregnant women was positively connected with PFOA. However, the available evidence was insufficient to establish the impacts of PFAS exposure on alterations in other thyroid hormones. Notably, this result is generally consistent with the results of previous meta-analysis on the effects of PFAS exposure on thyroid hormones in pregnant women [28]. The above findings suggest that the effects of PFAS exposure on human thyroid health may be consistent in pregnant women and the general population (men and non-pregnant women). Further analysis showed that when the sample size, region, age, BMI and other factors were considered, more significant associations were found between PFAS exposure and thyroid hormones.

The available data advanced the possibility that BMI influences the association between PFAS exposure and thyroid hormones [36,52]; thus, we conducted a subgroup analysis depending on whether the data in the paper were adjusted for BMI. In the group without BMI adjustment, it was found that PFAs were significantly correlated with FT3, FT4. However, no significant association was observed in the adjustment of BMI group. The relationship between thyroid hormone levels and weight is clearly recognized, with hyperthyroidism accompanied by weight loss and hypothyroidism by weight gain [53,54]. Some studies have confirmed that individuals outside the normal range of BMI have relatively abnormal thyroid hormone levels [34,55]. This indicates BMI was a confounding factor in the relationship between PFAS exposure and thyroid hormone. Moreover, a cell experiment study has shown that PFAS can stimulate the proliferation and differentiation of adipocytes [56]. It is a possibility that PFAS have an impact on body weight [57].

Previous studies have shown that environmental exposure significantly effects thyroid health [58]. Through subgroup analysis, this study found that the study region may be one key factor influencing PFAS exposure on thyroid health. We found that regarding the effects of PFAS exposure on thyroid hormone levels in Europe and North America, no significant effect was found in Asia. Diet is one of the pathways of environmental exposure to PFAS in humans [59]. Eating habits differ in different geographical locations and cultures. The food category with the highest average concentration of PFAS was "meat and meat products" [60]. Global per capita annual consumption of meat from 2021 to 2023 shows that the top three consuming regions are North America, Oceania, and Europe, accounting for 78.5 kg, 51.4 kg, and 55.6 kg, respectively. Residents of North America and Europe may be exposed to higher concentrations of PFAS, increasing the risk of changes affecting thyroid hormones [61].

In addition, our subgroup analysis also considered participants >19 years old and <19 years old in order to explore the effect of PFAS exposure on thyroid hormone levels. We found that exposure to PFOA and PFNA had a positive correlation with thyroid hormone levels in adolescents (<19). One study found that in areas where drinking water is highly contaminated with PFAS, thyroid hormone levels in adolescents (<19) are significantly affected, especially in pre-adolescent children (2–12) [36]. Adolescence is a stage of continuous body and brain developments, and this makes adolescents more sensitive to thyroid-disrupting chemicals than the adult population [62].

We discovered a positive effect between PFOA and FT3 when data were extracted from studies with sample sizes > 500. No significant correlation was found between PFOA exposure and FT3 with the sample sizes < 500, which indicated that sample size might be a reason for the heterogeneity of the results. In addition, we found no significant effect in PFAS on thyroid hormone levels in subgroups stratified based on sex; a potential possibility for this is that some unknown confusing factors were disturbed.

In subgroup analysis, it was shown that PFOA, PFNA, PFDA, and PFHxS have an association with thyroid hormone; no association was found between PFOS and thyroid hormone. The five PFAS were structurally similar, and the presence or absence of association results may be due to differences in exposure dose [63]. A study of Chinese adults showed that the changing levels of thyroid hormone (T3, T4) plateaued when the amount of PFAS exceeded a critical exposure threshold (about 0.5–10 ng/mL) [32]. Of the 14 studies included in this study, PFAS concentrations ranged from 0.001 to 1 μg/L in five studies [26,34,46,48,49], from 0.1 to 10 μg/L in three studies [44,45,47], and from 1 to 100 μg/L in six studies [32,33,35,43,50,51]. This suggests that differences in PFAS concentrations across the included studies may have contributed to the partial associations observed in the study results. In addition, in two recent studies exploring the relationship between PFAS and health outcomes, a non-monotonic dose–response relationship was found between PFOA (a common PFAS) and diabetes risk. This indicated that the association of exposure dose is not a simple monotonic relationship but a more complex pattern of change [64,65]. In the subgroup analysis of this study, we found a positive correlation between PFAS (PFOA, PFNA) and thyroid hormone, and a negative correlation between PFAS (PFDA, PFHxS) and thyroid hormone. The relationship between PFAS and thyroid hormone levels exhibits significant complexity and diversity, potentially demonstrating a non-monotonic dose–response relationship. Different PFAS showed varying associations with thyroid hormone levels. Subgroup analysis suggests that PFAS may exert potential toxicological effects on thyroid hormones through multiple mechanisms, necessitating further in-depth research to elucidate their specific mechanisms of action and dose–response relationships.

PFAS has the potential to influence thyroid levels in a variety of ways. Investigations have demonstrated that PFAS can bind with transthyretin (TTR) and thyroxine-binding globulin (TBG). TTR and TBG are two major thyroid hormone distributor proteins in human plasma, playing important roles in stabilizing the TH levels [66,67]. The combination of PFAS and distributor proteins can alter the key points of the thyroid axis, disturbing the thyroid hormone levels [68]. Additionally, it has been confirmed that iodide is an essential constituent of thyroid hormones, and NIS-mediated iodide uptake plays a pivotal role in their biosynthesis [69]. PFAS impairs iodine uptake by thyroid cells through the competitive inhibition of sodium iodide symporter (NIS) [70]. Some studies indicate that PFAS induces oxidative damage, disrupting normal immune function [71,72]. PFAS can increase the generation of reactive oxygen species (ROS) in vivo [73]. The accumulation of oxygen free radicals may inhibit thyroid peroxidase (TPO) activity, thereby interfering with thyroid hormone production and contributing to the development of hypothyroidism [74].

Still, there are limitations to this systematic review and meta-analysis. Firstly, according to our standard screening literature, the number of studies on specific PFAS in thyroid hormone levels is small, which may lead to heterogeneity between studies. Although subgroup analysis was performed, the leading causes of heterogeneity remain unclear. Secondly, the included studies were cross-sectional. When observing the relationship between exposures and outcomes, they were often subject to interference from multiple confounding factors. These factors may be simultaneously associated with exposure and health outcomes, thereby masking or distorting the associations. Therefore, a cautious and rigorous attitude should be adopted towards the conclusions of this study. Finally, we only stratified subgroups based on whether BMI was adjusted in the original literature, without considering other adjustment factors. If other adjustment factors are considered, the number of eligible articles will be small, which may lead to a less obvious significance in the results and some key information being ignored. Further large cohort studies with adequate and reliable exposure data should be conducted to better understand the association between PFAS exposure and thyroid hormone levels. In addition, with sufficient data, multiple comprehensive adjustment factors should be considered.

5. Conclusions

This study revealed a stable association between PFOA and FT3 in men and non-pregnant women. Subgroup analysis showed that sample size, region, BMI, and age were confounding factors affecting the association between exposure to PFAS and thyroid hormone changes. In particular, the correlation is more significant in studies with larger sample sizes and in studies from Europe and North America. In addition, it is of great concern that adolescents were more sensitive to PFAS exposure in men and non-pregnant women, which provides an important direction for follow-up research and related health risk assessment.

Supplementary Materials: The following supporting information can be downloaded at https://www.mdpi.com/article/10.3390/toxics13030214/s1: Figure S1: Sensitivity analysis; Figure S2: Egger's Test; Figure S3: Funnel plot; Table S1: Quality Assessment; Table S2: Subgroup associations of PFOA exposure with thyroid health effects; Table S3: Subgroup associations of PFNA exposure with thyroid health effects; Table S4: Subgroup associations of PFDA exposure with thyroid health effects; Table S5: Subgroup associations of PFOS exposure with thyroid health effects; Table S6: Subgroup associations of PFHxS exposure with thyroid health effects.

Author Contributions: B.Z. and M.Z.: methodology, formal analysis, investigation, data curation, writing—original draft, writing—review and editing, conceptualization, software; X.C.: methodology, investigation, data curation; C.L. (Chunyu Liu): methodology, investigation; C.L. (Chaofei Li), Y.Q., and X.L.: writing—review, resources, editing; S.L. and Y.C.: visualization, resources, supervision; P.L.: writing—review and editing, supervision, validation, project administration, resources, funding acquisition. All authors have read and agreed to the published version of the manuscript.

Funding: This research was funded by the Tianjin Research Program, grant number (24ZYCGCG00540, 24YFXTHZ00170), and Fujian Research Program, grant number (2023C0019).

Data Availability Statement: The original data presented in the study are included in the article/Supplementary Materials; further inquiries can be directed to the corresponding authors.

Conflicts of Interest: Chaofei Li, Sha Li and Yanying Chen are employed by Zhonghuan (Fujian) Environmental Technology Co., Ltd. Yu Qiu is employed by Fujian Jinhuang Environmental Protection Technology Co., Ltd. They declare no conflict of interest with Bin Zhang, Meizi Zhao, Xiangru Cong, Chunyu Liu, Xiaoxue Li and Penghui Li.

References

1. Chaves, C.; Bruinstroop, E.; Refetoff, S.; Yen, P.; Anselmo, J. Increased Hepatic Fat Content in Patients with Resistance to Thyroid Hormone Beta. *Thyroid* **2021**, *31*, 1127–1134. [CrossRef]
2. Koibuchi, N.; Jingu, H.; Iwasaki, T.; Chin, W.W. Current perspectives on the role of thyroid hormone in growth and development of cerebellum. *Cerebellum* **2003**, *2*, 279–289. [CrossRef]
3. Koibuchi, N. The Role of Thyroid Hormone on Cerebellar Development. *Cerebellum* **2008**, *7*, 530–533. [CrossRef]
4. Bloise, F.F.; Cordeiro, A.; Ortiga-Carvalho, T.M. Role of thyroid hormone in skeletal muscle physiology. *J. Endocrinol.* **2018**, *236*, R57–R68. [CrossRef]
5. Sun, Y.; Teng, D.; Zhao, L.; Shi, X.G.; Li, Y.Z.; Shan, Z.Y.; Teng, W.P.; Thyroid Disorders, Iodine Status and Diabetes Epidemiological Survey Group (TIDE). Impaired Sensitivity to Thyroid Hormones Is Associated with Hyperuricemia, Obesity, and Cardiovascular Disease Risk in Subjects with Subclinical Hypothyroidism. *Thyroid* **2022**, *32*, 376–384. [CrossRef]
6. Kim, M.J.; Kim, S.; Choi, S.; Lee, I.; Moon, M.K.; Choi, K.; Park, Y.J.; Cho, Y.H.; Kwon, Y.M.; Yoo, J.; et al. Association of exposure to polycyclic aromatic hydrocarbons and heavy metals with thyroid hormones in general adult population and potential mechanisms. *Sci. Total Environ.* **2021**, *762*, 9. [CrossRef]

7. Liu, S.S.; Zhao, G.D.; Li, J.; Zhao, H.X.; Wang, Y.F.; Chen, J.W.; Zhao, H.D. Association of polybrominated diphenylethers (PBDEs) and hydroxylated metabolites (OH-PBDEs) serum levels with thyroid function in thyroid cancer patients. *Environ. Res.* **2017**, *159*, 1–8. [CrossRef]
8. Zheng, L.; Wang, Z.C.; Yang, R.; Chen, W.N.; Zhang, J.; Li, R.X.; Lv, W.M.; Lin, B.; Luo, J.J. The interference between effects of PFAS exposure on thyroid hormone disorders and cholesterol levels: An NHANES analysis. *Environ. Sci. Pollut. Res.* **2023**, *30*, 90949–90959. [CrossRef]
9. Takaguchi, K.; Nishikawa, H.; Mizukawa, H.; Tanoue, R.; Yokoyama, N.; Ichii, O.; Takiguchi, M.; Nakayama, S.M.M.; Ikenaka, Y.; Kunisue, T.; et al. Effects of PCB exposure on serum thyroid hormone levels in dogs and cats. *Sci. Total Environ.* **2019**, *688*, 1172–1183. [CrossRef]
10. Lau, C.; Anitole, K.; Hodes, C.; Lai, D.; Pfahles-Hutchens, A.; Seed, J. Perfluoroalkyl acids: A review of monitoring and toxicological findings. *Toxicol. Sci.* **2007**, *99*, 366–394. [CrossRef]
11. Zhang, B.; Zhang, H.E.; Ren, Q.; He, B.; Zhang, Y.; Jiang, Z.W. Fabrication of Corrosion-Resistant Superhydrophobic Coatings and Impermeable Porous Structures Using Fluorinated Microemulsions Containing Thermally Decomposable Surfactants. *Coatings* **2024**, *14*, 1176. [CrossRef]
12. Galezowska, G.; Kolecka, K.; Cieszynska-Semenowicz, M.; Redko, V.; Gajewska, M. Screening of perfluoroalkyl substances and their environmental impact in sequencing batch reactors combined with nature-based solutions. *Ecol. Eng.* **2024**, *209*, 11. [CrossRef]
13. Chen, D.; Hu, X.H.; Chen, C.H.; Gao, Y.M.; Zhou, Q.H.; Feng, X.; Xu, X.H.; Lin, D.H.; Xu, J. Impacts of Perfluoroalkyl Substances on Aqueous and Nonaqueous Phase Liquid Dechlorination by Sulfidized Nanoscale Zerovalent Iron. *Environ. Sci. Technol.* **2024**, *58*, 11193–11202. [CrossRef]
14. Panieri, E.; Baralic, K.; Djukic-Cosic, D.; Djordjevic, A.B.; Saso, L. PFAS Molecules: A Major Concern for the Human Health and the Environment. *Toxics* **2022**, *10*, 44. [CrossRef]
15. Sodani, K.; Ter Braak, B.; Hartvelt, S.; Boelens, M.; Jamalpoor, A.; Mukhi, S. Toxicological mode-of-action and developmental toxicity of different carbon chain length PFAS. *Toxicol. Lett.* **2025**, *405*, 59–66. [CrossRef]
16. Aimuzi, R.; Luo, K.; Huang, R.; Huo, X.N.; Nian, M.; Ouyang, F.X.; Du, Y.T.; Feng, L.P.; Wang, W.Y.; Zhang, J.; et al. Perfluoroalkyl and polyfluroalkyl substances and maternal thyroid hormones in early pregnancy. *Environ. Pollut.* **2020**, *264*, 8. [CrossRef]
17. Ryu, S.; Burchett, W.; Zhang, S.M.; Modaresi, S.M.S.; Areiza, J.A.; Kaye, E.; Fischer, F.C.; Slitt, A.L. Species-Specific Unbound Fraction Differences in Highly Bound PFAS: A Comparative Study across Human, Rat, and Mouse Plasma and Albumin. *Toxics* **2024**, *12*, 253. [CrossRef]
18. Mussabek, D.; Ahrens, L.; Persson, K.M.; Berndtsson, R. Temporal trends and sediment-water partitioning of per- and polyfluoroalkyl substances (PFAS) in lake sediment. *Chemosphere* **2019**, *227*, 624–629. [CrossRef]
19. Witt, C.C.; Gadek, C.R.; Cartron, J.L.E.; Andersen, M.J.; Campbell, M.L.; Castro-Farías, M.; Gyllenhaal, E.F.; Johnson, A.B.; Malaney, J.L.; Montoya, K.N.; et al. Extraordinary levels of per- and polyfluoroalkyl substances (PFAS) in vertebrate animals at a New Mexico desert oasis: Multiple pathways for wildlife and human exposure. *Environ. Res.* **2024**, *249*, 14. [CrossRef]
20. Cioni, L.; Nikiforov, V.; Coelho, A.; Sandanger, T.M.; Herzke, D. Total oxidizable precursors assay for PFAS in human serum. *Environ. Int.* **2022**, *170*, 9. [CrossRef]
21. Cappelli, F.; Bamai, Y.A.; Van Hoey, K.; Kim, D.; Covaci, A. Occurrence of short- and ultra-short chain PFAS in drinking water from Flanders (Belgium) and implications for human exposure. *Environ. Res.* **2024**, *260*, 11. [CrossRef] [PubMed]
22. Lu, Y.; Guan, R.N.; Zhu, N.L.; Hao, J.H.; Peng, H.Y.; He, A.E.; Zhao, C.Y.; Wang, Y.W.; Jiang, G.B. A critical review on the bioaccumulation, transportation, and elimination of per- and polyfluoroalkyl substances in human beings. *Crit. Rev. Environ. Sci. Technol.* **2024**, *54*, 95–116. [CrossRef]
23. He, Q.R.; Yang, Q.K.; Wu, L.; He, Y.H.; Zeng, N.; Wang, Z.L. Neurotoxic effects of per- and polyfluoroalkyl substances (PFAS) mixture exposure in mice: Accumulations in brain and associated changes of behaviors, metabolome, and transcriptome. *J. Hazard. Mater.* **2025**, *489*, 12. [CrossRef]
24. Ojo, A.F.; Peng, C.; Ng, J.C. Assessing the human health risks of per- and polyfluoroalkyl substances: A need for greater focus on their interactions as mixtures. *J. Hazard. Mater.* **2021**, *407*, 14. [CrossRef]
25. Rickard, B.P.; Rizvi, I.; Fenton, S.E. Per- and poly-fluoroalkyl substances (PFAS) and female reproductive outcomes: PFAS elimination, endocrine-mediated effects, and disease. *Toxicology* **2022**, *465*, 20. [CrossRef]
26. Freire, C.; Vela-Soria, F.; Castiello, F.; Salamanca-Fernández, E.; Quesada-Jiménez, R.; López-Alados, M.C.; Fernandez, M.F.; Olea, N. Exposure to perfluoroalkyl substances (PFAS) and association with thyroid hormones in adolescent males. *Int. J. Hyg. Environ. Health* **2023**, *252*, 9. [CrossRef]
27. Chrousos, G.P. Stress and disorders of the stress system. *Nat. Rev. Endocrinol.* **2009**, *5*, 374–381. [CrossRef]
28. Zhang, L.; Liang, J.Y.; Gao, A. Contact to perfluoroalkyl substances and thyroid health effects: A meta-analysis directing on pregnancy. *Chemosphere* **2023**, *315*, 12. [CrossRef]

29. Zhang, S.Y.; Lei, X.N.; Zhang, Y.; Shi, R.; Zhang, Q.L.; Gao, Y.; Yuan, T.; Li, J.; Tian, Y. Prenatal exposure to per- and polyfluoroalkyl substances and childhood adiposity at 7 years of age. *Chemosphere* **2022**, *307*, 8. [CrossRef]
30. Matilla-Santander, N.; Valvi, D.; Lopez-Espinosa, M.J.; Manzano-Salgado, C.B.; Ballester, F.; Ibarluzea, J.; Santa-Marina, L.; Schettgen, T.; Guxens, M.; Sunyer, J.; et al. Exposure to Perfluoroalkyl Substances and Metabolic Outcomes in Pregnant Women: Evidence from the Spanish INMA Birth Cohorts. *Environ. Health Perspect.* **2017**, *125*, 11. [CrossRef]
31. Chen, W.L.; Bai, F.Y.; Chang, Y.C.; Chen, P.C.; Chen, C.Y. Concentrations of perfluoroalkyl substances in foods and the dietary exposure among Taiwan general population and pregnant women. *J. Food Drug Anal.* **2018**, *26*, 994–1004. [CrossRef]
32. Xing, Y.A.; Li, Z.; Wang, J.H.; Qu, Y.L.; Hu, Q.P.; Ji, S.S.; Chang, X.C.; Zhao, F.; Lv, Y.B.; Pan, Y.T.; et al. Associations between serum per- and polyfluoroalkyl substances and thyroid hormones in Chinese adults: A nationally representative cross-sectional study. *Environ. Int.* **2024**, *184*, 10. [CrossRef]
33. Xie, L.N.; Wang, X.C.; Su, L.Q.; Ji, S.S.; Gu, W.; Barrett, H.; Dong, X.J.; Zhu, H.J.; Hou, S.S.; Li, Z.H.; et al. The association between per-/polyfluoroalkyl substances in serum and thyroid function parameters: A cross-sectional study on teenagers living near a Chinese fluorochemical industrial plant. *Sci. Total Environ.* **2024**, *920*, 11. [CrossRef]
34. Ji, K.; Kim, S.; Kho, Y.; Paek, D.; Sakong, J.; Ha, J.; Kim, S.; Choi, K. Serum concentrations of major perfluorinated compounds among the general population in Korea: Dietary sources and potential impact on thyroid hormones. *Environ. Int.* **2012**, *45*, 78–85. [CrossRef]
35. Shrestha, S.; Bloom, M.S.; Yucel, R.; Seegal, R.F.; Wu, Q.; Kannan, K.; Rej, R.; Fitzgerald, E.F. Perfluoroalkyl substances and thyroid function in older adults. *Environ. Int.* **2015**, *75*, 206–214. [CrossRef]
36. Li, Y.; Xu, Y.Y.; Fletcher, T.; Scott, K.; Nielsen, C.; Pineda, D.; Lindh, C.H.; Olsson, D.S.; Andersson, E.M.; Jakobsson, K. Associations between perfluoroalkyl substances and thyroid hormones after high exposure through drinking water. *Environ. Res.* **2021**, *194*, 10. [CrossRef]
37. Shamseer, L.; Moher, D.; Clarke, M.; Ghersi, D.; Liberati, A.; Petticrew, M.; Shekelle, P.; Stewart, L.A.; Prisma, P.G. Preferred reporting items for systematic review and meta-analysis protocols (PRISMA-P) 2015: Elaboration and explanation. *BMJ-Br. Med. J.* **2015**, *349*, 25. [CrossRef]
38. Wang, Z.Y.; Cousins, I.T.; Scheringer, M.; Hungerbuehler, K. Hazard assessment of fluorinated alternatives to long-chain perfluoroalkyl acids (PFAAs) and their precursors: Status quo, ongoing challenges and possible solutions. *Environ. Int.* **2015**, *75*, 172–179. [CrossRef]
39. Brennan, N.M.; Evans, A.T.; Fritz, M.K.; Peak, S.A.; von Holst, H.E. Trends in the Regulation of Per- and Polyfluoroalkyl Substances (PFAS): A Scoping Review. *Int. J. Environ. Res. Public Health* **2021**, *18*, 900. [CrossRef]
40. Nhu, H.D.; Tri, D.V.; Luu, T.L.; Trippel, J.; Wagner, M. Degradation of 29 per- and poly-fluoroalkyl substances (PFAS) in water using fenton-assisted electrochemical oxidation process. *Sep. Purif. Technol.* **2025**, *362*, 13. [CrossRef]
41. Li, W.T.; Liu, X.Y.; Mao, H.; Wang, S.L. Concentration, distribution, and bioconcentration of short- and long-chain perfluoroalkyl substances in the water, suspended particulate matter, and surface sediment of a typical semi-enclosed bay. *Sci. Total Environ.* **2023**, *890*, 13. [CrossRef] [PubMed]
42. Schneck, A. Examining publication bias-a simulation-based evaluation of statistical tests on publication bias. *PeerJ* **2017**, *5*, 21. [CrossRef] [PubMed]
43. Bloom, M.S.; Kannan, K.; Spliethoff, H.M.; Tao, L.; Aldous, K.M.; Vena, J.E. Exploratory assessment of perfluorinated compounds and human thyroid function. *Physiol. Behav.* **2010**, *99*, 240–245. [CrossRef] [PubMed]
44. Byrne, S.C.; Miller, P.; Seguinot-Medina, S.; Waghiyi, V.; Buck, C.L.; von Hippel, F.A.; Carpenter, D.O. Exposure to perfluoroalkyl substances and associations with serum thyroid hormones in a remote population of Alaska Natives. *Environ. Res.* **2018**, *166*, 537–543. [CrossRef]
45. Caron-Beaudoin, É.; Ayotte, P.; Sidi, E.A.L.; McHugh, N.G.L.; Lemire, M.; Community of Lac Simon; Community of Winneway –Long Point First Nation; CSSS Tshukuminu Kanani of Nutashkuan; Community of Unamen Shipu. Exposure to perfluoroalkyl substances (PFAS) and associations with thyroid parameters in First Nation children and youth from Quebec. *Environ. Int.* **2019**, *128*, 13–23. [CrossRef]
46. Gallo, E.; Amidei, C.B.; Barbieri, G.; Fabricio, A.S.C.; Gion, M.; Pitter, G.; Daprà, F.; Russo, F.; Gregori, D.; Fletcher, T.; et al. Perfluoroalkyl substances and thyroid stimulating hormone levels in a highly exposed population in the Veneto Region. *Environ. Res.* **2022**, *203*, 9. [CrossRef]
47. Rodríguez-Carrillo, A.; Salamanca-Fernández, E.; den Hond, E.; Verheyen, V.J.; Fabelová, L.; Murinova, L.P.; Pedraza-Díaz, S.; Castaño, A.; García-Lario, J.; Remy, S.; et al. Association of exposure to perfluoroalkyl substances (PFAS) and phthalates with thyroid hormones in adolescents from HBM4EU aligned studies. *Environ. Res.* **2023**, *237*, 11. [CrossRef]
48. Tan, K.; Zhang, Q.Q.; Wang, Y.J.; Wang, C.F.; Hu, C.F.; Wang, L.; Liu, H.L.; Tian, Z.Q. Associations between *per-* and polyfluoroalkyl substances exposure and thyroid hormone levels in the elderly. *Sci. Total Environ.* **2024**, *920*, 9. [CrossRef]

49. Tillaut, H.; Monfort, C.; Giton, F.; Warembourg, C.; Rouget, F.; Cordier, S.; Laine, F.; Gaudreau, E.; Garlantezec, R.; Saint-Amour, D.; et al. Persistent organic pollutant exposure and thyroid function among 12-year-old children. *Neuroendocrinology* **2023**, *113*, 1232–1247. [CrossRef]
50. Webster, G.M.; Rauch, S.A.; Ste Marie, N.; Mattman, A.; Lanphear, B.P.; Venners, S.A. Cross-Sectional Associations of Serum Perfluoroalkyl Acids and Thyroid Hormones in US Adults: Variation According to TPOAb and Iodine Status (NHANES 2007-2008). *Environ. Health Perspect.* **2016**, *124*, 935–942. [CrossRef]
51. Wen, L.L.; Lin, L.Y.; Su, T.C.; Chen, P.C.; Lin, C.Y. Association Between Serum Perfluorinated Chemicals and Thyroid Function in US Adults: The National Health and Nutrition Examination Survey 2007-2010. *J. Clin. Endocrinol. Metab.* **2013**, *98*, E1456–E1464. [CrossRef] [PubMed]
52. Blake, B.E.; Pinney, S.M.; Hines, E.P.; Fenton, S.E.; Ferguson, K.K. Associations between longitudinal serum perfluoroalkyl substance (PFAS) levels and measures of thyroid hormone, kidney function, and body mass index in the Fernald Community Cohort. *Environ. Pollut.* **2018**, *242*, 894–904. [CrossRef] [PubMed]
53. Song, E.; Ahn, J.; Oh, H.S.; Jeon, M.J.; Kim, W.G.; Kim, W.B.; Shong, Y.K.; Kim, T.Y. Sex-Dependent Association between Weight Change and Thyroid Dysfunction: Population-Level Analysis Using the Korean National Health and Nutrition Examination Survey. *Eur. Thyroid J.* **2019**, *8*, 202–207. [CrossRef]
54. Qiu, Y.K.; Liu, Q.Y.; Luo, Y.H.; Chen, J.D.; Zheng, Q.Z.; Xie, Y.P.; Cao, Y.P. Causal association between obesity and hypothyroidism: A two-sample bidirectional Mendelian randomization study. *Front. Endocrinol.* **2024**, *14*, 13. [CrossRef]
55. Canova, C.; Di Nisio, A.; Barbieri, G.; Russo, F.; Fletcher, T.; Batzella, E.; Dalla Zuanna, T.; Pitter, G. PFAS Concentrations and Cardiometabolic Traits in Highly Exposed Children and Adolescents. *Int. J. Environ. Res. Public Health* **2021**, *18*, 12881. [CrossRef]
56. Watkins, A.M.; Wood, C.R.; Lin, M.T.; Abbott, B.D. The effects of perfluorinated chemicals on adipocyte differentiation *in vitro*. *Mol. Cell. Endocrinol.* **2015**, *400*, 90–101. [CrossRef]
57. Kinkade, C.W.; Rivera-Nunez, Z.; Thurston, S.W.; Kannan, K.; Miller, R.K.; Brunner, J.; Wong, E.Y.; Groth, S.; O'Connor, T.G.; Barrett, E.S. Per- and polyfluoroalkyl substances, gestational weight gain, postpartum weight retention and body composition in the UPSIDE cohort. *Environ. Health* **2023**, *22*, 16. [CrossRef]
58. Leko, M.B.; Gunjaca, I.; Pleic, N.; Zemunik, T. Environmental Factors Affecting Thyroid-Stimulating Hormone and Thyroid Hormone Levels. *Int. J. Mol. Sci.* **2021**, *22*, 6521. [CrossRef]
59. Vorst, K.L.; Saab, N.; Silva, P.; Curtzwiler, G.; Steketee, A. Risk assessment of per- and polyfluoroalkyl substances (PFAS) in food: Symposium proceedings. *Trends Food Sci. Technol.* **2021**, *116*, 1203–1211. [CrossRef]
60. Knutsen, H.K.; Alexander, J.; Barregård, L.; Bignami, M.; Brüschweiler, B.; Ceccatelli, S.; Cottrill, B.; Dinovi, M.; Edler, L.; Grasl-Kraupp, B.; et al. Risk to human health related to the presence of perfluorooctane sulfonic acid and perfluorooctanoic acid in food. *EFSA J.* **2018**, *16*, 284. [CrossRef]
61. Xie, Y.; Berntsen, H.F.; Zimmer, K.E.; Ropstad, E.; Verhaegen, S.; Connolly, L. Luteolin protects against adipogenic and lipogenic potency induced by human relevant mixtures of persistent organic pollutants (POPs) in the 3T3-L1 model. *Food Chem. Toxicol.* **2023**, *173*, 10. [CrossRef] [PubMed]
62. Lanphear, B.P. The Impact of Toxins on the Developing Brain. *Annu. Rev. Public Health* **2015**, *36*, 211–230.
63. Guo, P.F.; Warren, J.L.; Deziel, N.C.; Liew, Z. Exposure range matters: Considering nonlinear associations in the meta-analysis of environmental pollutant exposure using examples of per- and polyfluoroalkyl substances and birth outcomes. *Am. J. Epidemiol.* **2025**, *9*, kwae309. [CrossRef]
64. Mancini, F.R.; Rajaobelina, K.; Praud, D.; Dow, C.; Antignac, J.P.; Kvaskoff, M.; Severi, G.; Bonnet, F.; Boutron-Ruault, M.C.; Fagherazzi, G. Nonlinear associations between dietary exposures to perfluorooctanoic acid (PFOA) or perfluorooctane sulfonate (PFOS) and type 2 diabetes risk in women: Findings from the E3N cohort study. *Int. J. Hyg. Environ. Health.* **2018**, *221*, 1054–1060. [CrossRef] [PubMed]
65. Dunder, L.; Salihovic, S.; Elmståhl, S.; Lind, P.M.; Lind, L. Associations between per- and polyfluoroalkyl substances (PFAS) and diabetes in two population-based cohort studies from Sweden. *J. Expo. Sci. Environ. Epidemiol.* **2023**, *33*, 748–756. [CrossRef]
66. Dharpure, R.; Pramanik, S.; Pradhan, A. In silico analysis decodes transthyretin (TTR) binding and thyroid disrupting effects of per- and polyfluoroalkyl substances (PFAS). *Arch. Toxicol.* **2023**, *97*, 755–768. [CrossRef]
67. Shen, Y.; Bovee, T.F.H.; Molenaar, D.; Weide, Y.; Nolles, A.; Mitrovic, C.B.; van Leeuwen, S.P.J.; Louisse, J.; Hamers, T. Optimized methods for measuring competitive binding of chemical substances to thyroid hormone distributor proteins transthyretin and thyroxine binding globulin. *Arch. Toxicol.* **2024**, *98*, 3797–3809. [CrossRef]
68. Degitz, S.J.; Olker, J.H.; Denny, J.S.; Degoey, P.P.; Hartig, P.C.; Cardon, M.C.; Eytcheson, S.A.; Haselman, J.T.; Mayasich, S.A.; Hornung, M.W. *In vitro* screening of *per*- and polyfluorinated substances (PFAS) for interference with seven thyroid hormone system targets across nine assays. *Toxicol. Vitro* **2024**, *95*, 12. [CrossRef]
69. Riesco-Eizaguirre, G.; Santisteban, P.; De la Vieja, A. The complex regulation of NIS expression and activity in thyroid and extrathyroidal tissues. *Endocr.-Relat. Cancer* **2021**, *28*, T141–T165. [CrossRef]

70. Conti, A.; Strazzeri, C.; Rhoden, K.J. Perfluorooctane sulfonic acid, a persistent organic pollutant, inhibits iodide accumulation by thyroid follicular cells in vitro. *Mol. Cell. Endocrinol.* **2020**, *515*, 10. [CrossRef]
71. Santhanam, S.D.; Ramamurthy, K.; Priya, P.S.; Sudhakaran, G.; Guru, A.; Arockiaraj, J. A combinational threat of micro- and nano-plastics (MNPs) as potential emerging vectors for per- and polyfluoroalkyl substances (PFAS) to human health. *Environ. Monit. Assess.* **2024**, *196*, 31. [CrossRef]
72. Di Nisio, A.; Rocca, M.S.; De Toni, L.; Sabovic, I.; Guidolin, D.; Dall'Acqua, S.; Acquasaliente, L.; De Filippis, V.; Plebani, M.; Foresta, C. Endocrine disruption of vitamin D activity by perfluoro-octanoic acid (PFOA). *Sci. Rep.* **2020**, *10*, 12. [CrossRef] [PubMed]
73. Wielsoe, M.; Long, M.H.; Ghisari, M.; Bonefeld-Jorgensen, E.C. Perfluoroalkylated substances (PFAS) affect oxidative stress biomarkers *in vitro*. *Chemosphere* **2015**, *129*, 239–245. [CrossRef] [PubMed]
74. Kochman, J.; Jakubczyk, K.; Bargiel, P.; Janda-Milczarek, K. The Influence of Oxidative Stress on Thyroid Diseases. *Antioxidants* **2021**, *10*, 1442. [CrossRef] [PubMed]

MDPI AG
Grosspeteranlage 5
4052 Basel
Switzerland
Tel.: +41 61 683 77 34

Toxics Editorial Office
E-mail: toxics@mdpi.com
www.mdpi.com/journal/toxics

www.ingramcontent.com/pod-product-compliance
Lightning Source LLC
Chambersburg PA
CBHW061521210926
51850CB00008B/1997